A SPECIAL ISSUE OF
COGNITIVE NEUROPSYCHOLOGY

The Cognitive Neuropsychology of False Memories

edited by

Daniel L. Schacter

Harvard University, Cambridge, USA

Psychology Press Ltd, Publishers
27 Church Road
Hove
East Sussex
BN3 2FA
UK

British Library Cataloguing-in-Publication Data

A catalogue record for this book is available from the British Library

ISBN: 0-86377-693-0

Typeset by Quorum Technical Services Ltd, Cheltenham
Printed and bound in the United Kingdom by Henry Ling Ltd, Dorchester

Contents

---

* This book is also a special issue of the journal *Cognitive Neuropsychology* which forms Issues 3, 4 and 5 of Volume 16 (1999). The page numbers used here are taken from the journal and so begin on p. 193.

COGNITIVE NEUROPSYCHOLOGY, 1999, 16 (3/4/5), 193–195

THE COGNITIVE NEUROPSYCHOLOGY OF FALSE MEMORIES: INTRODUCTION

Daniel L. Schacter
Harvard University, Cambridge, USA

This special issue of Cognitive Neuropsychology is devoted to one of the most intensively investigated topics in recent memory research: the analysis of false memories. Experimental and theoretical studies of memory have long been informed by analyses of errors, distortions, and illusions in remembering (for reviews, see Estes, 1997; Johnson, Hashtroudi, & Lindsay, 1993; Roediger, 1996; Schacter, 1995). Within cognitive psychology, Sir Frederic Bartlett's monograph, *Remembering*, is generally recognised as a key source of modern research on memory distortions (Bartlett, 1932). Bartlett pioneered the use of errors and distortions as a tool for probing reconstructive aspect of memory. His approach enjoyed a revival during the 1970s, when a number of researchers developed new techniques for exploring memory distortions, and conceptualised them in the context of schema theories that were heavily influenced by Bartlett's thinking (Alba & Hasher, 1983). During the 1990s, there has been renewed interest in memory errors and distortions, sparked in part by a heated debate concerning the accuracy of traumatic memories recovered in psychotherapy (e.g., Loftus, 1993; Read & Lindsay, 1997). It is in the context of this debate that the term "false memory" has come into common usage in psychological research. False memories refer to recollections that are in some way distorted or, in extreme cases, involve remembering events that never happened at all.

Cognitive neuropsychologists, like cognitive psychologists, have long been aware of, and interested in, the occurrence of false memories. Until recently, relevant research was comprised mainly of descriptive case studies of patients who produced confabulations about past experiences. During the past few years, however, there has been a marked increase in experimental research and theorising concerning the cognitive neuropsychology of false memories. New methods for systematically eliciting and analysing confabulation have been developed, and research has extended beyond the domain of confabulation to investigate experimentally different kinds of memory distortions and illusions in a variety of populations. In addition, electrophysiological and neuroimaging techniques have been applied to the analysis of false memories. This recent surge of research has—much in the spirit of Bartlett—attempted to use the occurrence of memory distortions as a window into the nature of basic memory processes (for review, see Schacter, Norman, & Koutstaal, 1998).

The papers in this special issue are characterised by a variety of methodological and conceptual approaches. Kopelman provides an opening overview of cognitive neuropsychological research on false memories, and relates this work to theoretical, clinical, and legal issues. The next four papers involve detailed case studies of brain-damaged patients. Dab, Claes, Morais, and Shallice report a series of experiments indicating impaired search and intact monitoring or verification processes in a case of confabulation. Dab et al. discuss the observed pattern of preserved and impaired abilities in the context of several recent theoretical accounts of confabulation and related memory distortions.

Requests for reprints should be addressed to Daniel L. Schacter, Department of Psychology, Harvard University, Cambridge, MA 02138, USA.

Supported by grant AG08441 from the National Institute on Aging.

Parkin, Ward, Bindschaedler, Squires, and Powell describe a patient with left frontal lobe damage who exhibits exceptionally high levels of false recognition. Their experiments indicate that encoding deficits play an important role in this patient's heightened false recognition.

Rapcsak, Reminger, Glisky, Kaszniak, and Comer describe two patients with frontal lobe damage who exhibit increased false recognition of faces on both anterograde and retrograde memory tests. They conclude that these patients fail to invoke effortful strategies that can normally be used to suppress false recognition. Ward, Parkin, Powell, Squires, Townshend, and Bradley describe a patient who shows elevated false recognition of faces and names of unfamiliar people. Ward et al. establish the specificity of the deficit, relate the impairment to component processes that have been postulated in theoretical models of person recognition, and conclude that inflated false recognition results from a failure in top-down regulation of the person recognition system.

Four papers focus on groups of brain-damaged patients. The articles by Koutstaal, Schacter, Verfaellie, Brenner, and Jackson, and by Melo, Winocur, and Moscovitch examine false recognition and recall in amnesic patients. Previous research delineated conditions in which amnesic patients are more or less susceptible than controls to false memory effects, and related these findings to theoretical distinctions between memory for general or gist information on the one hand and memory for detailed, specific information on the other. The papers by Koutstaal et al. and Melo et al. extend and refine the earlier findings, point toward possible differences among subgroups of amnesic patients, and also help to specify the conditions under which amnesic patients show greater or lesser susceptibility to false memory effects.

Balota, Cortese, Duchek, Adams, Roediger, McDermott, and Yerys examine false recall and recognition in patients with Alzheimer's disease. They use a "converging semantic associates" procedure initially developed by Deese (1959), recently revived and modified by Roediger and McDermott (1995), that produces high levels of false recall and recognition in healthy people (this procedure was also used by Melo et al.). Balota et al. report evidence that, relative to their own level of veridical recall and recognition, Alzheimer's patients are more susceptible to false recall and recognition than are normal older adults. However, in absolute terms, Alzheimer's patients showed reduced levels of false recognition and similar levels of false recall compared to healthy elderly controls. Dalla Barba, Nedjam, and Dubois examined relations among confabulation, executive functions, and source memory in Alzheimer's patients. They found that confabulation arises with respect to the future as well as the past, and conclude that it results from a disorder of what they term "temporality".

Four papers focus on false memories in normal ageing. One of the more intriguing findings from recent research is that older adults are sometimes more susceptible to false memories than are younger adults, a finding that is replicated in the normal elderly controls studied by Balota et al. Using a variant of the Roediger and McDermott false recognition procedure that involves repeated study and testing, Kensinger and Schacter report that young adults reduce false recognition with repeated study/test trials whereas older adults do not. They relate this finding to the theoretical distinction between memory for gist and specific information. Jacoby also provides evidence that older adults can be more susceptible to false memories than younger adults, using a novel procedure in which subjects are biased to produce false memories by misinformation that is presented after an initial learning trial. Jacoby discusses his results and related findings in terms of an accessibility bias that influences performance independently of recollective processes.

The articles by Kensinger and Schacter and by Jacoby both consider the contribution of impaired recollection of source information to age-related increases in false memories. Mather, Johnson, and De Leonardis extend research on source monitoring and ageing into a novel domain: stereotype reliance. They show that older individuals, who are characterised by poor memory for the exact source of information, tend to rely more on pre-existing stereotypes when trying to remember who said what than do younger adults. They also report evidence that these effects are related to performance on tasks sensitive to frontal lobe dysfunction. Similarly, Rubin, Van Petten, Glisky, and Newberg found that older adults' susceptibility to illusory memory conjunctions, where people falsely recognise as "old" re-combinations of previously studied items, is related to performance on frontal-sensitive tasks. They also report a separate study using event-related potentials that shows that brain activity during true recognition differs from that observed during false recognition of illusory conjunctions.

Dodhia and Metcalfe investigate two types of false memories—one involving misleading post-event information (Loftus, Miller, & Burns, 1978), the other involving false recognition of semantic associates in a variant of the Roediger and McDermott procedure—in the context of a formal computational model (CHARM). They demonstrate how the model can help to explain some of the effects they observe, but also present data concerning the suppression of false memories that are difficult for the model to handle. In discussing how the model needs to be altered to account for the observed patterns of data, Dodhia and Metcalfe provide a further illustration of how the investigation of false memory phenomena can be revealing at a theoretical level.

Taken together, the findings and ideas from the papers in the special issue constitute a compelling case that the study of memory errors, distortions, and illusions from a cognitive neuropsychological perspective can provide useful insights into basic memory processes (for further discussion and illustration, see Schacter, in press). They thus suggest that further development of the cognitive neuropsychology of false memories will be an informative and enlightening enterprise.

REFERENCES

Alba, J.W., & Hasher, L. (1983). Is memory schematic? *Psychological Bulletin, 93*, 203–231.

Bartlett, F.C. (1932). *Remembering*. Cambridge: Cambridge University Press.

Deese, J. (1959). On the prediction of occurrence of particular verbal intrusions in immediate recall. *Journal of Experimental Psychology, 58*, 17–22.

Estes, W.K. (1997). Processes of memory loss, recovery, and distortion. *Psychological Review, 104*, 148–169.

Johnson, M.K., Hashtroudi, S., & Lindsay, D.S. (1993). Source monitoring. *Psychological Bulletin, 114*, 3–28.

Loftus, E.F. (1993). The reality of repressed memories. *American Psychologist, 48*, 518–537.

Loftus, E.F., Miller, D.G., & Burns, H.J. (1978). Integration of verbal information into a visual memory. *Journal of Experimental Psychology: Human Learning and Memory, 4*, 19–31.

Read, J.D., & Lindsay, D.S. (Eds.) (1997). *Recollections of trauma: Scientific research and clinical practice*. New York: Plenum Press.

Roediger, H.L., III. (1996). Memory illusions. *Journal of Memory and Language, 35*, 76–100.

Roediger, H.L., III, & McDermott, K.B. (1995). Creating false memories: Remembering words not presented in lists. *Journal of Experimental Psychology: Learning, Memory and Cognition, 21*, 803–814.

Schacter, D.L. (1995). Memory distortion: History and current status. In D.L. Schacter (Ed.) *Memory distortion: How minds, brains, and societies reconstruct the past.* (pp. 1–43). Cambridge, MA: Harvard University Press.

Schacter, D.L. (in press). The seven sins of memory: Insights from psychology and cognitive neuroscience. *American Psychologist*.

Schacter, D.L., Norman, K.A., & Koutstaal, W. (1998). The cognitive neuroscience of constructive memory. *Annual Review of Psychology, 49*, 289–318.

COGNITIVE NEUROPSYCHOLOGY, 1999, 16 (3/4/5), 197–214

VARIETIES OF FALSE MEMORY

Michael D. Kopelman
King's College, University of London, UK

False memories have been described in many different contexts, but their characteristics and underlying mechanisms have seldom been compared or debated. Those reviewed in the present paper include: spontaneous confabulation in brain disease, false recognition cases, delusional memories and other delusions in psychosis, "confabulations" in schizophrenia, "internalised" false confessions for crime, apparently false or distorted memories for child abuse, pseudologia fantastica, the acquisition of new identities or "scripts" following fugue or in multiple personality, and momentary confabulation in healthy subjects. It is suggested that these should be viewed as different types of false memory, and that confabulations and delusions should be kept conceptually distinct. However, they can all be characterised within a general model of memory and executive function, provided that social factors and some notion of "self" (here called a "personal semantic belief system") are included in the model.

INTRODUCTION

Neuropsychological discussion of false memories has traditionally confined itself to those confabulations that can arise in organic amnesia and/or frontal lobe disease. However, the notions of "false memory" and "confabulation" have recently been broadened to encompass a much wider range of disorders. In part, this results from neuropsychologists applying their methods in new contexts, including psychiatric and forensic settings, but also it results from social concerns about the implications of false memories. Questions arise concerning whether the false memories that occur in these various contexts represent the same or differing phenomena, whether they should all be called "confabulation," and whether their underlying mechanisms/deficits have anything in common. This issue has not been debated, to date, by those employing the term "confabulation" within these new contexts, and the purpose of the present paper is to review these varieties of false memory and to pose these questions.

SPONTANEOUS CONFABULATION IN FRONTAL DISORDERS AND AMNESIA

Spontaneous Confabulation

This is the form of false memory most familiar to neuropsychologists, and consequently it will be reviewed only briefly. It can be regarded as a kind of template, against which to compare the other types of false memory. In "spontaneous"confabulation, there is a persistent, unprovoked outpouring of erroneous memories, as distinct from "momentary" or "provoked" confabulation, in which fleeting

Requests for reprints should be addressed to Michael D. Kopelman, Neuropsychiatry and Memory Disorders Clinic, Division of Psychiatry and Psychology, King's College, University of London, St Thomas's Campus, London SE1 7EH, UK.

The author is grateful to Dr. Kate Leafhead for reading an early draft of this paper and to the editor and Professors Art Shimamura and Martin Conway for helpful referee comments.

intrusion errors or distortions are seen in response to a challenge to memory, such as a memory test (Berlyne, 1972; Kopelman, 1987a). Spontaneous confabulation arises most commonly in autobiographical or other aspects of episodic memory (Dalla Barba, 1993a; Dalla Barba, Cappelletti, Signorini, & Denes, 1997), but it can occur in semantic memory as well (Dalla Barba, 1993b; Kopelman, Ng, & Van den Bourke, 1997; Moscovitch & Melo, 1997). Spontaneous confabulation has usually been attributed to executive dysfunction, resulting from frontal lobe pathology (Baddeley & Wilson, 1986; Kapur & Coughlan, 1980; Luria, 1976; Moscovitch & Melo, 1997; Stuss, Alexander, Liberman, & Levine, 1978), but confusional states and/or metabolic disturbance can also produce executive dysfunction and confabulation (DeLuca & Cicerone, 1991; Kopelman et al., 1997). There have been a number of recent attempts to provide a more specific explanation of what goes wrong in spontaneous confabulation. These have taken the form of either (1) an emphasis on disrupted "editing" functions, or (2) an emphasis on temporal context or other source monitoring deficits.

Disrupted Editing Processes

Moscovitch (1989) postulated a deficit in the strategic component of retrieval processes, such that loose rules of plausibility and association are left to guide memory retrieval, and the resulting "memories" are not edited or suppressed (inhibited) in a normal fashion. Somewhat similarly, Conway and Tacchi (1996) discussed a failure in the executive evaluation of accessed memories, and Kopelman (1987a) attributed spontaneous confabulation to "the completely incoherent and context-free retrieval of memories and associations." Burgess and Shallice (1996a) proposed deficits in a description process, an editor process, and a mediator process, which all contribute differently to the clinical phenomena of confabulations. The "descriptor" produces a specification of the type of trace that would satisfy the demands of a retrieval task, and "noisy" specification will increase the chance of an inappropriate representation being produced as a candidate memory. The "editor" checks that the output of the long-term storage system fits with previously retrieved memory elements and also with the overall task requirements. When the "editor" is impaired, confabulators will respond to a question without giving it adequate consideration or checking and self-correcting themselves (compare Mercer, Wapner, Gardner, & Benson, 1977). The "mediator" controls cognitive (strategic and problem solving) operations concerning the adequacy or plausibility of retrieved memory elements under strategic control: Impairment results in reasoning errors and in the presence of bizarre or "fantastic" responses. This model is in essence very similar to Moscovitch and Melo's (1997) formulation that confabulation is the product of impaired cue-retrieval (cues can be ambiguous, resulting in retrieval errors in normal subjects but especially if memory is impaired), faulty strategic search (producing misleading cues and, thereby, inappropriate memories), and defective monitoring (the resulting errors are not edited out).

Schacter, Norman, and Koutstaal (1998) have recently proposed a general "constructive memory framework" emphasising both encoding operations (initial binding of the distributed features of an episode together as a coherent trace with sufficient pattern separation of similar episodes) and retrieval processes (formation of a sufficiently focused retrieval description with which to probe memory stores, plus post-retrieval monitoring and verification). If episodes are not stored in a manner that allows them to be accessed separately at retrieval *or* if retrieval cues are not specific enough ("focused") *or* if criterion-setting is lax, memory distortion or confabulation is likely to result.

Context and Source Monitoring Deficits

The second major approach places emphasis upon temporal context memory impairments, resulting in a confusion about the temporal ordering of memory fragments (Schnider, von Däniken, &

Gutbrod, 1996), or upon an impairment in the functioning of "temporal consciousness" (Dalla Barba et al., 1997) or, more broadly, upon a deficit in source monitoring (Johnson, 1991; Johnson, Hashtroudi, & Lindsay, 1993; Schacter, Harbluk, & McLachlan, 1984). This is, of course, neither a new idea nor completely unrelated to the editing deficits just considered. Korsakoff (1889) himself placed emphasis upon, and gave examples of, temporal confusions resulting in confabulations, and this idea has been taken up by many others (e.g. Moll, 1915; Talland, 1965; Van der Horst, 1932; Victor, Adams, & Collins, 1971). In a neat study, Schnider et al. (1996) found that a small group of "spontaneous confabulators" could be differentiated from other amnesic patients and healthy controls on the basis of their errors on a temporal context memory task, but not on other memory or executive tasks. In Dalla Barba's (1993a; Dalla Barba et al., 1997) variant of this hypothesis, "temporal consciousness" is intact but malfunctioning, in that confabulating patients are aware of a past, present, and future (unlike severely amnesic patients) but, in making temporal judgements, they employ only the most stable elements from their long-term memory stores. Asked what they did yesterday or will do tomorrow, the patients reply with the well-established routines or habits of a lifetime, however irrelevant to their present situation. More generally, Johnson and colleagues (Johnson, 1991; Johnson et al., 1993) have argued that confabulation may result from a wider range of source (context) or reality (differentiating the "real" from the imagined) monitoring deficits which, in turn, could be secondary to impairments in encoding, retrieval, motivation, or judgement processes.

Two recent studies (Johnson, O'Connor, & Cantor, 1997; Kopelman et al., 1997) provide some support for this viewpoint, but they also make it clear that temporal or source monitoring deficits alone cannot account for all instances of confabulation (compare Moscovitch & Melo, 1997). In the Kopelman et al. (1997) study, an analysis of a severely confabulating patient's errors suggested that many confabulations (particularly in episodic memory) may plausibly have resulted from the conflation and inappropriate retrieval of "real" memory fragments out of temporal sequence, but that others resulted from perseverations (particularly in semantic memory) or from the patient giving instantaneous, ill-considered, and unchecked responses to immediate environmental and social cues. The Johnson et al. (1997) study failed to discriminate between a severely confabulating patient and three other patients with frontal lesions in terms of performance on several measures of source monitoring. Johnson et al. concluded that confabulation may reflect an interaction between a vivid imagination, an inability to retrieve autobiographical memories systematically, and source monitoring deficits.

Social Context

In the light of the discussion to follow, it is worth emphasising that the social context may influence or even be causative in some instances of confabulation (Johnson, 1991; Kopelman et al., 1997), and Conway and Tacchi (1996) argued that a subject's current preoccupations and motivations can influence the content of confabulation. Kopelman (1997) mentioned the example of a man who was the innocent victim of a bombing, during which he sustained a fairly severe head injury. This man was attended in hospital for the first 24 hours by very fierce-looking armed police officers but, by the time he came out of his confused state and post-traumatic amnesia (which was after approximately 72 hours), the police had gone. During the course of the following week, the patient started to retrieve a few "fragments" of memory from within the amnesic gap, but he said that he had difficulty determining when and where some of these memories had arisen: for example, he had a memory of looking up at a vehicle on a dark night, but he was unsure when and in what city this had occurred. However, some months later, he gave a graphic description of the police's response to him in hospital. Although this might conceivably have been a retrieved fragment of memory, the man's semi-comatose state and severe confusion during the first 24 hours of his hospitalisation make it much more likely that this was a confabulation—based on what his relatives and friends had told him about the admittedly very tense situation when he arrived in hospital.

False Recognition

A related issue concerns three case studies of patients who showed a high rate of false recognition responses on cognitive testing (Delbecq-Derouesné, Beauvois, & Shallice, 1990; Parkin, Bindschaedler, Harsent, & Metzler, 1996; Schacter, Curran, Gallucio, Milberg, & Bates, 1996). All these patients had frontal lobe lesions (bilateral, right-, and left-sided respectively). One patient was reported to confabulate (Delbecq-Derouesné et al., 1990); the second (Schacter et al., 1996) did not engage in "extensive" spontaneous confabulation, and did not show confabulations when administered the "confabulation batteries" developed by Dalla Barba (1993a) and Moscovitch (1995); in the third case (Parkin et al., 1996), no comment was made, although the particular pathology (ruptured anterior communicating artery aneurysm) is often associated with confabulation in the early stages. In two of these patients (Schacter et al., 1996; Parkin et al., 1996), the pathological false recognition appeared to be particularly evident when novel material was presented from previously studied semantic categories, but it was also present in response to nonstudied words, pseudowords, faces, and environmental sounds. It was suggested that false alarms arose when the test items were "generally" (Schacter) or "incidentally" (Parkin) consistent with the class, category, or characteristics of a study list, and the patients failed to recollect the identity of particular items: in such circumstances, both patients showed an over-reliance on familiarity (Schacter et al., 1996; Parkin et al., 1996). However, unlike confabulating patients, these three patients showed a relative preservation of recall for everyday experiences. As also discussed by Delbecq-Derouesné et al. (1990), what remains unclear is whether such cases provide a "model" for one particular component of the deficits found in confabulating patients, or whether theirs is a qualitatively distinct disorder.

DELUSIONAL MEMORIES, CONFABULATIONS, AND DELUSIONS IN PSYCHIATRIC PATIENTS

Delusional Memory

Delusional memory is the closest analogue in psychiatric patients of confabulation in neurological cases. A delusional memory consists of either a true memory that gives rise to a deluded interpretation or (more commonly) a false memory arising in the context of a psychosis (Buchanan, 1991; Kopelman, 1997). Kopelman (1987b) argued that the clinical phenomena of delusional memories can closely resemble those of spontaneous confabulations, resulting from frontal lobe disease. By definition, a delusional memory is held as an absolute conviction, not amenable to argument, and not culturally explicable. Delusional memories are usually intensely preoccupying, and often bizarre. Similar features were described in spontaneous confabulation by Baddeley and Wilson (1986), and it is often only the context that distinguishes the clinical features of a delusional memory from those of confabulation, i.e. psychosis rather than organic amnesia and/or frontal lobe disease (Buchanan, 1991; Kopelman, 1987b, 1997).

However, there may be certain respects in which delusional memories differ from spontaneous confabulations. The first is that they may be more elaborate and systematised, and sometimes they occur in people who are otherwise functioning normally without other complaints (Baddeley, Thornton, Chua, & McKenna, 1996; Kopelman, Guinan, & Lewis, 1995). Kopelman (1997) gave the example of a garage mechanic who claimed in 1981 that he had planned and carried out a well-publicised murder involving a London aristocrat 8 years' earlier. This man's account was very convincing, and he had been living a well-integrated and apparently normal life until his intense preoccupations with the "murder" resulted in a hospital admission, in which other "first rank" symptoms of schizophrenia became evident. The "memory" subsided to a considerable extent on treatment with neuroleptic medication, although it never completely disappeared. Likewise, Kopelman et al. (1995) described a 47-year-old clerical worker, who had been studying for a PhD in English literature and who was extremely articulate about Chaucerian and Shakespearean works. This woman claimed that, in the summer of 1970, she had been working on a fruit-picking farm, when she encountered an internationally famous orchestral conductor, who also happened to be working there. She claimed that he fell in love with her and pursued her, and that they had been communicating by "telepathy" ever since. There is no evidence that the meeting had ever occurred or that there had been any relationship (an instance of the so-called de Clérambault syndrome), but this "memory" remained intensely preoccupying for years thereafter.

In the Kopelman et al. (1995) case, a number of cognitive tests were carried out. Consistent with her educational accomplishments, this patient was found to have a verbal IQ of 131, and she did not show any evidence of executive or frontal dysfunction. In the latter respect, she was unlike virtually all patients with spontaneous confabulation described in the literature. Somewhat similarly, David and Howard (1994) described four patients with delusional memories: A limited range of cognitive tests were performed, but these included the cognitive estimates task (Shallice & Evans, 1978), on which none of the patients showed any evidence of executive dysfunction. However, David and Howard (1994) obtained some evidence that the perceptual characteristics of their patients' delusional memories were stronger than those of real memories, and they argued that this misled an "evaluation system" to accept the delusional memories as real, despite their inherent implausibility. Nevertheless, delusional memories cannot be simply bright or vivid perceptions. It is likely that some interaction between a person's mental state, self-beliefs, and expectations results in the abnormal perceptual qualities and the deluded interpretation of these memories. This will be considered further later.

"Confabulation" in Schizophrenia

Nathaniel-James and Frith (1996) have recently investigated "confabulation" in schizophrenic patients, requiring their patients to recall a fable/story, and then to identify the correct moral from it. They found a significantly increased rate of intrusion errors or "momentary" confabulations in the schizophrenic patients' recall, compared with that of healthy controls. This remained true even after attempting to control post hoc for the level of recall performance by examining confabulations in two matched sub-groups of subjects. The authors found a significant association with performance on one executive test (the Hayling test; Burgess & Shallice, 1996b), but not with two more traditional executive tests (card-sorting, verbal fluency). Correlations with anterograde memory tests were not reported. Nathaniel-James and Frith argued that the schizophrenic patients appeared to be reorganising and reconstructing the original story material, resulting in new ideas. They contrasted this observation with the findings in Korsakoff and Alzheimer patients by Kopelman (1987), arguing that these patients' confabulations were qualitatively different in that they tended to introduce irrelevant or unrelated material into the story. In a more detailed investigation of three of their patients, Nathaniel-James, Foong, and Frith (1996) found that schizophrenic patients were unable to distinguish plausible from implausible sentences and stories or to correct their errors after listening to a tape-recording of their own recall of the fables. They found that all three confabulating patients performed poorly on measures of response suppression (the Hayling test) and response monitoring (a continuous series task; Gurd, 1995). Nathaniel-James and colleagues concluded that confabulation in schizophrenic patients appears to be related to an inability to monitor and suppress inappropriate responses and also (to a lesser extent) to "formal thought disorder," and they argued that faults occur both at input, where narrative material is encoded in a disorganised manner, and at output, where this disorganisation is compounded by a faulty editing process (Nathaniel-James & Frith, 1996; Nathaniel-James et al., 1996).

A difficulty with these studies is that it is not entirely clear how far the schizophrenics' intrusion errors might simply reflect (1) the impaired anterograde memory found in schizophrenic patients (Cutting, 1979; McKenna et al., 1990) and (2) the particular delusional beliefs that preoccupied their patients. Although Nathaniel-James and Frith (1996) addressed these issues, their matching for level of memory performance was post-hoc, and an experimental manipulation to control for the level of performance would be desirable. Second, a detailed analysis of the extent to which the "confabulation" related to delusional themes was not given. Finally, the qualitative contrast with the performance of Korsakoff and Alzheimer patients in the Kopelman (1987a) study was not entirely justified, since the nature of the confabulations in the amnesic patients varied from subject-to-subject (some reorganised and reconstructed the story). The most striking difference was that the amnesic patients' responses were much briefer than the schizophrenics', presumably reflecting the severity of their memory disorder—which is why experimental matching of recall memory is needed in this type of study. In brief, whilst the Nathaniel-James and Frith argument is very interesting, it remains possible that the "confabulations" of schizophrenics are simply momentary intrusion errors and distortions, resulting from a faulty memory (as discussed later), coloured by the preoccupying delusional beliefs of these patients.

Delusions

The preceding section raises the question of the relationship between delusions and memory and executive function but, before considering this, it is necessary to distinguish between delusions in general and delusional memories, which are a very specific type of delusion. Delusions are common in psychiatric patients, whereas delusional memories are very rare. Delusions can be interpreted in terms of memory dysfunction, but it is by no means unequivocal that they are best understood as memory phenomena: Their content can be very varied, and they can arise either secondarily to an hallucination or to an affective state, or as a deluded interpretation of a "real" perception, or out of a particularly perplexed psychological state (known as delusional mood or delusional atmosphere), or they may emerge "out of the blue" (autochthonous delusions) (Schneider, 1959; Fish, 1967; Gelder, Gath, & Mayou, 1989; Kopelman, 1994). For example, relatively common delusions—for instance, that one's thoughts are being controlled, or that one has a special religious mission, or that spies are lining up outside the house—do not necessarily have a memory component. By contrast, delusional memory is by definition a memory phenomenon.

Baddeley et al. (1996) have investigated the relationship of delusions to memory and executive function by comparing the cognitive performance of five schizophrenic patients, who were currently experiencing delusions, with that of five other schizophrenic patients who were no longer experiencing delusions. These authors found no or minimal differences between these two groups across a number of standard executive, episodic, and semantic memory tasks. Moreover, the deluded schizophrenic patients performed *better* than the comparison group on the autobiographical incident component of the Autobiographical Memory Interview (Kopelman, Wilson, & Baddeley, 1989, 1990). This difference was mainly accounted for by the tendency of the nondeluded patients to produce generic memories, or no memories at all, rather than recall of specific incidents. However, it was also noted that, although the rate of production of personal memories by the deluded patients was relatively normal, they did tend to produce some bizarre responses. As in studies of delusional memory (David & Howard, 1994; Kopelman et al., 1995), the authors found no evidence that delusions were associated with a specific deficit in executive function, either by itself or in association with memory impairment. They also noted that delusions tended to be relatively fixed, compared with the shifting and changing nature of many confabulations. Baddeley et al. (1996) concluded that the delusional beliefs of schizophrenic patients, although often bizarre, did not simply reflect a breakdown in executive function or autobiographical memory.

On the other hand, delusional misidentification syndromes are often associated with the concurrence of bilateral frontal lobe pathology and right posterior lesions (Ellis & Young, 1990; Young, Leafhead, & Szulecka, 1994; Young, Reid, Wright, & Hellawell, 1993). In these cases, there can be a link with confabulation. Box, Laing, and Kopelman (in press) have recently described a young woman who suffered a severe head injury, resulting in pathology to the right ventro-medial frontal cortex with some involvement of the left ventro-medial and the right dorso-lateral regions as well. There was also a right parietal infarct. The patient showed fleeting confabulations, which were succeeded by a more stable Fregoli (misidentification) delusion, in which the patient believed that her mother was occupying the bed opposite, followed in turn by the deluded belief that a nephew was inhabiting the hospital. These psychiatric features arose in the context of severe memory, perceptual, and executive dysfunctions, which outlasted the abnormal beliefs by several months. The findings were interpreted in terms of an initial deficit in the executive "specification" and "verification" of memories, the specification dysfunction resolving more rapidly than the problem in verification. It was argued that the co-occurrence of spontaneous confabulation and delusional misidentification probably resulted from the bilateral ventro-medial frontal pathology, but that neuropsychological theory also needs to take account of how these abnormal ideas emerge, evolve, and wane through time.

Confabulation and Delusions

In summary, there is a strong case for keeping the notions of confabulation, delusional memory, and delusion conceptually separate. Although delusional memories share many characteristics with spontaneous confabulation, they differ in that delusional memories appear to be thematic and unrelated to executive dysfunction, whereas confabulations are fluctuating and multifaceted as well as virtually always related to executive dysfunction (Baddeley et al., 1996; Kopelman et al., 1995). Furthermore, it is very important to distinguish between delusional memory, which is rare and by definition a memory phenomenon, and delusions in general, which are common and not necessarily related to memory. In general, empirical evidence suggests that delusions occur independently of any memory or executive dysfunction (Baddeley et al., 1996; Kopelman et al., 1995). Delusions constitute abnormal beliefs about oneself and/or about the external world, which may arise for a variety of reasons. In very specific instances, deluded self-beliefs can interact with the contents of perception or fantasy to produce a delusional memory (see earlier). Moreover, very occasionally, certain specific forms of delusion, such as delusional misidentification, may coincide with or even appear to evolve from spontaneous confabulations, because of common underlying (frontal) pathology (Benson & Stuss, 1990; Box et al., in press).

FALSE CONFESSIONS AND MEMORIES IN FORENSIC SETTINGS

False Confessions

False confession to an offence is an instance in which false or faulty memory can have devastating consequences to oneself. Gudjonsson. and colleagues (Gudjonsson, 1992; Gudjonsson & MacKeith, 1988; Gudjonsson & Lebegue, 1989) have described a series of people who have made false confessions and, in many cases, subsequent evidence has confirmed that the confessor could not have committed the crime. A striking feature of these accounts is that the subject can become very convinced and convincing about what was alleged to have happened.

Gudjonsson and MacKeith (1988) described four circumstances in which people make voluntary false confessions—a morbid desire for publicity or notoriety; a desire to aid or protect a real criminal; the belief of a guilt-ridden individual that confessing to a crime will relieve him or her of guilt about some real or imagined previous transgression; and the inability of a person with a psychiatric disorder to distinguish between reality and fantasy. In addition, there are coerced confessions that, in some cases, become internalised, i.e. the subject eventually comes to believe what he or she has "confessed." For example, Gudjonsson and MacKeith (1990) described a 17-year-old man, who made a very detailed confession, which he repeated on several occasions, concerning the murder of two frail and elderly neighbours. After being held in custody for

1 year, he was released by a Court when somebody else pleaded guilty to the murders and was convicted. The latter person always insisted he had acted alone, and his self-incriminating admissions were supported by other evidence. The authors identified a number of factors which had resulted in a "coerced-internalised" type of confession by the initial suspect.

More recently, Gudjonsson, Kopelman, and MacKeith (in press) have described a case of false confession in which the degree of coercion by the police was minimal, although there were errors of omission (failure to call a lawyer or doctor early enough) as well as serious mistakes by the medical and legal teams involved. A 17-year-old man had voluntarily walked into a police station to try to ascertain in his own mind whether or not he had committed a particularly brutal murder. The young man had been interviewed by police in routine enquiries, and he spent the following evening preoccupied with "visions" of the victim's face, and he determined to go to the police station the next day to make up his mind whether or not he had committed the murder. During the course of the next 24 hours, the young man's statements progressed from "it might have been me" and "I don't know if I killed her or not. I keep seeing her", through "I must have done it because I can see a picture of her", to "I am sure I killed her ... I know I did it." Ultimately, this resulted in a written "confession." In this case, the man continued to equivocate, and he went to trial, unsure what he would plead, but wanting to see the evidence to help him make up his mind regarding his own guilt. He was convicted and served 25 years in prison before his conviction was quashed on the basis of fresh psychological and psychiatric evidence, but during the intervening years he made at least two unequivocal "confessions."

Gudjonsson and MacKeith (1982) have introduced the concept of a "memory distrust syndrome," in which people develop a fundamental distrust of their own memories and become vulnerable to making a false confession. This can be seen as a form of source amnesia (Johnson et al., 1993; Schacter et al., 1984) because the distrust makes subjects more susceptible to relying on external sources of information, and they become confused concerning whether memories have been generated internally or from external sources. Gudjonsson (1992) has described a number of contexts in which a memory distrust syndrome may develop, and he uses the term "confabulation" to describe the false memories that result. Factors such as depression and low self esteem may make a subject especially vulnerable to this process (Gudjonsson et al., in press).

Because of this phenomenon, Gudjonsson and colleagues have conducted a series of investigations examining the predispositions to confabulation when recalling prose passages from the Gudjonsson Suggestibility Scale (Gudjonsson, 1987). They have investigated forensic psychiatric patients from regional secure units (Smith & Gudjonsson, 1995a,b) as well as Icelandic juvenile offenders (Gudjonsson & Sigurdsson, 1995). They have found that frank intrusion errors ("fabrications") were not correlated with distortions in memory, that confabulation was not strongly correlated with memory, intelligence, self-esteem, or compliance, and that confabulation did not correlate with scores from a reality monitoring task (Johnson & Raye, 1981; Bentall, Baker, & Havers, 1991). In one study, there were significant correlations with rate of forgetting, anxiety, and suggestibility scores (Smith & Gudjonsson, 1995a), but the association with suggestibility did not emerge in another study (Gudjonsson & Sigurdsson, 1995). Smith and Gudjonsson (1995a) concluded that a subject's uncertainty and expectations are factors contributing to suggestibility and that they may also influence confabulation, but that other factors must also contribute to confabulation.

A major problem with these latter studies obviously concerns how far momentary confabulations in story recall can be used as a model for false confessions in major crime. On the other hand, it seems plausible from the case-studies that such confessions are produced by a combination of external coercion, internal self-doubt (from low self-esteem and/or depression), and source memory errors, resulting in faulty attribution. The case studies also suggest that the strength with which these faulty attributions are held can vary from continuing uncertainty to absolute conviction.

Recovered Memory for Childhood Sexual Abuse

Whereas the false memories of confessors cause damage to themselves, the allegedly false accusations and memories in child sexual abuse cases can result in considerable harm to others. This controversial topic has been extensively reviewed elsewhere (Conway, 1997; Read & Lindsay, 1997; Schacter, Coyle, Fischbach, Mesulam, & Sullivan, 1995). Lindsay and Read (1994, p. 328) concluded that:

> One of the most unnerving implications of the cognitive psychological research reviewed in this paper is that people can be very confident in their memories and beliefs and, at the same time, very wrong. People can believe they are remembering events in their own lives when those events never happened.... We believe that our concern about the possibility of illusory memories of childhood sexual abuse is better grounded in reality than the beliefs of people who deny the fallibility of memory and argue for the unqualified acceptance of all reports of recovered memories of childhood events.

On the other hand, there are many studies indicating a widespread prevalence of (remembered) child sexual abuse (e.g. Mullen, Martin, Anderson, Romans, & Herbison, 1993; Romans, Martin, Anderson, O'Shea, & Mullen, 1995), and Oliver (1993) drew attention to cases of documented abuse (not necessarily sexual), which were not reported in subsequent self-report surveys, some of which Oliver attributed to "memory blockages." Pope and Hudson (1995) reviewed studies that attempted to test whether memories of childhood sexual abuse can be repressed, finding only four investigations bearing on this issue—Herman and Schatzow (1987); Briere and Conte (1993); Loftus, Polonsky, and Fullilove (1994); and Williams (1994). They criticised these studies on the basis that *either* the original abuse had not been corroborated *or* the findings were heavily dependent on self-report, in which case a report of past forgetting needed to be corroborated. On the basis of these observations, the authors concluded that "present evidence is insufficient to permit the conclusion that individuals can 'repress' memories of childhood sexual abuse," and the implication was that "recovered memories" must be "false." On the other hand, given the difficulty of corroborating past abuse or past forgetting, there was suggestive evidence within the cited studies that subsamples of the subjects, who reported abuse, might indeed have experienced forgetting at some time in the past (for example, 19% in the Loftus et al., 1994 study). Moreover, Schooler and colleagues (Schooler, Ambadar, & Bendiksen, 1997; Schooler, Bendiksen, & Ambadar, 1997) have described a number of cases where the recovery of memories for trauma or abuse appears to have been corroborated, and there was at least some evidence of previous forgetting.

Shimamura (1997) documented the evidence that highly emotional or traumatic experiences can enhance memory storage transiently but in a fragmented form, in which "free-floating" memory fragments are poorly located in temporal and spatial context. On the basis of what is known about frontal and medial temporal mechanisms in memory (Shimamura, 1994, 1997), such memory fragments would be especially vulnerable both to forgetting and to distortions and augmentations such that, if memory were reinstated, it would be very unlikely to be either accurate or complete. A somewhat similar argument (Schacter, 1996; Schacter, Norman, & Koutstaal, 1997) is that, in some subjects, memories for abuse are never actually completely forgotten, but they are retained in a vague, unelaborated form, because they have seldom or never been rehearsed; such memories would be vulnerable to the normal processes of decay and interference, together with the use of conscious avoidance or suppression. Appropriate cueing might result in re-retrieval of these memories, but the "weak trace" would make them very vulnerable to distortion. It is also very plausible that false memories for sexual abuse may be much more likely to arise in particular social contexts (Kopelman, 1997), which might be a seed-bed of dispute and misunderstanding, sexual ambiguity, and misinterpreted cues, sometimes (but not necessarily) fanned by over-interpretative therapist interventions.

OTHER INSTANCES OF FALSE MEMORY IN PSYCHIATRIC PATIENTS

There are other, rare instances in which false memories arise in psychiatric patients, associated with the adoption of a false identity or identities. For example, occasional patients are seen who create a web of fantasies, lies, and untruths around themselves, almost compulsively. This phenomenon is known as "pseudologia fantastica" (or, sometimes, "pathological lying"), which Fish (1967) classified as a form of confabulation. This occurs in people who do not have known brain disease or frontal lobe dysfunction, although they are often of low IQ. For example, the present author once saw a young man, not very bright and originally from a family of travellers, who talked endlessly about being a pop star, about other stars he knew, and about his show business activities, despite the fact that it soon became clearly apparent that he led a fairly mundane life in South London and he had come to attention after being charged with a minor offence. Nevertheless, he appeared to believe his own stories, including his statement that he was "world-wide famous in Streatham." Fish claims that some such subjects "enjoy dressing up in uniforms and posing as officers in the armed forces, while others pass themselves off as secret service agents." He comments that "as many secret service agents are immature, histrionic individuals, it may be difficult to distinguish these patients from the real thing"(!).

There may be certain resemblances between such patients and those who develop an apparently prolonged psychogenic amnesia, following a typical fugue episode, or even those with multiple personality (dissociative identity) disorder. Kopelman, Christensen, Puffet, and Stanhope (1994) described a patient who experienced a typical fugue state lasting 7 days, but who then continued to report autobiographical amnesia for a further period of almost 18 months. In the meantime, the patient had established herself with a new name, a new home, a new job, a new relationship (and eventually marriage), and in a new country—a completely novel identity and way of life. Subsequently, it was found that she had (at least partially) been simulating her amnesia from about 3 months after the onset, despite her excellent performance on most laboratory-designed tests for "simulation." This does not mean that this patient was completely or deliberately malingering in the sense of being fully aware of what she was doing: She was extremely convincing, and she gave the impression of being someone who had come to believe her own "scripts" (Conway, 1990; Schank & Abelson, 1977). Interestingly, there were instances when this patient was able to recognise something (such as the hotel she had initially stayed at in London) or "knew" something (for example, that photographs must be of her relatives) without being able to remember or consciously recollect anything else about them; this is similar to phenomena widely described in normal memory and organic amnesia (Gardiner & Parkin, 1990; Kopelman, 1995; Schacter, 1987). There are certain resemblances in the description by Markowitsch, Fink, Thöne, Kessler, and Heiss (1997) of a 37-year-old patient who experienced a fugue episode for 5 days whilst out cycling, ending up 200 miles south of his home, and who then continued to claim autobiographical amnesia for a period of at least 8 months following the initial episode. From the behaviour of the Kopelman et al. (1994) case, it is possible to see how multiple personality disorder (dissociative identity disorder) might evolve, if differing scripts were encouraged and reinforced by doctors and psychologists as well as the outside world (Merskey, 1992, 1995). If that were the case, it would be entirely consistent with the evidence of inter-personality transfer of implicit learning in the absence of inter-personality transfer of explicit memories, described by Kihlstrom and Schacter (1995).

In these cases, the salient feature is not so much how the new "memories" have emerged (sometimes following a short period of memory loss), but that the subject appears to believe these memories with some degree of conviction, and does not seem simply to be malingering. Conway and Tacchi (1996) argued that control processes evaluate patterns of activation arising in a long-term knowledge base, accepting or rejecting representations as being memories or not of an experienced event, according to whether or not they are compatible with some other aspect of control processes, i.e. the self. The self is defined as "a currently active set of personal plans and goals derived from more elaborate representations," which influences retrieval from autobiographical memory, but which is also constrained by the autobiographical knowledge base. Conway (1996; Conway & Tacchi, 1996) postulated that autobiographical memories are transitory mental constructions that are effortfully constructed and effortfully maintained: He argued that three broad layers of autobiographical knowledge have been identified—lifetime periods, general events, and event-specific knowledge. Lifetime periods refer to lengthy periods of time typically measured in years and they represent goals, plans, and themes of the self during these particular periods. Conceivably, in each of the above examples, a person's current conception of self or identity produces a shift in the organisation of these lifetime periods within autobiographical memory and either a selective failure to retrieve from certain lifetime periods relative to others (following fugue or in multiple personality) or biased and anomalous recall (pseudologia fantastica). Such selectivity of retrieval would also be comprehensible if autobiographical memory were organised along the lines proposed in Morton's "headed records" model (Morton, Hammersley, & Bekerian, 1985).

MOMENTARY CONFABULATION IN HEALTHY SUBJECTS

It should also be acknowledged that some of the intrusion errors and distortions that healthy subjects can make have the characteristics of confabulation. This was clearly indicated by Bartlett (1932, pp. 175, & 204–205) in discussing the intrusions and distortions that people make in story recall:

> Epithets are changed into their opposites; incidents and events are transposed; names and numbers rarely survive intact ...; opinions and conclusions are reversed ... At the same time, the subjects may be very well satisfied with their efforts believing themselves to have passed on all important features with little or no change ... Consider particularly the case in which a subject was remembering a story which he heard, say, five years previously, in comparison with a case in which he was given certain outline materials and constructs which he calls a new story ... In both cases, it was common to find the preliminary check, the struggle to get somewhere, the varying play of doubt, hesitation, satisfaction and the like, and the eventual building up of the complete story accompanied by the more and more confident advance in a certain direction. In fact ... remembering appears to be far more decisively an affair of construction rather than one of mere reproduction ... As has been shown again and again, condensation, elaboration and invention are common features of ordinary remembering.

Consistent with this, Hammersley and Read (1986) found that healthy subjects were more vulnerable to interference effects from misleading information when recalling a story at 1 week's delay than at immediate recall, and that the misleading information was most likely to produce errors if it was presented shortly before the recall of the story. Similarly, Kopelman (1987a) compared recall of Logical Memory passages in healthy controls at a 1-week delay with that of Korsakoff and Alzheimer patients at immediate recall and 45 minutes' delay. This reduced the overall level of the healthy subjects' recall scores to nearer that of the amnesic patients, and 47% of the healthy subjects showed some evidence of momentary confabulation at the 1-week delay, compared with 50% of the Korsakoff sample and 44% of the Alzheimer group at immediate or 45 minutes' delay. Moreover, there were qualitative similarities between the intrusion errors produced by each group. Following the controversy concerning false memory for childhood abuse, recent research has produced copious evidence of similar intrusions and distortions in experimental tasks by both adults and children (for review, see e.g. Lindsay & Read, 1994; Read & Lindsay, 1997; Schacter et al., 1998).

FALSE MEMORY AND CONFABULATION—ONE TYPE OR MANY?

Can these different types of false memory all be understood in terms of faulty biological systems and, if they can, are common mechanisms/deficits involved? At this stage, any theories must inevitably be tentative because of the lack of comparative neuropsychological studies on this topic.

In a neuroimaging study, Schacter, Reinman, et al. (1996) found that the left medial temporal (parahippocampal) memory system was activated during both accurate ("veridical") and faulty ("illusory") recognition of word stimuli. However, veridical recognition was associated with a significant blood flow increase in the left temporoparietal cortex, which was considered to reflect the retrieval of auditory or phonological information about previously hearing or rehearsing true targets, whereas illusory recognition was associated with activation in the anterior prefrontal cortex, orbito-frontal cortex, and the cerebellum, which was postulated as a critical pathway for the effortful processes involved in error detection. Schacter, Reiman, et al. also suggested that false recognition patients may well have a deficit in this error detection system as a result of their frontal lesions. The overlap between the brain systems activated by veridical and illusory memories helps to explain the salience of illusory memory in many circumstances.

These findings help to provide the beginnings of a model for the biological systems involved—see Fig. 1. We know that the medial temporal/diencephalic memory system plays a critical role in the encoding and consolidation as well as the retrieval of new memories, both from neuropsychological studies of lesion patients (Kopelman & Stanhope, 1997, 1998; Mayes & Downes, 1997; Milner, 1966; Squire, 1987) and from recent neuroimaging studies (e.g. Kopelman, Stevens, Foli, & Grasby, 1998; Montaldi, et al. 1998; Schacter, Alpert, Savage, Rauch, & Albert, 1996). The temporo-parietal phonological recognition circuits presumably exist within a larger episodic memory system, and the prefrontal/cerebellar error detection circuit within a frontal "verification" system, and both are postulated to receive their inputs from the medial temporal/diencephalic system. The model suggests that frontal control systems are important in the retrieval of autobiographical memories (Della Sala, Laiacona, Spinnler, & Trivelli, 1993; Kopelman, 1991, 1992; Kopelman, Stanhope, & Kingsley, in press; Shimamura, 1994, 1997). It also postulates a personal semantic belief system ("self") that interacts closely with both frontal control systems and the autobiographical memory store: This is supposed to be akin to Conway and Tacchi's (1996) notion of "self" but less closely tied to "plans." Can the varieties of false memory just reviewed be understood within the context of such a model, which is derived from a variety of ideas well-established in neuropsychology?

As discussed earlier, spontaneous confabulation is likely to result from a combination of memory specification (description; focused retrieval) and verification (editing; monitoring) deficits within the frontal/executive system. The temporal context memory and source monitoring deficits, well described in confabulating patients, probably contribute to both specification and verification errors. "Strategic search" can be seen as the outcome of planning and organisation upon context and trace specification (see Fig. 1). In these terms, the false recognition cases may reflect an isolated and partial impairment of verification (error detection). By contrast, momentary or "provoked" confabulation arises where the trace itself is "weak" for whatever reason, which may be impaired "binding" or pattern separation (Schacter et al., 1998), a long delay until retrieval (Kopelman, 1987a), or an impairment in the medial temporal/diencephalic memory system as in schizophrenia (McKenna et al., 1990): In each case, faulty retrieval from the episodic memory store results, but this is not necessarily associated with executive dysfunction.

Delusional memories are much more difficult to account for in the absence of evidence of memory or executive dysfunction. David and Howard (1994) postulated that the sensory and phenomenological characteristics of delusional memories are hyper-intense, distorting the operation of a "comparator" which compares "incoming memories or fantasies", with the contents of semantic memory. That would suggest that any malfunction must be in the early processing of the "input," and is therefore consistent with the intact operation of frontal control or executive systems (Kopelman et al., 1995). However, as already discussed, the hyper-intense properties of the "input" probably reflect modulation in terms of a person's self-beliefs, mental state, and expectations: Within

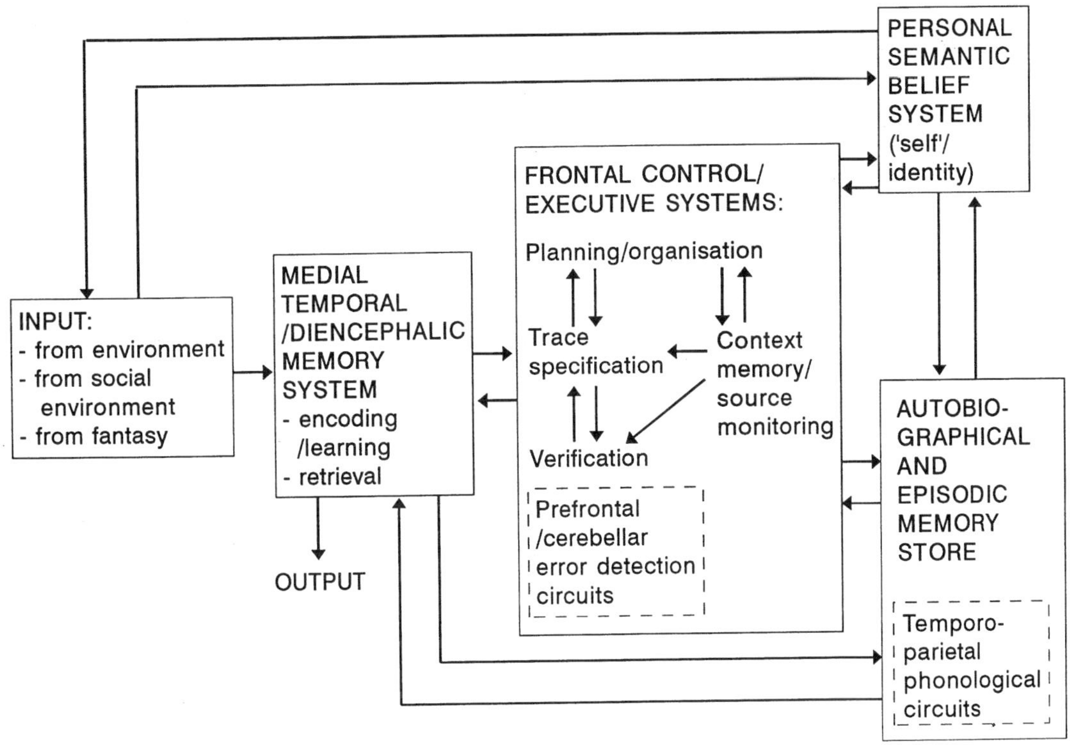

Fig. 1. *Systems involved in generation of false memories/confabulations.*

the present model (Fig. 1), this can be viewed as an amplifying effect from the personal semantic belief system to the input.

With regard to delusions in general, Frith (1992) has postulated deficits in the monitoring of action, and his ideas could easily be incorporated into a model of frontal control/executive systems. However, as Baddeley et al. (1996) have pointed out, this hypothesis is not consistent with the evidence of intact executive function in patients with delusions. The nature of delusions is an extensive topic that goes beyond the scope of the present paper (Baddeley et al., 1996; Frith, 1992; Garety & Hemsley, 1994), but delusions are not necessarily memory phenomena; they arise in varying circumstances that may not have a common underlying basis; and it seems probable that the mechanism or mechanisms giving rise to delusions differ from the processes that produce confabulation. Theories of delusions and theories of confabulation need to be kept clearly and conceptually distinct, despite the occasional overlap of these phenomena (Box et al., in press).

The internalised confessions of some offenders, "recovered" or distorted memories of childhood abuse, and the adoption of fantasised personal "scripts" (pseudologia fantastica), new scripts (following fugue episodes), or multiple scripts (dissociative identity disorder) reflect biases introduced from the social environment at "input" (e.g. coerced confessions, child sexual abuse) and/or from the personal semantic belief system (e.g. cases of altered identity) upon frontal control systems and autobiographical memory retrieval. In false confession, source memory errors arising in the context of social coercion and poor self-esteem (a form of personal self-belief) give rise to the faulty attribution. In identity disorders, it is possible that the influence of the personal semantic belief system results in biased or selective retrieval from autobiographical memory. In this connection, it is important to note that extreme or very stressful social circumstances can also influence the content, or even the occurrence, of confabulation in patients with frontal lobe disorder (Conway & Tacchi, 1996; Johnson, 1991; Kopelman, 1997).

CONCLUSIONS

A variety of situations in which false memories may arise has been reviewed. The main factors involved may be brain damage affecting frontal control and executive systems (spontaneous confabulation), a weak memory trace (momentary confabulation), anomalous processing of input modulated by personal self-beliefs (delusional memories), social coercion and source memory errors, usually in the context of low self-esteem (false confession), and anomalous, biased, or selective retrieval from autobiographical memory (pseudologia fantastica, fugue, multiple personality). Some of these phenomena may result characteristically from a combination of factors (e.g. the absence of rehearsal and a particular social context in cases of apparently false or distorted memories for child sexual abuse). In others, an interaction between social and biological factors may occasionally be important (the confabulations produced by brain damaged patients in very stressful or extreme situations). Although all these phenomena can be described and characterised within a general model of memory and executive function, provided that social factors and some notion of "self" (called here a "personal semantic belief system") are introduced, different components of the model have been highlighted in the generation of particular instances of false memory. It follows that these phenomena are probably best viewed as different types of false memory, with varying underlying mechanisms, and that the term "confabulation" is perhaps most useful if confined to its current conventions (brain disease and instances of "momentary" confabulation): In particular, confabulations and delusions need to be kept conceptually distinct. However, the relative dearth of neuropsychological studies comparing false memory phenomena means that the specific processes involved require further investigation.

REFERENCES

Baddeley, A.D., Thornton, A., Chua, S.E., & McKenna, P. (1996). Schizophrenic delusions and the construction of autobiographical memory. In D.C. Rubin (Ed.), *Remembering our past: Studies in autobiographical memory*. Cambridge: Cambridge University Press.

Baddeley, A.D., & Wilson, B. (1986). Amnesia, autobiographical memory, and confabulation. In D.C. Rubin (Ed.), *Autobiographical memory*. Cambridge: Cambridge University Press.

Bartlett, F.C. (1932). *Remembering: A study in experimental and social psychology*. Cambridge: Cambridge University Press.

Benson, D.F., & Stuss, D.T. (1990). Frontal lobe influences on delusions: A clinical perspective. *Schizophrenia Bulletin*, *16*, 403–411.

Bentall, R.P., Baker, A.B., & Havers, S. (1991). Reality monitoring and psychotic hallucinations. *British Journal of Clinical Psychology*, *30*, 213–222.

Berlyne, N. (1972). Confabulation. *British Journal of Psychiatry*, *120*, 31–39.

Box, O., Laing, H., & Kopelman, M. (in press). The evolution of spontaneous confabulation, delusional misidentification, and a related delusion in a case of severe head injury. *Neurocase*.

Briere, J., & Conte, J. (1993). Self-reported amnesia for abuse in adults molested as children. *Journal of Traumatic Stress*, *6*, 21–31.

Buchanan, A. (1991). Delusional memories: First-rank symptoms? *British Journal of Psychiatry*, *159*, 472–474.

Burgess, P.W., & Shallice, T. (1996a). Confabulation and the control of recollection. *Memory*, *4*, 359–411.

Burgess, P.W., & Shallice, T. (1996b). Response suppression, initiation and strategy use following frontal lobe lesions. *Neuropsychologia*, *34*, 263–273.

Conway, M.A. (1990). *Autobiographical memory: An introduction*. Buckingham, UK: Open University Press.

Conway, M.A. (1996). Autobiographical memories and autobiographical knowledge. In D.C. Rubin (Ed.), *Remembering our past: Studies in autobiographical memory* (pp. 67–93). Cambridge: Cambridge University Press.

Conway, M.A. (Ed.). (1997). *Recovered memories and false memories*. New York: Oxford University Press.

Conway, M.A., & Tacchi, P.C. (1996). Motivated confabulation. *Neurocase*, *2*, 325–339.

Cutting, J. (1979). Memory in functional psychosis. *Journal of Neurology, Neurosurgery, and Psychiatry*, *42*, 1031–1037.

Dalla Barba, G. (1993a). Confabulation: Knowledge and recollective experience. *Cognitive Neuropsychology*, *10*, 1–20.
Dalla Barba, G. (1993b). Different patterns of confabulation. *Cortex*, *29*, 567–581.
Dalla Barba, G., Cappelletti, J.Y., Signorini, M. & Denes, G. (1997). Confabulation: Remembering "another" past, planning "another" future. *Neurocase*, *3*, 425–436.
David, A.S., & Howard, R. (1994). An experimental phenomenological approach to delusional memory in schizophrenia and late paraphrenia. *Psychological Medicine*, *24*, 515–524.
Delbecq-Derouesné, J., Beauvois, M.F., & Shallice, T. (1990). Preserved recall versus impaired recognition. *Brain*, *113*, 1045–1074.
Della Sala, S., Laiacona, M., Spinnler, H., & Trivelli, C. (1993). Impaired autobiographical recollection in some frontal patients. *Neuropsychologia*, *31*, 823–840.
DeLuca, J., & Cicerone, K.D. (1991). Confabulation following aneurysm of the anterior communicating artery. *Cortex*, *27*, 417–423.
Ellis, H.D., & Young, A.W. (1990). Accounting for delusional misidentifications. *British Journal of Psychiatry*, *157*, 239–248.
Fish, F. (1967). *Clinical psychopathology: Signs and symptoms in psychiatry*. Bristol: John Wright & Sons.
Frith, C.D. (1992). *The cognitive neuropsychology of schizophrenia*. Hove, UK: Lawrence Erlbaum Associates Ltd.
Gardiner, J.M., & Parkin, A.J. (1990). Attention and recollective experience. *Memory and Cognition*, *18*, 579–583.
Garety, P.A., & Hemsley, D.R. (1994). *Delusions: Investigations into the psychology of delusional reasoning* (reprinted, 1997). Hove, UK: Psychology Press.
Gelder, M., Gath, D., & Mayou, R. (1989). *Oxford textbook of psychiatry*. Oxford: Oxford University Press.
Gudjonsson, G. H. (1987). A parallel form of the Gudjonsson Suggestibility Scale. *British Journal of Clinical Psychology*, *26*, 215–221.
Gudjonsson, G.H. (1992). *The psychology of interrogations, confessions, and testimony*. Chichester, UK: John Wiley & Sons.
Gudjonsson, G.H., Kopelman, M.D., & MacKeith, J.A.C. (in press). Unreliable admissions to homicide: A case of misdiagnosis of amnesia and misuse of abreaction technique. *British Journal of Psychiatry*.
Gudjonsson, G.H., & Lebegue, B. (1989). Psychological and psychiatric aspects of a coerced-internalized false confession. *Journal of the Forensic Science Society*, *29*, 261–269.
Gudjonsson, G.H., & MacKeith. J.A.C. (1982). False confessions. Psychological effects of interrogation. A discussion paper. In A. Trankell (Ed.), *Reconstructing the past: the role of psychologists in criminal trials* (pp. 253–269). Deventer, The Netherlands: Kluwer.
Gudjonsson, G.H., & MacKeith, J.A.C. (1988). Retracted confessions: Legal, psychological and psychiatric aspects. *Medicine, Science and the Law*, *28*, 187–194.
Gudjonsson, G.H., & MacKeith, J.A.C. (1990). A proven case of false confession: Psychological aspects of the coerced-compliant type. *Medicine, Science and the Law*, *30*, 329–335.
Gudjonsson, G.H., & Sigurdsson, J.F. (1995). The relationship of confabulation to the memory, intelligence, suggestibility, and personality of juvenile offenders. *Nordic Journal of Psychiatry*, *49*, 373–378.
Gurd, J.M. (1995). Mechanisms of word retrieval: Neuropsychological investigations of patients with Parkinson's disease. In B. De Gelder, & H. Morais (Eds.), *Speech and reading: A comparative approach* (pp. 339–351) Hove, UK: Lawrence Erlbaum Associates Ltd.
Hammersley, R., & Read, J.D. (1986). What is integration? Remembering a story and remembering false implications about the story. *British Journal of Psychology*, *77*, 329–41.
Herman, J.L., & Schatzow, E. (1987). Recovery and verification of memories of childhood sexual trauma. *Psychoanalytic Psychology*, *4*, 1–14.
Johnson, M.K. (1991). Reality monitoring: Evidence from confabulation in organic brain disease patients. In G.P. Prigatano & D.L. Schacter (Eds.), *Awareness deficit after brain injury: Clinical and theoretical issues*. New York: Oxford University Press.
Johnson, M.K., Hashtroudi, S., & Lindsay, D.S. (1993). Source monitoring. *Psychological Bulletin*, *114*, 3–28.
Johnson, M.K., O'Connor, M., & Cantor, J. (1997). Confabulation, memory deficits, and frontal dysfunction. *Brain and Cognition*, *34*, 189–206.
Johnson, M.K., & Raye, C.L. (1981). Reality monitoring. *Psychological Review*, *88*, 67–85.
Kapur, N., & Coughlan, A.K. (1980). Confabulation and frontal lobe dysfunction. *Journal of Neurology, Neurosurgery and Psychiatry*, *43*, 461–463.
Kihlstrom, J.F., & Schacter, D.L. (1995). Functional disorders of autobiographical memory. In A.D. Baddeley, B.A. Wilson, & F.N. Watts (Eds.), *Hand-*

book of memory disorders (pp. 337–364). Chichester, UK: John Wiley & Sons.
Kopelman, M.D. (1987a). Two types of confabulation. *Journal of Neurology, Neurosurgery and Psychiatry, 50*, 1482–1487.
Kopelman, M.D. (1987b). Amnesia: Organic and psychogenic. *British Journal of Psychiatry, 150*, 428–442.
Kopelman, M.D. (1991). Frontal lobe dysfunction and memory deficits in the alcoholic Korsakoff syndrome and Alzheimer-type dementia. *Brain, 114*, 117–137.
Kopelman, M.D. (1992). The "new" and the "old": Components of the anterograde and retrograde memory loss in Korsakoff and Alzheimer patients. In L.R. Squire & Butters (Eds.), *The neuropsychology of memory* (2nd edition, pp. 130–146). New York: Guilford Press.
Kopelman, M.D. (1994). Structured psychiatric interview: Psychiatric history and assessment of the mental state. *British Journal of Hospital Medicine, 52*, 93–98.
Kopelman, M.D. (1995). The assessment of psychogenic amnesia. In A. Baddeley, B. Wilson, & F. Watts (Eds.), *Handbook of memory disorders*, (pp. 427–448). Chichester, UK: John Wiley & Sons.
Kopelman, M.D. (1997). Anomalies of autobiographical memory: Retrograde amnesia, confabulation, delusional memory, psychogenic amnesia, and false memories. In. J.D. Read & D.S. Lindsay (Eds.), *Recollections of trauma: Scientific research and clinical practice*, (pp. 273–303).New York: Plenum Press.
Kopelman, M.D., Christensen, H., Puffett, A., & Stanhope, N. (1994). The Great Escape: A neuropsychological study of psychogenic amnesia. *Neuropsychologia, 32*, 675–691.
Kopelman, M.D., Guinan, E.M., & Lewis, P.D.R. (1995). Delusional memory, confabulation, and frontal lobe dysfunction: A case study in de Clérambault's syndrome. *Neurocase, 1*, 71–77.
Kopelman, M.D., Ng. N., & Van den Brouke, O. (1997). Confabulation extending across episodic memory, personal and general semantic memory. *Cognitive Neuropsychology, 14*, 683–712.
Kopelman, M.D., & Stanhope, N. (1997). Rates of forgetting in organic amnesia following temporal lobe, diencephalic, or frontal lobe lesions. *Neuropsychology, 11*, 343–356.
Kopelman, M.D., & Stanhope, N. (1998). Recall and recognition memory in patients with focal frontal, temporal lobe and diencephalic lesions. *Neuropsychologia, 36*, 785–796.
Kopelman, M.D., Stanhope, N., & Kingsley, D.E.P. (in press). Retrograde amnesia in patients with diencephalic, temporal lobe, or frontal lesions. *Neuropsychologia*.
Kopelman, M.D., Stevens, T.G., Foli, S., & Grasby, P. (1998). PET activation of the medial temporal lobe in learning. *Brain, 121*, 875–887.
Kopelman, M.D., Wilson, B., & Baddeley, A.D. (1989). The Autobiographical Memory Interview: A new assessment of autobiographical and personal semantic memory in amnesic patients. *Journal of Clinical and Experimental Neuropsychology, 11*, 724–744.
Kopelman, M.D., Wilson, B.A., & Baddeley, A.D. (1990). *The Autobiographical Memory Interview*. Bury St Edmunds, UK: Thames Valley Test Company.
Korsakoff, S.S. (1889). Psychic disorder in conjunction with peripheral neuritis. [Translated and republished by M. Victor & P.I. Yakovlev (1955).] *Neurology, 5*, 394–406.
Lindsay, D.S., & Read, J.D. (1994). Psychotherapy and memories of childhood sexual abuse: A cognitive perspective. *Applied Cognitive Psychology, 8*, 281–338.
Loftus, E.F., Polonsky, S., & Fullilove, M.T. (1994). Memories of childhood sexual abuse: Remembering and repressing. *Psychology of Women, 18*, 67–84.
Luria, A.R. 1976). *The neuropsychology of memory*. New York: John Wiley.
Markowitsch, H.J., Fink, G.R., Thöne, A., Kessler, J, & Heiss, W.-D. (1997). PET study of persistent psychogenic amnesia covering the whole life span. *Cognitive Neuropsychiatry, 2*, 135–158.
Mayes, A.R., & Downes, J.J. (1997). What do theories of functional deficit(s) underlying amnesia have to explain? *Memory, 5*, 3–36.
McKenna, P., Tamlyn, D., Lund, C., Mortimer, A., Hammond, S., & Baddeley, A.D. (1990). Amnesic syndrome in schizophrenia. *Psychological Medicine, 20*, 967–972.
Mercer, B., Wapner, W., Gardner, H., & Benson, D. (1977). A study of confabulation. *Archives of Neurology (Chicago), 34*, 429–433.
Merskey, H. (1992). The manufacture of personalities. The production of multiple personality disorder. *British Journal of Psychiatry, 160*, 327–340.
Merskey, H. (1995). Multiple personality disorder and false memory syndrome. *British Journal of Psychiatry, 166*, 281–283.
Milner, B. (1966). Amnesia following operation on the temporal lobes. In C.W.M. Whitty & O. Zangwill (Eds.), *Amnesia* (1st edition). London: Butterworths.

Moll, J.M. (1915). The amnesic or Korsakoff's syndrome with alcoholic aetiology: An analysis of 30 cases. *Journal of Mental Science*, *61*, 423–437.

Montaldi, D., Mayes, A.R., Barnes, A., Pirie, H., Hadley, D.M., Patterson, J., & Wyper, D.J. (1998). Associative encoding of pictures activates the medial temporal lobes. *Human Brain Mapping*, *6*, 85–104.

Morton, J., Hammersley, R.H., & Bekerian, P.A. (1985). Headed records: A model for memory and its failures. *Cognition*, *20*, 1–23.

Moscovitch, M. (1989). Confabulation and the frontal system: Strategic versus associative retrieval in neuropsychological theories of memory. In H.L. Roedinger & F.I. Craik (Eds.), *Varieties of memory and consciousness: Essays in honour of Endel Tulving*. Hillsdale, NJ: Lawrence Erlbaum Associates Inc.

Moscovitch, M. (1995). Confabulation. In D.L. Schacter, J.T. Coyle, G.D. Fischbach, M.M. Mesulam, & L.E. Sullivan (Eds.), *Memory distortion*. Cambridge MA: Harvard University Press.

Moscovitch, M., & Melo, B. (1997). Strategic retrieval and the frontal lobes: Evidence from confabulation and amnesia. *Neuropsychologia*, *35*, 1017–1034.

Mullen, P.E., Martin, J.L. Anderson, J.C., Romans, S.E., & Herbison, G.P. (1993). Childhood sexual abuse and mental health in adult life. *British Journal of Psychiatry*, *163*, 721–732.

Nathaniel-James, D.A., Foong, J., & Frith, C.D. (1996). The mechanisms of confabulation in schizophrenia. *Neurocase*, *2*, 475–483.

Nathaniel-James, D.A., & Frith, C.D. (1996). Confabulation in schizophrenia: Evidence of a new form? *Psychological Medicine*, *26*, 391–399.

Oliver, J.E. (1993). Intergenerational transmission of child abuse: Rates, research, and clinical implications. *American Journal of Psychiatry*, *150*, 1315–1324.

Parkin, A.J., Bindschaedler, C., Harsent, L., & Metzler, C. (1996). Pathological false alarm rates following damage to the left frontal cortex. *Brain and Cognition*, *32*, 14–27.

Pope, H.G. Jr., & Hudson, J.I. (1995). Can memories of childhood sexual abuse be repressed? *Psychological Medicine*, *25*, 121–126.

Read, J.D., & Lindsay, D.S. (Eds). (1997). *Recollections of trauma: Scientific research and clinical practice*. New York: Plenum Press.

Romans, S.E., Martin, J.L., Anderson, J.C., O'Shea, M.L., & Mullen, P.E. (1995). Factors that mediate between child sexual abuse and adult psychological outcome. *Psychological Medicine*, *25*, 127–142.

Schacter, D.L. (1987). Implicit memory: History and current status. *Journal of Experimental Psychology: Learning, Memory and Cognition*, *13*, 501–518.

Schacter, D.L. (1996). *Searching for memory: The brain, the mind and the past*. New York: Harper Collins.

Schacter, D.L., Alpert, N.M., Savage, C.R., Rauch, S.L., & Albert, M.S. (1996). Conscious recollection and the human hippocampal formation. *Proceedings of the National Academy of Science, USA*, *93*, 321–325.

Schacter, D.L., Coyle, J.T., Fischbach, G.D., Mesulam, M.-M., & Sullivan, L.E. (Eds). (1995). *Memory distortion: How minds, brains and societies reconstruct the past*. Cambridge, MA: Harvard University Press.

Schacter, D.L., Curran, T., Galluccio, L., Milberg, W.P., & Bates, J.F. (1996). False recognition and the right frontal lobe: A case study. *Neuropsychologia*, *34*, 793–808.

Schacter, D.L., Harbluk, J.L., & McLachlan, D.R. (1984). Retrieval without recollection: An experimental analysis of source amnesia. *Journal of Verbal Learning and Verbal Behavior*, *23*, 593–611.

Schacter, D.L., Norman, K.A., & Koutstaal, W. (1997). The recovered memories debate: A cognitive neuroscience perspective. In M.A. Conway (Ed.), *Recovered memories and false memories*. New York: Oxford University Press.

Schacter, D.L., Norman, K.A., & Koutstaal, W. (1998). The cognitive neuroscience of constructive memory. *Annual Review of Psychology*, *49*, 289–318.

Schacter, D.L., Reiman, E., Curran, T., Yun, L.S., Bandy, D., McDermott, K.B., & Roediger, H.L. III. (1996). Neuroanatomical correlates of veridical and illusory recognition memory: Evidence from positron emission tomography. *Neuron*, *17*, 267–274.

Schank, R.C., & Abelson, R.P. (1977). *Scripts, plans, goals, and understanding*. Hillsdale, NJ: Lawrence Erlbaum Associates Inc.

Schneider, K. (1959). *Clinical psychopathology* (5th ed.). (Translated by M.W. Hamilton.) New York: Grune & Stratton.

Schnider, A., von Däniken, C., & Gutbrod, K. (1996). The mechanisms of spontaneous and provoked confabulations. *Brain*, *119*, 1365–1375.

Schooler, J.W., Ambadar, Z., & Bendiksen, M. (1997). A cognitive corroborative case study approach for investigating discovered memories of sexual abuse. In J.D. Read & D.S. Lindsay (Eds.), *Recollections of trauma: Scientific evidence and clinical practice* (pp. 379–387). New York: Plenum Press.

Schooler, J.W., Bendiksen, M., & Ambadar, Z. (1997). Taking the middle line: Can we accommodate both fabricated and recovered memories of sexual abuse? In M.A. Conway (Ed.), *Recovered memories and false memories.* New York: Oxford University Press.

Shallice, T., & Evans, M.E. (1978). The involvement of the frontal lobes in cognitive estimates. *Cortex, 14,* 294–303.

Shimamura, A.P. (1994). Memory and frontal lobe function. In M.S. Gazzaniga (Ed.), *The cognitive neurosciences* (pp. 803–813). Cambridge MA: MIT Press.

Shimamura, A.P. (1997). Neuropsychological factors associated with memory recollection: What can science tell us about reinstated memories? In J.D. Read, & D.S. Lindsay (Eds.) *Recollections of trauma: Scientific research and clinical practice.* New York: Plenum Press.

Smith, P., & Gudjonsson, G. (1995). The relationship of mental disorder to suggestibility and confabulation among forensic inpatients. *Journal of Forensic Psychiatry, 6,* 499–515.

Smith, P., & Gudjonsson, G.H. (1995). Confabulation among forensic inpatients and its relationship with memory, suggestibility, compliance, anxiety, and self-esteem. *Personality and Individual Differences, 19,* 517–523.

Squire, L.R: (1987). *Memory and brain.* Oxford: Oxford University Press.

Stuss, D.T., Alexander, M.P., Liberman, A., & Levine, H. (1978). An extraordinary form of confabulation. *Neurology, 28,* 1166–1172.

Talland, G.A. (1965). *Deranged memory.* New York: Academic Press.

Van der Horst, L. (1932). Über die Psychologie des Korsakowsyndroms. *Monatsschrift für Psychologie und Neurologie, 83,* 65–84.

Victor, M., Adams, R.D., & Collins, G.H. (1971). *The Wernicke-Korsakoff syndrome* (1st ed.) Philadelphia., PA: F.A. Davis Co.

Williams, L.M. (1994). Recall of childhood trauma: A prospective study of women's memories of child sexual abuse. *Journal of Consulting and Clinical Psychology, 62,* 1167–1176.

Young, A.W., Leafhead, K.M., & Szulecka, M.K. (1994). The Capgras and Cotard delusions. *Psychopathology,* 27, 226–231.

Young, A.W., Reid, I, Wright, S., & Hellawell, D.J. (1993). Face-processing impairments and the Capgras delusion. *British Journal of Psychiatry, 162,* 695–698.

COGNITIVE NEUROPSYCHOLOGY, 1999, 16 (3/4/5), 215–242

CONFABULATION WITH A SELECTIVE DESCRIPTOR PROCESS IMPAIRMENT

Saskia Dab
Université Libre de Bruxelles and Fonds National de la Recherche Scientifique, Bruxelles, Belgium

Thierry Claes
Hôpital Erasme, Bruxelles, Belgium

José Morais
Université Libre de Bruxelles, Belgium

Tim Shallice
University College London and Scuola Internazzional di Studi Avanzzati, Trieste, Italy

Confabulation is usually assumed to result from a deficit in either the memory verification processes alone or in both the search and the verification processes. The present study concerns a patient who, in contrast to other patients, displayed confabulations but had preserved memory verification abilities. She exhibited only a selective impairment of the search processes. Recognition abilities were preserved, and cued recall was better than free recall. On the latter task, she recalled fewer correct items and produced more intrusions than control subjects. The patient had normal performance in several tests usually assumed to tap "executive functions." It is thus concluded that an impairment in verification, regardless of whether it is specific or not to memory, is not a necessary component of confabulations. The case is discussed in relation to two memory control processes models (Burgess & Shallice, 1996a; Moscovitch, 1989, 1995 ; Moscovitch & Melo, 1997), to the Source Monitoring Framework (Johnson, Hashtroudi, & Lindsay, 1993), and to the Constructive Memory Framework (Schacter, Norman, & Koutstaal, 1998). We proposed new hypotheses about possible deficits in the search process so as to account for the difference between amnesic patients with and without confabulations.

INTRODUCTION

The term confabulation has been variously defined and used in several situations ranging from minor distortions (e.g. Kopelman, 1987) to implausible and fantastic accounts (Stuss, Alexander, Lieberman, & Levine, 1978) and sometimes includes perseverative responses (e.g. Shapiro, Alexander, Gardner, & Mercer, 1981). A general definition can be that confabulations are "erroneous memories, either false in themselves or resulting from true memories misplaced in context and inappropriately retrieved or interpreted" (Kopelman, Guinan, & Lewis, 1995; for a more extended speci-

Requests for reprints should be addressed to Saskia Dab, Université Libre de Bruxelles, Laboratoire de Psychologie Expérimentale, 50 Av. Franklin Roosevelt, 1050 Bruxelles, Belgium (Fax: 00-32-2-650.22.09. E-mail: sasdab@ulb.ac.be).

We are grateful to Luc Foulon for part of the controls' testing and of the preparation of task materials; to Patrick Fery for very useful comments; to Josiane Lechat for help in analysing the CT scan. We would also like to kindly thank PAD, the three institutes that enabled us to start and to follow the investigation carried on with her: the Service de Neurologie de l'Hôpital Erasme, the Centre Neurologique Williams Lenox, and the Centre de Jour pour Adultes Cérébro-Lésés La Braise, Marcia Johnson, and an anonymous reviewer for their very helpful comments on an earlier draft.

fication of characteristics, see Burgess & Shallice, 1996a; Moscovitch, 1989, 1995; Talland, 1965). In this paper, the term confabulation refers to a memory error that cannot be due to a pure failure of language such as verbal comprehension or verbal production impairment. Studies on confabulations mainly involve the verbal modality (e.g. Berlyne, 1972; Dalla Barba, Cipolotti, & Denes, 1990; Kopelman, 1987; Talland, 1965), but can also concern nonverbal knowledge (e.g. Joslyn, Grundvig, & Chamberlain, 1978; Kern, Van Gorp, Cummings, Brown, & Osato, 1992) or behaviour (e.g. Baddeley & Wilson, 1986; Moscovitch, 1989).

Confabulation was first described in Korsakoff patients (see Talland, 1965), but it is accepted that patients with a variety of aetiologies can confabulate, such as: anterior communicating artery aneurysm (ACoA) patients (e.g. DeLuca, 1993; DeLuca & Cicerone, 1991; Kapur & Coughlan, 1980; Shapiro, et al., 1981; Stuss et al., 1978), closed-head injury patients (e.g. Baddeley & Wilson, 1986, 1988; Shapiro et al., 1981; Stuss et al., 1978), normal pressure hydrocephalus patients (Mercer, Wapner, Gardner, & Benson, 1977), Wernicke's encephalopathy patients (Mercer et al., 1977), and Alzheimer patients (Kern et al., 1992; Kopelman, 1987; Mercer et al., 1977). Confabulatory patients are often assumed to have a frontal syndrome, even though some of the patients described had no apparent deficit on so called "frontal" tasks (e.g. Delbecq-Derouesné, Beauvois, & Shallice, 1990; Kapur & Coughlan, 1980; Papagno & Muggia, 1996; Schnider, von Däniken, & Gutbrod, 1996; patient 16).

Various accounts of confabulations that occur in neurological patients have been proposed. Among the earlier theories were the compensatory explanation, i.e. patients confabulate to compensate for their memory deficit (e.g. Feinberg, 1980), and the disorientation explanation, i.e. patients confabulate because their temporal frame of reference is disrupted (e.g. Schnider, Gutbrod, Hess, & Schroth, 1996; Van der Horst, 1932, cited by Talland, 1965). Going beyond the general assumption that confabulation is a deficit in memory processes, two main types of interpretations have been proposed in recent years: the memory control processes (e.g. Burgess & Shallice, 1996a; Moscovitch, 1989, 1995; Moscovitch & Melo, 1997; Shallice, 1988) and the source memory accounts (Johnson, 1991; Johnson et al., 1993). These two approaches were combined together in a recent theoretical framework proposed by Schacter, Norman, and colleagues: the constructive memory framework (Norman & Schacter, 1996; Schacter et al., 1998).

According to the memory control interpretation, confabulation arises at the retrieval rather than at the encoding or storage stages of memory. The main argument is that patients also confabulate about events or information that they knew prior to the occurrence of their lesion, when encoding and storage processes can be assumed to be normal (Moscovitch, 1995). It has also been proposed that confabulation can consist of new incorrect autobiographical representations replacing autobiographical traces that have deteriorated, which suggests degraded representation rather than failure of access (Dalla Barba et al., 1990).

This interpretation has been articulated in most detail in two versions. Burgess and Shallice (1996a) proposed a theory of autobiographical retrieval based on the model of retrieval of Norman and Bobrow (1979; Conway, 1990; Morton, Hammersley, & Bekerian, 1985; Shallice, 1988). To summarise their position, three types of processes are held to be engaged in the retrieval of autobiographical information: the *descriptor* processes, the *memory editor* processes, and the *mediator* processes. The descriptor processes provide a description of the characteristics of the memory trace that is to be retrieved in order to satisfy task demands. It is presupposed that multiple levels of descriptors can activate different regions within the long-term memory storage system. The memory editor processes continuously check the memory output, both with respect to the task demands and to previously retrieved memories. They evaluate if the retrieved memory elements are compatible with each other, with the previously retrieved elements, with the overall descriptor, and with task requirements. These editor processes are specifically devoted to the memory domain and are not under direct strategic control. The mediator processes are a set of cognitive problem-solving processes involved in reasoning. They provide the necessary cognitive abilities to evaluate the plausibility of a particular conjunction of retrieved memory elements. If an incompatibility is detected and not resolved, a respecification is provided and new descriptors are set. The mediator processes are not thought to be specific to the memory domain.

If the descriptor process is impaired, then the patient might for instance activate too wide a region of the memory store, and so elements from different memories could be retrieved together. For example, RW (Delbecq-Derouesné et al., 1990) replaced a piece of information by a related piece from another story in the recall of short stories (Burgess & Shallice, 1996a). However, if only the descriptor process is impaired, then the patient should have a relatively preserved cued recall as in this task a description is explicitly provided and therefore the rate of confabulatory responses should decrease compared to free recall. With an impaired memory editor process, however, the patient should have difficulty in verifying, evaluating, checking, and correcting memory output, as well as in inhibiting incorrect responses; in particular, one should observe a lack of self-correction. Finally, an impaired mediator process would lead to poor plausibility judgements, hypothesis testing, and reasoning.

Moscovitch's (1989, 1995; Moscovitch & Melo, 1997) version of the memory control processes interpretation is based on a theory that distinguishes two kinds of retrieval processes: the *ecphoric system* and the *strategic system*. The ecphoric system, also called the associative/cue-dependent retrieval system, is held to be quite automatic and is engaged when a specific cue interacts with information stored in memory. The output of this interaction is either the memory that has been sought or the material for subsequent strategic search. The strategic processes, by contrast, are active, effortful, goal-directed, and intelligent. They have a role in both the early and the late stages of the search-and-retrieval process. At the early or pre-ecphoric stage, strategic processes are involved in framing the memory problem, in initiating and organising the memory search on the basis of the available knowledge by constraining the search using general and personal knowledge. At the late or post-ecphoric stage, once the memory trace is retrieved, other strategic processes monitor this output by evaluating, verifying, and checking the retrieved memory elements. These strategic processes also place the retrieved memory elements into their proper temporal and spatial context, as memory is randomly stored and not organised in its chronological context.

According to Moscovitch and Melo (1997), confabulation results from the association of the following deficits: (1) the faulty output from the ecphoric retrieval system, (2) an impaired strategic pre-ecphoric search process, which accounts for omissions but also increases the probability of retrieving a faulty output, and (3) defective monitoring. The first two conditions are necessary but not sufficient to produce confabulation: they give rise to omissions and distortions that are recognised and edited. Confabulation only occurs if the monitoring is defective.

As accepted by either of these interpretations, both semantic and episodic knowledge are prone to confabulations. However, confabulation is said to be more apparent or frequent when episodic knowledge is concerned, because the retrieval of episodic memory is more likely to make greater demands on strategic processes than is the retrieval of semantic memory (see Moscovitch & Melo, 1997, for an extended discussion).

Unlike Burgess and Shallice (1996a), who clearly postulate two distinct types of retrieval processes—the descriptor processes (search) and the editing processes (verification)—Moscovitch (1989) did not make such a distinction, although he endowed the strategic retrieval processes with two different roles. But, according to Moscovitch and Melo (1997), the different aspects of retrieval are mediated by different processes, so that the search and monitoring processes should, in principle, be dissociable from each other.

Some evidence for this dissociation can be found in the neuropsychological literature. Recently, Hanley, Davies, Downes, and Mayes (1994) described a patient with a selective deficit in the search processes. ROB is an ACoA patient who displayed normal recognition despite very impoverished recall, even when a procedure for matching the difficulty level between the two types of test was used. The patient did not confabulate at the time of the investigation. According to Hanley et al., ROB had an impairment in the system that implements strategic search. The authors suggested that another system is responsible for the verification of candidate memories, the impairment of which leads to both difficulty in recognition and confabulation, as it occurred in RW, the patient described by Delbecq-Derouesné et al. (1990). Thus, according to Hanley et al. whereas confabulatory amnesics have a monitoring deficit, amnesic patients with impaired retrieval who do not confabulate have a search deficiency.

Moscovitch and Melo's (1997) position is slightly different: Amnesic patients who do not confabulate have a specific search deficit whereas confabulators have both a search and a monitoring impairment. With a specific deficit in memory search, omissions should occur in recall. With an additional monitoring deficit, confabulations would be produced. Hanley et al.'s (1994) findings are consistent with this hypothesis.

In the second type of theoretical interpretation of confabulation, "source" information is considered as a core element to explain the presence of the symptom. According to the *source monitoring framework* (SMF) (Johnson et al., 1993, p. 3) source monitoring "refers to the set of processes involved in making attributions about the origins of memories, knowledge. and beliefs." Retrieval includes the activation of memory records, their evaluation and attribution "to particular sources through decision processes performed during remembering." In a number of papers Johnson and her colleagues have proposed that SMF involves a whole variety of processes (e.g. generating retrieval cues, weighting features, setting criteria, heuristic matches to expectations about properties of various sources, reasoning about consistency, plausibility, etc., together with processes affecting encoding: see, e.g., Johnson, 1997; Johnson et al., 1993; Johnson, Kounios, & Nolde, 1996). Thus, deficits in source monitoring may result from impairment in attribution processes as well as from disruption in encoding qualitative characteristics of events. However, earlier versions of the theory put rather strong emphasis on comparison of already activated information with criteria. This may make the most natural account of confabulation given in the theory from the perspective of retrieval processes: One in which such errors arise from an impairment at a late stage.

This interpretation of the SMF account of confabulations would contrast with Burgess and Shallice's (1996a), Moscovitch's (1989, 1995), and Moscovitch and Melo's (1997) point of view that a verification problem cannot be sufficient to account for confabulations. That the search process is impaired in confabulatory patients is suggested by the fact that, in these patients, the prompting technique leads to the production of both correct and incorrect responses at recall to a greater extent than is the case in amnesic patients without confabulation and in control subjects (Moscovitch & Melo, 1997). Moreover, as their first response confabulatory patients produce a considerable number of memory errors, whereas normal subjects only produce a few (Burgess & Shallice, 1996a).

In Schacter, Norman, and colleagues' account the initial stage of the recall processes is assumed to be involved, more precisely an impairment at the level of focusing processes (Schacter et al., 1998). In the *constructive memory framework* (CMF), memories do not constitute accurate records of past experience, but rather are the result of constructive processes prone to errors, distortions, and illusions. A memory of a new event is conceptualised by a pattern of different features representing different aspects of the event. These features are widely distributed in different regions of the brain so that no single location contains the complete pattern of the event. To be efficient, such a system needs to solve several problems. At the encoding stage, the different features of an event must be linked together to form a coherent and bound representation. Moreover, an event must be represented sufficiently separately from the other events; this implies *pattern separation processes*. Similar problems arise at the retrieval stage because retrieval cues can potentially match stored information that does not constitute the sought-after information. To avoid such difficulty, a first step in the retrieval processes involves processes that form a refined description of the characteristics of the sought-after event: the focusing processes (very similar to the description processes postulated by Burgess & Shallice, 1996a). When a description is formed, it activates a subset of features of an event and, by the *pattern completion processes*, activation spreads through the remaining features constituting the event. Finally, a decision must be taken to determine if the retrieved information forms an episodic trace, in opposition to fantasy or generated images. Monitoring processes must reinstall the context of the event. In this respect, Schacter and colleagues' view is similar to the one proposed by Johnson: A central problem of the retrieval stage is to link information to their source. On the one hand, source information would play a role in both the search and monitoring processes. Indeed, according to Norman and Schacter (1996), both the search and monitoring processes depend on the contextual information associated to an event, and both processes rely on the application of contextual constraints. These authors go as far as to claim (op. cit., p. 241) that "strategic retrieval and monitoring reflect two different uses of the same computational machinery. Therefore it may not be necessary to assign strategic retrieval and monitoring to separate neural circuits."

Thus this conception is very similar to the first one proposed by Moscovitch (1989) who postulated the existence of a single strategic system that would intervene at both a pre- and a post-ecphoric stage. However, as we discussed previously, neuropsychological findings are, instead in favour of a dissociation between the two types of processes.

The impairments that Schacter and colleagues consider to be responsible for the production of confabulations are very similar to the ones contemplated by Burgess and Shallice (1996a) or by Moscovitch and Melo (1997): a deficit in both the focusing and the monitoring processes, with a possible pattern completion processes impairment. What differs from the conception of Burgess and Shallice is the consideration of different types of impairment as regards the search process (focusing/descriptor processes). The search processes can break down in two distinct ways. On the one hand, brain damage can eliminate completely the ability to generate contextual constraints (outright failure). In this case, the subject would be unable to generate a representation of the contextual constraints that define the sought-after episode. On the other hand, the contextual constraints would not be sufficiently adequately specified and, therefore, would fail to discriminate between the sought-after trace and competing episodes (unfocusing, defocusing, or blurring impairment). Confabulations, intrusions, and false recognitions would result from this type of impairment. However, clearly stated by Schacter et al. (1998, p. 311) is, the additional involvement of a monitoring deficit: "if these processes were unimpaired, patients would be able to reject nontarget information."

We describe here a case study of a patient who exhibited confabulations after brain damage and whose pattern of performance suggests a selective impairment of the search or descriptor processes but who had apparently preserved verification abilities. Thus, contrary to the predictions derived from the models of autobiographical memory described earlier, confabulation—at least in a milder form—can occur without any marked verification deficit, regardless of whether this impairment occurs alone or is combined with a search deficit.

The investigation was carried out in two stages: a clinical and exploratory phase while PAD was at the hospital, followed by a more elaborated experimental study 1 year post-surgery, when the patient was at home, and later in a day centre. In the first part of the investigation, the patient's cognitive abilities and behaviour changed across time due to spontaneous recovery. In the second phase, however, she was clinically stable.

CASE HISTORY

The patient investigated, PAD, is a 40-year-old right-handed woman who left high school at the age of 15 and worked first as a secretary, then as a shop assistant in a bakery and in a newspaper shop. She later remained unemployed for several years. She lived on her own with her child, who is now 11 years old. She has no history of psychiatric disorder. She was admitted to the Hospital Erasme in

Brussels in November 1995 because of a rupture of the anterior communicating artery that was repaired by neurosurgery. She was in coma for about 3 weeks. The latest CT scan (November 1996, 1 year post-surgery) showed lesions localised to the left frontal hemisphere in the territory of the left anterior artery that affected the whole medial surface of the frontal lobe and of the cingulate anterior of the central sulcus (see Figs. 1 and 2).

PAD exhibited a normal intellectual level. On the Raven's Progressive Matrices, she performed at an IQ 108 level. On the WAIS, she had Verbal and Performance IQs of 99 and 96, respectively. There was some variation between subtest scores, which ranged from scale score 13 (Digit Span) to scale score 7 (Picture Arrangement). She had normal digit span and preserved language abilities: naming (Bachy-Languedoc, 1989: 44/45), comprehension (Token Test; De Renzi & Faglioni, 1978: 36/36), oral expression, writing, and reading were all normal.

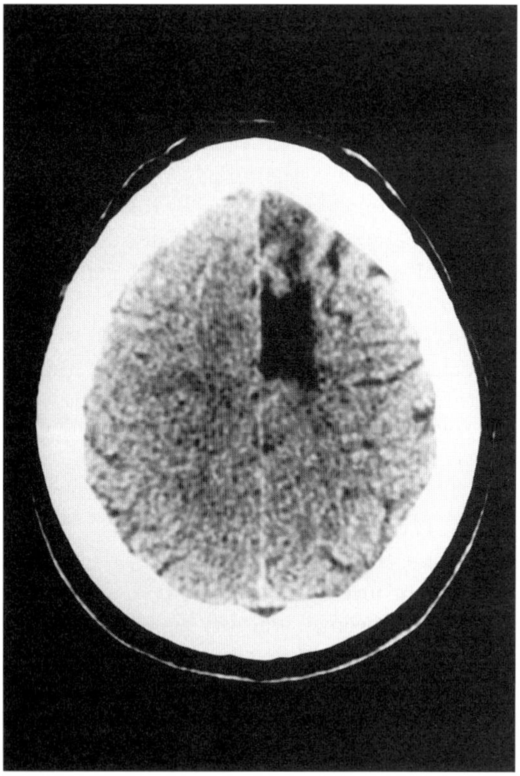

Fig. 1. *CT scan of PAD 1 year post-onset (left-right reverse).*

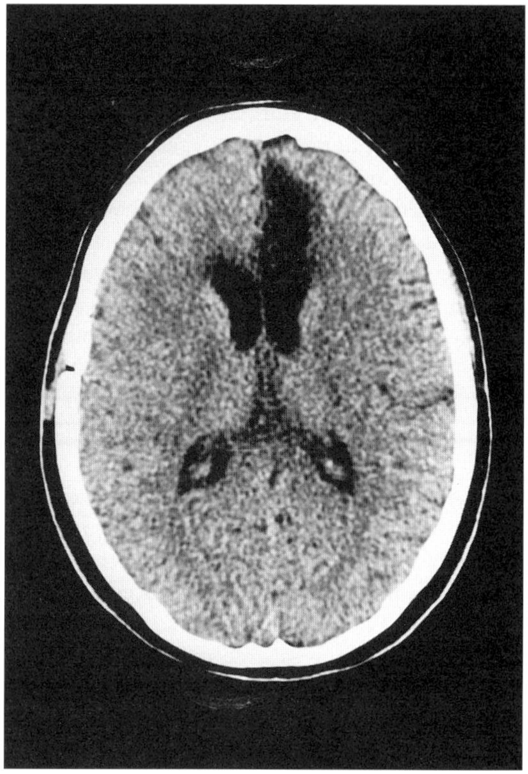

Fig. 2. *CT scan of PAD 1 year post-onset (left-right reverse).*

On a variety of tests assumed to be sensitive to frontal lesions, PAD's performance was markedly impaired 2 months after surgery. However, she scored in the normal range 1 month later (see Table 1).

It is worth noting that, although PAD's performance was normal in most of the tests sensitive to frontal lesions, she displayed behavioural changes that are often observed in patients with frontal lesions: She remained apathetic, severely anasognosic according to the staff from the day centre where she stayed, and did not seem able to take care of herself or of her child satisfactorily.

PAD's long-term memory was impaired and remained so in spite of both an improvement with time and satisfactory performance on some tasks. During the first phase of investigation, PAD

Table 1. *Performance on First and Second Administration of Tests Sensitive to Frontal Lobe Lesions*

	PAD		
	First Administration	*Second Administration*[a]	*Normal Data Mean (SD)*
Verbal Fluency; Cardebat et al. (1990)	Letter P = 5 Letter R = 6 Animals = 9 + 3 errors Fruits = 6 + 2 errors	Letter P = 17 Letter R = 15 Animals = 17 Fruits = 19	Letter P = 20.6 (± 6.00) Letter R = 19.0 (± 6.4) Animals = 30.1 (± 11.4) Fruits = 19.9 (± 3.32)
Tower of London; Shallice (1982)	Tests administration had to be stopped because the patient could not perform the task.	3N = 3.5 5N = 6 5I+ = 9.3 5I− = 8.31	3N = 3.4 (± 1.2) 5N = 8.2 (± 3.5) 5I+ = 8.0 (± 3.2) 5I− = 8.3 (± 2.6)
Stroop Test	Reading = 85sec Colour Naming = 140sec Interference = automatic reading activity uninhibited: PAD read all the items	Reading = 44sec Colour Naming = 64sec Interference = 108sec	Reading = 42.8sec (± 8.2) Colour Naming = 72.3sec (± 23.0) Interference = 119.5sec (± 39.3)
Trail Making Test: Kennedy (1981)	Part A: 40sec: between percentile 10 and 25. Part B: more than 5min., 6 errors: inferior to percentile 10	Part A: 55sec: between percentile 10 and 25. Part B: 75sec: between percentile 50 and 75	
WCST; Nelson (1976): normal data; Fery (personal communication)	Test administration had to be stopped because the patient could not perform the task. Nine perseveration errors out of 19 items.	Number of categories = 6 Errors = 1	Number of categories = 5.3 (± 1.6) Errors = 5.7 (± 8.4)
Six Elements Test; Shallice & Burgess (1991)	Number of subtasks tackled: 4 Max time on any subtask: 7min 10sec.	Numbers of subtasks tackled: 5 Max time on any subtask: 5min 20sec	Number of subtasks tackled: 5.7 (± 0.5) Max time on any subtask: 5.4 (± 0.53)

[a] 3N: problems to be solved in 3 movements, neutral; 5N: 5 movements, neutral; 5I+: 5 movements, positive inducer; 5I−: 5 movements, negative inducer.

showed marked confabulatory behaviour, with some reduplicative phenomena (e.g. mistaking the building she could see from the window in her hospital room for the high school she went to when she was teenager; very often confusing one of the psychologists for somebody she used to know). Although confabulations decreased with time, they were still apparent when she left the hospital 4 months post-surgery. Confabulations were observed in both oral (when the patient was asked to answer questions as well as when she talked freely) and written language. The patient kept a diary during her stay in the hospital in which she also noted events that never occurred, e.g. "I had a surgery to my knee."

On the Wechsler Memory Scale-Revised (1991), administered 4 months post-surgery, she obtained relatively satisfactory scores: Verbal MQ = 95, Visual MQ = 86, Full scale MQ = 85, except on the delayed tasks in which she was markedly impaired: delayed MQ = 54 (e.g. Logical Memory I and II: 25 and 16, Verbal Paired Associates I and II: 23 and 8, Visual Reproduction I and II: 36 and 14). On the personal semantic part of the Autobiographical Interview (Kopelman, Wilson, & Baddeley, 1990; adapted for French version by

Coyette & Van der Linden, 1998), the patient was below the controls (Kopelman et al., 1990), but the most altered performance concerned the recall of post-lesion information (Childhood: 13.5, Early Adult: 12 and Recent Life: 4—in each case, out of a maximum of 21). The episodic part of the test was not analysed because it contained too many confabulatory elements and, therefore, was not scorable. Indeed, the patient's recalls were incoherent, obviously incorrect, and contained reduplicative phenomena involving the examiner. For instance, when asked to tell the examiner about a wedding she had been to, PAD told her it was the place where they first met! When told this was not the case, the patient seemed surprised and asked if the examiner was indeed Yolande, the sister of a friend of her's.

On the Semantic Buschke Test (Grober & Buschke, 1987; French version: Coyette, Van der Linden, Calicis & Wijn, 1998), all free recall scores (4, 0, 1, 0 out of 16) were under the minimal level (5, 8, 11, 12). The semantic cues helped the patient to recall more items, but performance was still poor (6, 7, 7, 9 out of 16). She produced a total of 44 intrusions in all free and cued recall tests combined. The yes/no recognition performance was also grossly altered (14/16 correct responses and 13/16 false positives; corresponding controls minimal level: 15 and 0). The results of the California Verbal Learning Test (CVLT; Delis, Kramer, Kaplan, & Ober, 1987; French version: Deweer, et al.,1998) are presented in Table 2. Only two recall scores were 2SDs below the normal mean (from normal data: Deweer, et al., 1998): short and long delay free recalls. She also made more false positives than controls on the yes/no recognition part of the test.

To investigate PAD's premorbid identification abilities, we used a test of recognition of famous and nonfamous faces. She correctly recognised 19/20 famous people and correctly rejected 20/20 unknown people. To investigate her performance on an effortful search for semantic information, a test of geographical knowledge was used. Using a map of Belgium, the patient was asked, first, to give the names of the surrounding countries; then, being presented with the names of the 11 most famous Belgian towns, she was invited to complete the blanks on the map that correspond to these towns. She was impaired on both countries and Belgian town names, showing a considerable number of confabulations[1]. For instance, she indicated the country to the east of Belgium as being England rather than Germany!

One year post-surgery, PAD still confabulated, if relatively mildly in comparison to the errors produced earlier. For instance, when asked to describe the neuropsychologist with whom she was working regularly at the hospital, she produced a description that did not correspond to him at all. Or, when asked to recall the previous testing session, she often incorrectly answered by recalling tasks from earlier sessions the examiner had had with her or from testing sessions she had had with another examiner. Similar examples were observed when asked to recall the lunch she had had on the previous day.

On the Rivermead Behavioural Memory Test (1994), she obtained a so-called "poor memory" score (PAD's profile score = 18/24; normal range: 22–24/24; and PAD's screening score = 8–12/12; normal range: 10–12/12). On list learning tests, free recall was impaired, but cued recall and recognition were normal. Thus, on the "Free and Cued Recall Task" (Semantic Buschke: Grober & Buschke, 1987; French version: Coyette et al., 1998), three out of four free recall scores were below the normal range (scores: 8, 7, 10, 10 out of 16; the lower bound of normal scores: 5, 8, 11, 12). We observed three intrusions in free recall. However, all but one item could be recalled when the patient was given the semantic cue (28/29). The yes/no recognition was perfect. On the Selective Reminding Test (Classic Buschke, 1974), she recalled fewer items (mean = 8.4) than the controls (mean = 14 ± 0.68) and displayed very poor list learning (20.2%, controls = 82.8% ± 11.3%). She

[1] These errors could not be due to a lack of geographical knowledge because we reassessed the same competence several months later and her performance markedly improved, suggesting that her errors were due to a failure in recollecting the correct information rather than to a lack of knowledge.

Table 2. *Performance on First and Second Administration of the California Verbal Learning Test*

	PAD		
	First Administration	*Second Administration*	*Normal Data Mean (± SD)*
Total recall from trial 1–5	46	57	55.5 (± 9.1)
List B (interference trial)	8	11	6.6 (± 1.4)
Short delay free recall	2	7	11.0 (± 2.7)
Short delay cued recall	9	12	11.4 (± 2.1)
Long delay free recall	6	10	11.8 (± 2.3)
Long delay cued recall	7	12	12.2 (± 1.9)
All recalls intrusions	11	8	4.0 (± 4.7)
Recognition—hit	16	15	14.4 (± 2.0)
Recognition—false positive	4	3	0.6 (± 0.8)

Each trial has 16 items.

made 10 intrusions in free recall. Her performance on a forced-choice recognition task was perfect.

The California Verbal Learning Test was administered again and the cueing benefit was confirmed. The results are shown in Table 2. Performance was in the normal range except for the high rate of false alarms on the yes/no recognition. However, the hit rate was close to 100% and, therefore, there is no evidence of loss of sensitivity in the recognition test. An exceedingly high number of intrusions was still observed in the recall tests. To investigate whether or not her good recognition scores were due to a ceiling effect in the list learning tests previously mentioned, PAD was given a more difficult standardised recognition test: the Recognition Test for Words and Faces (Warrington, 1984). She scored 46/50 (control mean = 44.8) for the words subtest and 45/50 (control mean = 44.8) for the faces subtest. Her scores were higher than the mean score of patients with either left temporal injury (38.2) or left frontal injury (40.5). Overall, PAD's recognition abilities were indeed preserved.

We asked PAD to tell the tale of Little Red Riding Hood, assuming that the task taps well-known premorbid semantic knowledge. In recall, PAD made important mistakes, e.g. indicating that the wolf was eating Little Red Riding Hood when they first met in the forest and then wore Little Red Riding Hood's clothes. However, when given some negative feedback about the mistakes she made and some prompting (e.g. when the wolf and Little Red Riding Hood first met in the forest, the wolf did not eat Little Red Riding Hood. What happened instead?), PAD could tell parts of the story properly.

Summary of Clinical Neuropsychological Investigation

The patient presented with normal language, IQ, and short-term memory abilities from the beginning of investigation. She displayed normal performance on several frontal tasks from 3 months post-surgery onwards. However, her long-term memory remained impaired in spite of an improvement reflected in both more correct responses and fewer confabulations. Memory errors occurred more frequently on episodic than on semantic information. She was impaired in recall of both remote and recent events, but the recall of post-lesion events was the more impaired. The patient was more impaired on free than cued recall; by contrast, recognition was better and became normal 1 year post-surgery. The intrusions she made in the memory tests involved both extra-list and prior-list errors. Both prospective and source memory were impaired.

Taken together, the changes observed between some months and 1 year post-surgery were essentially quantitative. No major qualitative changes were noticed. Recognition and cued recall continued to be carried out better than free recall. Intrusions were still present in most of memory tasks.

PAD still produced confabulations although these were less apparent.

EXPERIMENTAL INVESTIGATIONS

In the experimental investigations, we addressed the following questions. Did PAD make confabulations in both the episodic and the semantic domains? Was her source and temporal order memory impaired? Can PAD's behaviour be interpreted as reflecting only a retrieval deficit or should one consider it as also involving an encoding deficit? Were the confabulations she produced the result of both a search and verification impairment or did they stem from a selective search deficit?

These questions were investigated in several tests that involve different kinds of memory processes. For instance, all learning tests involve, at least, encoding, storage, and retrieval and the retrieval phase generally implies search, activation, and verification. However, some processes are more involved in some tests than in others. For instance, the organisation of the search is more important in free recall than in cued recall or recognition. To shed light on the deficit that a given patient exhibits, a comparison of his/her performance across several types of tests is needed. This approach was adopted in the present study. Therefore, when we investigate verification in an AB-AC paradigm, we are aware that this test requires other memory processes, but we assume that this test is highly loaded in verification compared to other memory tests. This holds also for the other memory investigations developed and presented in this paper. When standardised normal results are available, the performance that PAD obtained was compared to them; when not, either four or six control subjects were tested who were matched for age, sex, and level of education. The mean age of the-six subjects was 39.5 (40.5 for the relevant four) and the range: 37 to 42 (38 to 42). Their mean number of years of education was 9 (also for the relevant four) (range: 8 to 10).

To decide whether PAD's performance was or was not normal, a criterion based on the range of the control subjects, sample was used. The usual two standard deviations from the mean was not adopted because many recall tasks show large standard deviations.

Episodic and Semantic Memory

Confabulation is often described as concerning mainly episodic memory (e.g. Dalla Barba, 1993a; Dalla Barba et al., 1990; Talland, 1965). However, it has been shown that semantic memory retrieval can also be prone to confabulation (e.g. Dalla Barba, 1993b; Delbecq-Derouesné et al., 1990; Moscovitch & Melo, 1997; Sandson, Albert, & Alexander, 1986). To investigate both the type and the evolution of confabulation in the patient, we used a questionnaire inspired by Dalla Barba's study (1993a). It contains questions on general and personal semantic memory, episodic memory, orientation in time and place, and "I don't know" episodic and semantic questions (questions for which the appropriate answer is "I don't know", e.g. 'What is the capital of Bolania?", 'What did you have for dinner the 13 of April 1992?"). The responses were scored as correct answer, confabulation (a commission error), or omission. The results are shown in Table 3.

An evolution was observed across the four administrations of the tests, namely an increasing number of correct answers and omissions, with a decreasing number of confabulations. The overall pattern of performance remained stable during the period: a much higher proportion of confabulations on questions tapping episodic memory than on those tapping semantic memory. However, on "I don't know" questions, there was almost no difference in the incidence of confabulations between episodic and semantic type questions. Compared to control subjects, PAD produced more confabulations: initially to all question categories, but by 1 year post-onset virtually limited to episodic questions only.

Source and Temporal Order Memory

Source Memory

Source memory was investigated because confabulation has also been characterised as a correct

Table 3. *Performance in Percentage across Each Section by PAD on Different Occasions and by Control Subjects*

	26/1/96	*13/2/96*	*29/2/96*	*13/11/96*	*Normal Range*
Personal Semantic Memory					
Correct response	75.0%	81.25%	81.25%	100.0%	Not scorable[a]
Confabulation: Any error	25.0%	18.75%	18.75%	0.0%	
Omission	0.0%	0.0%	0.0%	0.0%	
General Semantic Memory					
Correct responses	75.0%	87.5%	100.0%	100.0%	100%–100%
Confabulation: Any error	25.0%	12.5%	0.0%	0.0%	0%–0%
Omission	0.0%	0.0%	0.0%	0.0%	
Episodic Memory					
Correct response	0.0%	6.25%	6.25%	43.75%	Not scorable[a]
Confabulation: Any error	100.0%	62.5%	56.25%	31.25%	
Omission	0.0%	31.25%	37.5%	25.0%	
Orientation to Time and Place					
Correct response	70.0%	80.0%	70.0%	100.0%	100%–100%
Confabulation: Any error	30.0%	20.0%	20.0%	0.0%	0%–0%
Omission	0.0%	0.0%	10.0%	0.0%	
Episodic I Don't Know					
Correct response: I don't know	70.0%	80.0%	100.0%	100.0%	100%
Confabulation: Any error	30.0%	20.0%	0.0%	0.0%	0%
Semantic I Don't know					
Correct response: I don't know	81.0%	86.7%	100.0%	93.75%	87.5%–100%
Confabulation: Any error	19.0%	13.3%	0.0%	6.25%	0%–12.5%

[a]The controls' answers to personal semantic and episodic questions were not scorable because the examiners did not personally know the control subjects. Therefore, Kopelman and colleagues (1997) controls' scores were used. As their control subjects did not produce confabulations or omissions, it can be inferred that they obtained a ceiling score of 100% for these two question categories.

memory misplaced from its proper context, i.e. a so-called "source memory error". Moreover, source memory is assumed to depend upon frontal lobe functioning (e.g. Schacter, 1987; Schacter, Harbluck, & McLachlan, 1984; Shimamura, 1995; Shimamura, Janowsky, & Squire, 1991). This type of error was observed both in the recall of everyday life events and in list learning (as prior list intrusions). To investigate source memory, the task proposed by Janowsky, Shimamura, and Squire (1989) was used. In the first testing session, the patient was asked to learn some general facts ($N = 20$) likely to be unknown to the patient considering her level of education. In order to select facts unknown to the patient, each fact was first presented in the form of a question (e.g. "In which country is the Iriri river located?"). From 30 such questions, 20 unknown facts were selected and the corresponding answers were provided. The questioning was then repeated until the patient could retrieve the answer to each question. PAD needed 11 trials to recall the answer to all questions.

After an 11-day retention interval, both fact and source recall were tested. For this test phase, we used the 20 facts the patient had learned, 10 difficult new facts (questions that the patient was unlikely to know, e.g. "What is the capital of Kenya?") and 10 easy new facts (questions that the patient was likely to know, e.g. "What is the capital of England?"). The patient was first asked to answer all the questions, which were presented randomly. Then, she was asked to indicate where the information had been learned. An "extra-experimental source error" was noted if the patient reported that the information was learned outside the study when in fact it was previously learned during the previous session. An "experimental source error" was noted when the patient reported that the information was learned in the study when in fact it was not the case. In addition, she was asked to say which was the last time she heard that information. An 8 alternative forced-choice recognition task was administered for all 40 items.

Eleven days after the study phase, PAD could only recall 4 out of the 20 learned facts (20%). This performance is lower than that of the mean of the frontal patients tested by Janowsky et al. (1989) (40%). On recognition, she was much better, obtaining 70% correct responses for the old facts, a performance closer to the mean performance of the young control group from the Janowsky et al. study (74%). On the source memory judgements test, PAD correctly judged that the 20 old facts were learned from the experimenter on the previous session, but incorrectly attributed to this source 4 out of 10 difficult new facts. In other words, she only made experimental source errors (20%) and no extra-experimental ones. This pattern of performance is different from the one displayed by the frontal patients investigated by Janowsky et al., who made both types of source errors (15% extra-experimental and 20% experimental source errors) and from control subjects, who made experimental source errors alone, and very infrequently (2%). As PAD only produced one type of error, one could argue that she used a lax criterion in her decision. The correct response score could, thus, be overestimated and the error score underestimated. In this test, her "source memory" ability was impaired.

Temporal Order Memory

According to Moscovitch, the post-ecphoric strategic process is responsible for the temporal ordering of the randomly retrieved memory elements. This temporal order ability was investigated with two different types of material: historical facts and autobiographical facts. In the first version (inspired by Shimamura, Janowsky, & Squire's study, 1990), the subject was presented with 20 historical facts, each on a card, in random order (e.g. Kennedy's assassination, the knocking down of the Berlin Wall, the independence of the Congo) and asked to sort them according to their chronological order.

In this test, performance was assessed by means of a Spearman correlation measure between the actual chronological order of the historical events and the patient's judged order. It was .83 and .85 in the first and second administrations of the test, whereas the control subjects' (six in this test) correlation varied from .88 to .97.

A possible reason for the below-normal performance that PAD obtained in this test was her lack of knowledge of historical facts. In fact, her comments during the test would fit this hypothesis. To avoid this possible artefact, an autobiographical version was constructed with 31 important personal facts from the patient's life, e.g. her father's death, her nephews' births, her sisters' weddings. The personal order task was presented twice and the order given by the patient was the same across the two testing sessions. We administered the same task independently to her older sister: the Spearman correlation between PAD's and her sister's ordering of autobiographical facts was .99. This result is consistent with the hypothesis that her failure to achieve normal performance on the Historical version of the test was due to a lack of general knowledge rather than a temporal order memory impairment per se.

Performance on the source memory test had confirmed the clinical observation that PAD was making source errors in the recall of everyday life events. A different pattern was found in the temporal order tests. Although her performance was somewhat below the normal range for the ordering of historical facts, it seems that PAD's temporal order memory was relatively preserved. This conclusion is clearly supported by the very high correlation observed between PAD and her sister's ordering in the personal facts test.

Encoding vs. Retrieval Impairment

PAD's pattern of memory performance in clinical tests fits well with a retrieval impairment: good recognition, a large benefit from cueing in recall, and confabulations that also occur for events prior to the aneurysm rupture. However, as we tested PAD after her illness, it could be argued that her performance on the learning tests could also have resulted from an encoding deficit. To test this hypothesis and to attempt to differentiate between an impairment of retrieval and an impairment of both encoding and retrieval, the encoding and the retrieval conditions were manipulated in word list and story learning tests. A larger increase in the recall of correct responses, compared to the one exhibited by the control subjects, when cues were given at retrieval, would reflect a deficit in the retrieval processes. Likewise, a similar effect when cues were given at encoding would reflect a deficit in the encoding processes. This was tried using two procedures.

Memory Tests Following a Semantic Orienting Task

We know from the Semantic Buschke that semantic category information facilitates PAD's recall performance. To determine whether other semantic cues, for instance sentences, could lead as well to a better performance, a test based on the semantic orienting encoding procedure was used (inspired from Craik & Tulving, 1975). PAD was presented with 90 sentences, 1 at a time, on cards. Each card contained both a sentence with a missing word and, below, a target word. For each sentence, the patient was asked to say whether the target word would fit the sentence well. Half of the words were plausible or compatible with the context of the sentence, the other half did not, e.g. "it is on the ... that he learned the King's dead"—radio; "the ... snored all night long"—hat. In this test, 30 target words occurred once, and 30 occurred twice but with a different sentence each time. The patient was not informed that this sentence plausibility judgement test would be followed by a recall test. After a 1-minute delay, PAD was asked to recall as many target words as possible in 5 minutes. She was then presented with the sentences and asked to recall the corresponding target words, i.e. a cued recall task. This was followed by an old/new recognition test containing the 60 target words and 60 distractors.

PAD answered correctly to 89/90 sentences; the range of 4 control subjects varied from 87/90 to 90/90. This suggests that she performed the semantic orienting task correctly. The results of the recall and recognition tests are shown in Table 4.

Like the control subjects, PAD recalled more words in the cued condition compared to the free recall condition, especially when the words were compatible with the sentence. Overall, PAD's scores were within the normal range.

Story Learning Test

Finally, encoding and retrieval conditions were manipulated in a story learning test (the material and procedure were taken from Delbecq-Derouesné et al., 1990). Each story was tested on a different session. The cues consisted of precise questions about part of the story. Cues were provided or not at encoding and/or at retrieval. Four conditions were adopted: (1) with no semantic cues either in encoding or in retrieval conditions, (2) cues in the encoding condition, (3) cues in the retrieval condition, and (4) cues in both the encoding and the retrieval condition. To obtain the same rhythm in the uncued as in the encoding conditions, the experimenter inserted silences during the story presentation.

PAD'S performance was below that of the four controls for both free recall (52.8%; controls' range: 69.4–77.8%) and recall with cues given at encoding (27.5%; controls' range: 50.0–62.5%). Her correct responses (72.5% and 79.41%) scores were within the normal range (67.2–85% and 70.6–91.2%) only when the cues were given at retrieval only or at both encoding or retrieval. Overall, PAD produced more errors (9) than the control subjects (controls' range: 0–6). The error scores were higher than the maximal range when cues were not given at retrieval (3 and 5, controls' range: 0–2 in both cases), but normal when cues were available at retrieval (0 and 1, controls' range: 0–2 in both cases). To make more apparent the specificity of this cueing effect, Figs. 3 and 4 show, for the correct responses, the highest and lowest bound of the controls' scores as well as PAD's score when recall conditions are grouped in terms of presence versus absence of cues at encoding (Fig. 3) or at retrieval (Fig. 4). The data from the control subjects indicate an improvement with cues given at retrieval, but not with cues given at encoding. In PAD's case, a strong benefit from retrieval cues is observed: Cues given at retrieval brought her back into the normal range (see Fig. 4). Clearly, the presence of the cues helped PAD to retrieve more pieces of information and to prevent her

Table 4. *Performance on the Semantic Encoding Procedure Test (Inspired by Craik & Tulving, 1975)*

	Free Recall		*Cued Recall*		*Recognition*	
	CR	*ER*	*CR*	*ER*	*CR*	*ER*
Total Presented 1						
PAD	5/30		10/30	4/30	17/30	
Control range	1–6/30		8–17/30	2–10/30	16–22/30	
Total Presented 2						
PAD	5/60		23/60	5/60	26/60	
Control range	4–12/60		23–33/60	2–20/60	18–25/60	
Total Compatible						
PAD	8/45		30/45	5/45	26/30	
Control range	3-14/45		26–41/45	2-10/45	25–27/30	
Total Not Compatible						
PAD	2/45		3/45	4/45	17/30	
Control range	0–9/45		4–13/45	2-20/45	9-22/30	
Distractors						
PAD					53/60	7/60
Control range					50–58/60	2–10/60
Total						
PAD	10/90	4	33/90	9/90	96/120	
Control range	5–18/90	0–9	33–50/90	6–30/90	90–107/120	

CR = correct response; ER = intrusion errors.

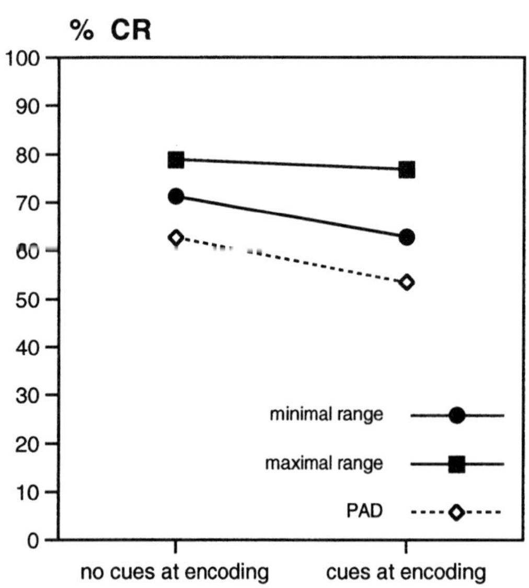

Fig. 3. *Percentage of correct responses dividing trials according to whether cues are or are not given at encoding.*

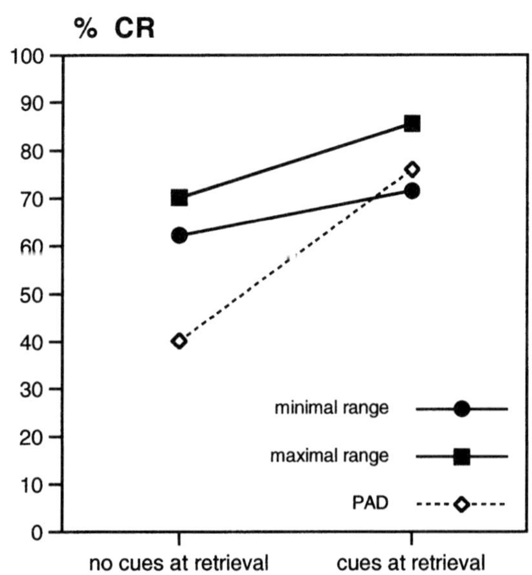

Fig. 4. *Percentage of correct responses dividing trials according to whether cues are or are not given at retrieval.*

from producing errors at this stage. This was not the case with the encoding cues.

Summary
In the word list learning task following a semantic encoding procedure, PAD behaved normally. But the results observed in the story learning task suggest a problem at retrieval. Indeed, the cues at encoding did not have a particular effect on performance but providing cues at retrieval gave a strong benefit to the patient, whose performance then became within the normal range. However, this was not observed in the retrieval following semantic orienting test. A possibility is that story recall required more effortful and strategic processes than did the semantic orienting test. The deficit was therefore easier to elicit in story than in word learning tasks.

Overall, the results suggest a specific impairment in the retrieval processes. The pattern of memory performance that PAD obtained in traditional clinical memory tests is also consistent with this conclusion: preserved recognition abilities, better cued than free recall, and the observation of errors for the retrieval of information that PAD knew prior to her illness.

Search and Memory Verification Processes

As has previously been suggested, PAD's impairment concerns the retrieval process. More precisely, it seems that this deficit takes place mainly at the earliest stage of retrieval: the search stage. It has been argued that preserved recognition and cued recall are, indeed, evidence for intact memory verification processes (e.g. Hanley et al., 1994; Parkin, Yeomans, & Bindschaedler, 1994). This would imply that PAD would have a selective deficit in the search processes. But, in our view, more evidence is needed to rule out a deficit conclusively in both the search and verification processes. PAD was therefore given further experimental tasks.

Memory Verification Processes
AB–AC Paradigm. Many verbal memory paradigms, e.g. free recall and retrieval (but not encoding), can be carried out essentially unaffected by the simultaneous carrying out of a demanding but routine task such as a serial choice reaction task, which does not produce structural interference when combined with the memory task (e.g. Baddeley, Lewis, Eldridge, & Thompson, 1984; Craik, Govoni, Naveh-Benjamin, & Anderson, 1996). This is not the case for recall of AB–AC pairs. A concurrent serial choice reaction time task produces a significant decline in the rate of correct recall and an increase in the number of inter-list confusion errors (Cinan & Shallice, 1998). The difference with, say, free recall can be explained by the greater monitoring requirements of retrieval in the AB–AC situation.

PAD's abilities to evaluate, verify, and reject incorrect memory information were investigated by means of an AB–AC paradigm (inspired by Kinsbourne & Winocur, 1980; Winocur & Weiskrantz, 1976). To intensify the monitoring demands the experiment was constructed with a first list containing 16 A–B pairs of words that was presented 4 times (examples of AB pairs in the semantically related and unrelated conditions are "mountain–ski" and "rain–money," respectively), with a 20-second counting backwards task between each presentation. The counting backwards task consisted in counting backwards in 3s from a given number, which varied across trials. After the fourth presentation, PAD was given the 16 A words and asked to perform a cued recall of the B words corresponding to the A words. A second list of 16 AC words was then presented once (for examples, AC pairs in the semantically related and unrelated conditions are "mountain–snow" and "rain–pencil," respectively), and, after a 20-second counting backward task, the patient was presented with the 16 A words and asked to recall the 16 corresponding C words. We finally administered a 3-alternative recognition task in which the patient had to choose the C word corresponding to the A word with the B and another word as distractors. The tests were replicated with different words, both in the semantically related and unrelated conditions.

It was assumed that in the C cued recall the subject has to reject the more salient, but incorrect, B response, because the AB associations have been presented four times whereas the AC words have been presented only once. The occurrence of a B error in the C cued recall test or in the recognition test would reflect inappropriate memory verification or checking processes. Results are presented in Table 5.

In the semantically related condition, the number of correct responses in all three conditions were within the normal range. The number of AB intrusions in the AC test was within the normal range in the first administration, but higher in the replication test. However, in the recognition condition, her AB errors were within normal range in both tests. We observed the same pattern of performance in the semantically unrelated conditions, except that PAD did not produce more AB errors than the control subjects in the AC tests. She was thus able to reject incorrect, although more salient, information when she had all the necessary information available.

Hayling Test. To assess whether PAD could inhibit automatic responses, the Hayling Test was used (Burgess & Shallice, 1996b; adapted for French version by Meulemans, Vincent, Andres, & Van der Linden, 1998). It taps response initiation (section A) and response suppression (section B) of the sentence's last word. In the first part of the test, the subject is asked to complete the sentence with an appropriate word (e.g. The captain wanted to stay with the sinking ... boat). In the second part of the test, the subject is asked to complete the sentence using a word unrelated to either the sentence or the word that could correctly fit the sentence (e.g. most cats see very well at ... banana). In section A, PAD's response latency (15sec) was within the normal range: the control subjects' (four control subjects in this test) latency was also 15sec (note that the procedure used for latency time gave a "1-second" measure when the latency time was 1sec or less). In the more critical section, PAD's latency (50sec) was below our control subjects' range (55–74sec). To analyse errors, we asked five independent judges to score the responses of PAD and of the control subjects. The score given by the majority of the judges was adopted. PAD's error score was within normal range (6; control subject, range 0–8; note, however, that the control subject who scored 0 was an outlier, and the other three control subjects' error score varied from 6–8). Furthermore, when compared to Burgess and Shallice's (1996b) data, PAD's error score was closer to the one of the controls than to those of anterior and bifrontal patients. PAD's performance thus suggests that she did not have a problem in verifying whether responses were appropriate.

Table 5. *Performance on Four AB–AC Paradigm Tests: Two Semantic and Two Unrelated Conditions*

	AB	*AC*	*Recognition*
Semantic Condition 1			
PAD correct responses	14	11	15
Normal range correct responses	9–16	4–14	8–16
PAD AB error		1	1
Normal range AB error		0–1	0–7
Semantic Condition 2			
PAD correct responses	15	11	13
Normal range correct responses	10–16	10–16	13–16
PAD AB error		4	3
Normal range AB error		0–3	0–3
Non-semantic Condition 1			
PAD correct responses	13	1	14
Normal range correct responses	2-14	0–9	8–16
PAD AB error		2	2
Normal range AB error		0–2	0–8
Non-semantic Condition 2			
PAD correct responses	11	1	16
Normal range correct responses	4–15	1–5	8–15
PAD AB error		0	0
Normal range AB error		0–0	0–6

Use of Semantic Information in the Memory Search Processes

Homogeneous and Heterogeneous Word Lists Learning Tasks. A new list learning test was designed in order to manipulate the number of semantic categories within a list. The task was run over 4 days, the first 2 and the last 2 sessions being run on 2 successive days. Three different 12-word lists were presented each day, and each list was presented 3 times (the word order varied from 1 list to another). Each list presentation was followed by a free recall test after counting backward for 20 seconds. Thus, the subject had to perform 9 free recalls each day. We used 2 different conditions. In the homogeneous condition, the lists consisted of

12 words from the same semantic category, e.g. a list of fruits, a list of flowers, and a list of vegetables. In the heterogeneous condition, the lists consisted of 12 mixed words from 3 different semantic categories, e.g. 4 fruit words, 4 vegetable words, and 4 flower words[2]. Two homogeneous and two heterogeneous conditions were run, in an AB–BA presentation paradigm, over 4 days. We used the same task in an unrelated word condition. It was assumed that, in the homogeneous condition, lists had different semantic category cues. In the heterogeneous condition it was the reverse: The three lists had the same semantic category cues. Therefore the prediction was that, if the patient used a general semantic category cue rather than both a general and some specific cues, more prior list intrusions would be found in the heterogeneous than in the homogeneous condition.

The results of PAD and of the six control subjects are shown in Table 6. PAD's correct response score was in the normal range for the heterogeneous but not for the other two conditions. She produced more prior-list and prior-day-list errors than did the control subjects. But her score was in the normal range for the number of extra-list errors in two out of three conditions. All intrusions were of a semantic type in both the homogeneous and heterogeneous conditions.

More correct responses were observed when the words came from a limited set of semantic categories than when the words were unrelated. There were more prior-list intrusions in the heterogeneous than in the homogeneous conditions. These results suggest that the semantic category information provided good assistance to the patient but also led to a great increase in the number of incorrect responses, as control subjects produced a very low number of intrusions. The semantic category information was guiding the errors produced—they were all of a semantic type in the homogeneous and heterogeneous conditions.

Table 6. *Performance on the Homogeneous and Heterogeous List Learning Test*

	Homogeneous	*Heterogeneous*	*Unrelated*
Control Responses			
PAD	137/216[a]	127/216	102/216
Control range	149–166	120–159	112–126
Prior List Errors			
PAD	2	11	3
Control range	0–1	1–9	0–6
Prior Day List Errors			
PAD	17	9	0
Control range	0–14	1–3	0
Extra-list Errors			
PAD	6	6	1
Control range	0–8	0–3	2–7

[a]216 correspond to 12 words in each list, 3 recalls per list, 3 lists per day, 2 different paradigms for a given condition: $12 \times 3 \times 3 \times 2 = 216$.

Release from Proactive Interference Test. To confirm the conclusions drawn from the previous tests, a release from proactive interference task was used (Wickens, 1970). In this situation, the subject was presented with four words from the same semantic category, e.g. four clothes, and was asked to perform a free recall test after a 20sec backward counting task. The same procedure was repeated for four trials. In the first three trials, the words were different but all came from the same semantic category. In the last trial, the words came from a different semantic category. The test contained eight sessions, with different words and different semantic categories in each session. Summing the results of the different sessions, what one typically observes with normal subjects is a decrease of correct responses from trial 1 to trial 3, i.e. a proactive interference build-up, and better performance on the last trial compared to the third one, i.e. release from proactive interference. This effect is assumed to reveal the use of the semantic category information in the search-and-retrieval process (Craik, 1979;

[2] Day 1: Heterogeneous condition: List 1: 4 fruits, 4 flowers, and 4 vegetables; List 2: 4 fruits, 4 flowers, and 4 vegetables; List 3: 4 fruits, 4 flowers, and 4 vegetables. Day 2: Homogeneous condition: List 1: 12 fruits, List 2: 12 vegetables; List 3: 12 flowers. Day 3: Homogeneous condition with weapons, kitchen utensils, and tools items. Day 4: Heterogeneous condition with weapons, kitchen utensils, and tools.

Watkins & Watkins, 1975; Wickens, Moody, & Dow, 1981).

If the patient used the semantic category information in the course of search and retrieval, she should exhibit the effect of release from proactive interference in the last trial, i.e. more correct responses in the last trial compared to the third trial, as normal subjects do. In Fig. 5, one can observe the release from proactive interference exhibited by control subjects and by PAD. Figure 6 shows that the patient produced more errors than the controls.

The number of correct responses produced by the patient is in the normal range. PAD exhibited the release from proactive interference effect (mean difference between the number of correct items recalled in trial 3 and in trial 4, $t = -3.81, p < 0.01$) as control subjects did ($t = -5.965, p < .005$). This result suggests that she used semantic category information in retrieval. However, she produced more incorrect responses than all the control subjects on three out of four trials.

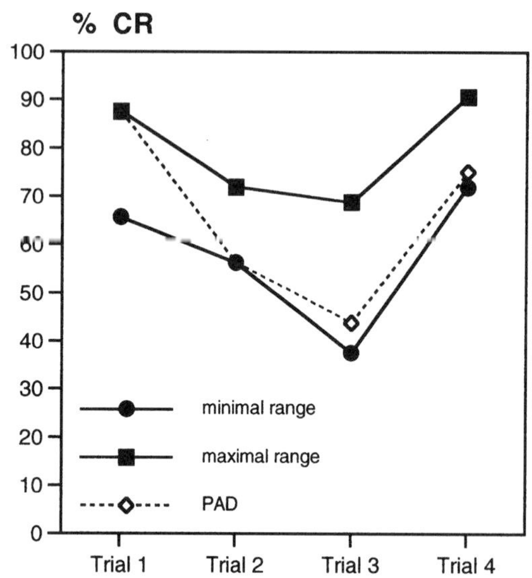

Fig. 5. *Percentage of correct responses in eight tests using the Release from Proactive Interference Paradigm.*

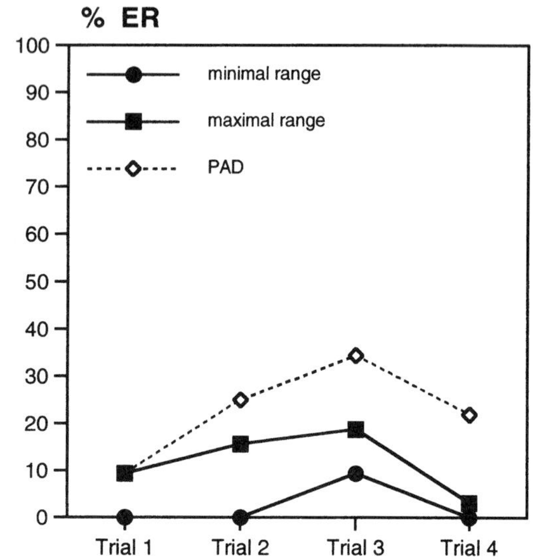

Fig. 6. *Percentage of intrusion errors in eight tests using the Release from Proactive Interference Paradigm.*

DISCUSSION

Summary of Investigations

PAD displayed normal intellectual level, short-term memory, and language abilities from the beginning of the investigation. Three months after surgery, she displayed normal performance on several frontal tasks. However, in the memory domain, she obtained normal performance in some of the tests, but displayed an impairment in others. These results can be summarised in the following way.

Normal Recognition. In the second period of investigation, recognition performance was consistently normal across different tests: the Free and Cued Recall Test (Semantic Buschke), the Selective Reminding Test (Classic Buschke), the Warrington Recognition Test for Words and Faces, the memory test following a semantic orienting task (Craik & Tulving), and the AB–AC paradigm test. The only recognition test where any abnormality was observed was the California Verbal Learning Test: The false alarm score was above the normal mean, but even here, the hit score was at ceiling.

Quantitative and Qualitative Free Recall Impairment. PAD's performance on free recall tasks was variable. In some tests, her scores were below the normal level. In the Free and Cued Recall Test, performance was under the minimal range for three out of four free recall tests. On the Selective Reminding Test, in which the to-be-learned material is not organised, the mean number of words recalled was below 8SD. However, in other tests, her scores were at a normal level (e.g. CVLT, the immediate logical memory subtest from the WMS-R, and the Craik and Tulving procedure test). One could suppose that this difference reflects a learning deficit rather than a retrieval impairment, because PAD is below the normal level when tested with a selective reminding procedure (Free and Cued Recall Test and Selective Reminding Test). Against this hypothesis is her normal mean improvement from trial 1 to trial 3 on the 18 lists assessed in the homogeneous heterogeneous unrelated task, which used a repeated presentation and test procedure. PAD's mean improvement was 3.61 and the corresponding control subjects' range varied from 3.11 to 4.61. Moreover, in the CVLT, she obtained a normal level free recall on the fifth trial from list 1. Both these last two data do not fit with a learning deficit.

Production of confabulations. PAD continued to produce confabulation 1 year after her stroke. There were everyday life memory confusions. In the episodic part of the questionnaire, she produced more than 31% of confabulatory responses; controls produced none in comparable circumstances (e.g. Kopelman, Ng, & Van Den Brouke, 1997). In verbal recall tests, she often produced an excessive number of errors, for instance in the homogeneous and heterogeneous task, the release from proactive paradigm, and the story learning test. Those memory errors reflect PAD's tendency to confabulate.

A quantitative and qualitative evolution of the confabulatory behaviour was observed: With time, PAD produced fewer errors and the memory distortions were of a milder type. Although there was a higher proportion of confabulations on questions tapping episodic memory than on those tapping semantic memory, no attempt to equate the strategic processing demands across episodic and semantic retrieval was made. Indeed, the errors that PAD produced in the recall of the Little Red Riding Hood tale could be considered as confabulations in a semantic test stressing strategic retrieval processes (see also Delbecq-Derouesné et al., 1990). The confabulations produced were usually semantically linked to the target items. PAD did not confabulate indiscriminately; rather the erroneous responses seem to have been prompted by the use of semantic information. For instance, in the homogeneous and heterogeneous task, she did not produce an abnormal number of incorrect responses in the unrelated condition, but did when the words came from a limited set of semantic categories—i.e. on the homogeneous and heterogeneous conditions.

Use of Semantic Information and Intact Cued Recall Performance. There is much evidence that PAD made excellent use of semantic information during retrieval. In fact, in the Free and Cued Recall Test (Grober & Buschke, 1987) PAD's performance was under the minimal range for three out of four free recalls, whereas, under the same semantic encoding condition, cued recall was performed at ceiling (28/29 words recalled with the cues). In the story learning test, the retrieval cues both enhanced the pieces of information retrieved and prevented her from making an abnormal number of errors. In the Wickens paradigm, she exhibited the usual release from proactive interference effect, suggesting that she relied on semantic information at retrieval. In the homogeneous and heterogeneous test, more correct responses were observed when the words came from a limited set of semantic categories (homogeneous condition: 137/216, and heterogeneous condition:127/216) than when the words were unrelated (unrelated condition: 102/216). Moreover, in this test, there were more prior list intrusions in the heterogeneous (11 prior list errors) than in the homogeneous conditions (2 prior list errors), i.e. when the semantic category information was the same for the three lists than when it was different across the lists. In the memory test following a semantic orienting task (Craik & Tulving), PAD's cued recall performance was within normal range when the word was compatible with the sentence but not when the sentence context was semantically unrelated to the word, suggesting that the semantic context had to be relevant to be used as an efficient cue at retrieval.

Relatively Preserved Normal Temporal Order Memory. PAD had preserved temporal order memory abilities. As it has previously been mentioned, although her score was below the minimal range for the historical facts version, the correlation between her estimate and the actual dates was very high (.83 and .85). However, the more convincing result is the score she obtained for the temporal ordering of personal facts. The Spearman correlation between PAD's and her sisters' ordering was .99. One cannot exclude the possibility that PAD did not perform as well for the historical facts as for the personal facts because in the former condition she did not know all the facts that she was asked to sort.

Variable Source Memory Abilities. In the source memory test (Janowsky et al., 1989), PAD made source memory errors, incorrectly judging four new facts (20%) as being derived from the previous sessions. Source memory errors were also observed in the misplacement or the condensation of information in the recall of everyday life events. The prior list errors found in several tests can also be viewed as source memory errors. However, the results that PAD obtained in the AB–AC paradigm test suggest that she had good source memory abilities. Indeed, in the recognition test she did not produce any more AB errors than control subjects.

Summary. In conclusion, although some of the scores obtained by PAD fit well with observations of previously described frontal patients, others do not. Confabulation has mostly been described in patients with frontal lesions. But not all patients with frontal lobe damage displayed confabulation (e.g. DeLuca, 1993 patients BC, GW, and DM; Schacter, Curran, Galluccio, Milberg, & Bates, 1996). PAD produced more confabulations for episodic than for general semantic memory, a result previously obtained (e.g. Dalla Barba, 1993a; Kopelman, et al., 1997). Preserved cued recall and impaired free recall on the one hand, and preserved or better recognition than recall on the other, have both been described previously in frontal patients (e.g. Hanley et al. 1994; Parkin et al.,1994; Volpe & Hirst, 1983). Source memory errors and temporal order memory impairment are usually assumed to be linked with frontal lobe dysfunction (e.g. Janowsky et al., 1989; Schacter, 1987; Schacter et al., 1984; Shimamura, 1995; Shimamura et al., 1991). In contrast with some other confabulators (e.g. Baddeley & Wilson, 1988; Conway & Tacchi, 1996; Fischer, Alexander, D'Esposito, & Otto, 1995; Moscovitch, 1989; Stuss et al., 1987) and some non-confabulating patients with frontal lobe damage (e.g. DeLuca, 1993; patients BC, GW and DM), PAD had normal performance in several tests assumed to be tapping "frontal function."

An Account of This Particular Pattern of Performance

An increasing number of conceptual accounts suggest that confabulation involves the control process, located primarily in prefrontal cortex, which are necessary for effective memory recall. In some old versions of this approach, the emphasis is specifically put on failure of verification or editing. However, more complex theories of the control processes tend to differentiate a few types of control processes. Two of these processes are, in the framework of Norman and Bobrow's theory (1979), the descriptor processes and the editing (verification) processes (Burgess & Shallice, 1996a; Shallice, 1988) and, in more traditional terminology, strategic search processes and monitoring processes (e.g. Moscovitch & Melo, 1997). Both processes should be impaired to give rise to confabulations (Burgess & Shallice, 1996a; Moscovitch, 1995; Moscovitch & Melo, 1997). In addition, there can be a contribution from abnormally faulty output from the associative cue-dependent processes (Moscovitch, 1989, 1995; Moscovitch & Melo, 1997), from the long-term storage systems (Burgess & Shallice, 1996a; Dalla Barba et al., 1990; Sandson et al., 1986), and from disturbed high-level mediator systems (e.g. Burgess & Shallice, 1996a), which have also been called executive functions (Baddeley & Wilson, 1986, 1988). In other accounts, confabulation results from a disruption in the decision processes that are involved in and responsible for source attribution (Johnson et al., 1993).

A Retrieval Processes Impairment

PAD had an impairment in the retrieval process rather than in the encoding or consolidation processes. As previously argued, some data are in favour of preserved encoding processes: the good performance observed in paired-associate learning tests, namely in the WMS-R and in the experimental AB–AC paradigm. In the latter, PAD could learn the AB pairs, even in the semantically unrelated condition (e.g. rain-money) in which PAD's performance was within normal range (she scored 13 and 11 out of 16 pairs of unrelated words; corresponding normal range: 2–14 and 4–15). Other data are in favour of impaired retrieval processes: the recall of incorrect information that occurred prior to the lesions (autobiographical interview, Little Red Riding Hood tale), the free recall impairment together with the good performance observed in recognition tests (see earlier), and the excellent benefit resulting from retrieval cueing (e.g. Semantic Buschke, Craik and Tulving's test, story learning test, see earlier).

Preserved Memory Verification Abilities

Several data suggest that PAD had preserved memory verification processes. The most striking finding is the consistently normal recognition performance that PAD obtained across several tasks (as in Hanley et al.'s study of ROB, 1994). However, confabulating patients are usually assumed to exhibit recall problems but not a recognition deficit, what would produce a problem for this argument. Moreover, the processes that follow a putative response in recall are presumably very similar to those operating in yes/no recognition after the item has been presented to the subject. In fact, recognition has not been systematically tested in many patients exhibiting confabulations (e.g. Baddeley & Wilson, 1986; Dalla Barba, 1993a; Mercer et al., 1977; Papagno & Muggia, 1996; Stuss et al., 1978) When recognition abilities were investigated, in nearly all cases confabulating patients produced abnormal performance (e.g. Baddeley & Wilson, 1988; Conway & Tacchi, 1996; Dalla Barba et al., 1990, 1997; Delbecq-Derouesné et al., 1990; Hodges & McCarthy, 1993; Johnson, O'Connor, & Cantor, 1997; Kopelman et al., 1997; Schnider, Gutbrod, et al., 1996; Schnider, von Däniken, et al., 1996). A few confabulators are suggested to have had normal recognition abilities. SB was one of them (Kapur & Coughlan, 1980), but he was assessed with forced-choice recognition tests only. HW (Moscovitch, 1989) was considered to have preserved recognition but the finding were not described in sufficient detail[3]. Intact recognition performance has been interpreted as reflecting unimpaired verification processes (e.g. Hanley et al., 1994; Schacter et al., 1996).

In addition, PAD's performance was within the normal range in the response suppression section (section B) of the Hayling test: Neither her latency nor her error score was higher than those of controls, suggesting that she did not have a verification problem. Most critically, the patient was able to reject incorrect but more salient information, when all the information that she needed to perform the task was available. In the AB–AC recognition paradigm, which normal subjects found difficult, she indeed had normal AC recognition scores (15, 13, 14, and 16 out of 16; corresponding normal range: 8–16, 13–16, 8–16, 8–15). More important, PAD did not produce more AB errors than control subjects in the AC recognition test (1, 3, 2, and 0 out of 16, corresponding normal range: 0–4, 0–3, 0–8, 0–4). Thus, when asked in the recognition test to choose the C word with the B word and another word as distractors, although the AB pairs were more salient because they had been presented four times while the AC pairs had been presented only once, PAD was able to reject the AB information correctly. It is worth noting that this finding has

[3] The patient HW obtained 12/16 on the CVLT recognition test. Note that according to the normal data that Schnider, Gutbrod, et al. (1996) used for their study, a performance of 12/16 in the recognition part of the CVLT corresponds to a level inferior to percentile 1. The other 14/14 recognition score cannot come from the WMS because the test does not involve any recognition subtest.

been replicated across four tests with different conditions (semantically and not semantically related pairs of words) and different materials (different words used in each of the four tests). Also consistent with preserved memory verification processes is the good performance in the temporal order memory tests, which are assumed to tap the post-ecphoric strategic processes (Moscovitch, 1995).

The most striking empirical finding made on PAD is that the patient was able to perform at a normal level on recognition tasks, including a demanding one dependent upon fine temporal dissociation, when recall tasks frequently lead to confabulation that reflects failure to discriminate the appropriate timing of the retrieved event; these include a recall task precisely paralleling the AB–AC recognition procedure. As far as we know, confabulation when comparable recognition tasks have been carried out accurately has not previously been recorded.

A Descriptor or Search Process Impairment

In the free recall task, one typically needs to set up appropriate descriptions to address the long-term memory store. In contrast, in the cued recall task, a description is provided, and in the recognition task one is presented with all the relevant information. Thus, a patient with a descriptor processes impairment only should have good performance on the recognition tests and relatively preserved cued recall. PAD's pattern of memory performance is consistent with these predictions.

What is the exact nature of the impairment? PAD was able to initiate a memory search and to set up memory descriptions. Indeed, she obtained normal performance in some of the free recall tests (Craik and Tulving's test and the California Verbal Learning Test, second administration). She used the semantic information, even when it was not explicitly given (see earlier). suggesting that the description processes rely on this feature. However, the semantic intrusions observed in several list learning tests suggest that the descriptions used by PAD might not be fully appropriate. In the homogeneous and heterogeneous tests, she made a greater number of intrusions than the controls, both from prior lists that were presented on the same day and from those presented on the previous day.

This implies that although the descriptions she articulated were well focused semantically they were not well focused in the temporal dimension. There was a subtle widening in the specification of what was required in memory. This result is especially striking when contrasted with the recognition results with the same material, which indicated that the temporal dimension could be monitored accurately in memory. In recall, where the description has to be self-generated she used too wide a specification. A similar pattern is observed in the release from proactive interference paradigm. PAD did not confabulate indiscriminately. Rather, her confabulations were prompted by the use of semantic category information to generate possibilities and by her failure to put more precise constraints in place during the search processing.

The prior list errors and the other so-called source memory errors could also result from a descriptor process impairment. An inappropriate or too-wide part of the long-term memory store could be activated because of inaccurate descriptions. For instance, when asked to say what she did on a previous testing session, PAD recalled tests from other sessions. In this case, her behaviour fitted with a too-general description being used (e.g. "what tests have I done?"). Again it was not specific enough to correctly focus temporally on the memory associated with the last testing sessions.

What does this imply as far as memory verification processes are concerned? Within the source memory framework many different processes are held to affect source monitoring (see Johnson, 1997, for review). However, many of these (e.g. comprehension errors, emotional focus, suggestion, social context) do not appear to be of much relevance in the present case. Others (e.g. the reviving or evaluating of additional supporting or disconfirming information [Craik, 1982] and inappropriately lax criteria) are relevant. Burgess and Shallice (1996a), in their protocol analysis of normal memory retrieval found there to be at least four different types of such processes. However, in their theory the most direct type of verification procedure is when the output of the memory stores is in conflict with the description itself. Even if intact, this type of verification procedure would not be able to check on a memory error that was the consequence of a description that was specified too widely. It is theoretically possible for a patient to exhibit memory errors with an undamaged verification process; note that normal subjects produce memory errors, and with poorly specified descriptions being used, the set of candidate errors would be much larger. In contrast with other such patients (e.g. those described by Baddeley & Wilson, 1988; Delbecq-Derouesné et al., 1990; Fischer et al., 1995) PAD's performance generally consistent with intact verification processes. However, without a more elaborate theory of the verification processes one cannot exclude the possibility that the tasks where confabulations occur are those where the monitoring needed to prevent errors requires quantitatively greater resources.

It can be counterintuitive that a patient with preserved memory verification abilities on direct testing exhibits confabulations. Indeed, traditionally in neuropsychology, whatever the domain of investigation, e.g. language, action, memory, or even neglect, commission errors are often seen as reflecting verification or inhibition impairments, whereas omission errors are seen as a problem of activation or initiation. This kind of explanation might be too simple a view, as suggested by the theories of Burgess and Shallice (1996a), Moscovitch and colleagues, (Moscovitch, 1989, 1995; Moscovitch & Melo, 1997) and Schacter, Norman, and colleagues (Norman & Schacter, 1996; Schacter et al., 1998): A verification impairment is not sufficient to account for florid commission errors in the memory domain. All these theories indeed emphasise the implication of a defective memory search in confabulations: a difficulty in specifying the memory to be sought for, a blurring of focus, or a difficulty in initiating and organising a memory search with the available knowledge.

However, although these theories clearly emphasise the impairment of an early retrieval stage, they do not explicitly consider that such a deficit alone could be enough to give rise to confabulation. Moscovitch and Melo's (1997) model, in particular, postulates that a deficit in at least three stages is necessary for confabulations to occur. It is worth noting that the possibility of a deficit restricted to the descriptor processes alone is not excluded, in principle, by the hypotheses included in the Burgess and Shallice (1996a) model. The memory editor processes check continuously the compatibility among the memory retrieved elements. Still, what is retrieved from the long-term stores is determined by the earlier description set-up. If all memory retrieved elements are compatible, although incorrect, the editor processes cannot detect the error. In this sense, it is theoretically possible to exhibit memory errors with preserved verification processes.

A patient with a very similar pattern of performance was previously described by Kapur and Coughlan (1980). SB was an ACoA patient who was investigated longitudinally during his spontaneous recovery. He first displayed spontaneous confabulations that were fictitious constructions, and only later produced provoked confabulations that were distortions of actual events and misplacements of events in an incorrect spatial and temporal context. This change in the pattern of his confabulations was paralleled by the improvement observed in tests assumed to be sensitive to frontal lesions, in which he first was impaired and later obtained normal performances. But no change was observed in other aspects of memory or other cognitive tests between these two periods. In the memory domain, he had preserved recognition abilities, displaying normal or near-normal scores on recognition tests. However, as far as we know, Kapur and Coughlan's findings had never been interpreted as reflecting preserved memory verification, possibly because there was no theoretical model available to account for these findings in the way suggested here. Indeed, it has been largely accepted that confabulation is mainly a problem of memory verification. Although SB has a similar pattern of memory performance, it is worth noting that he was tested with a forced-choice recognition test only. It is therefore not entirely convincing that SB had preserved memory verification abilities.

The empirical finding from Mercer et al. (1977), on the inverse relation between the latency to respond and the number of self-corrections observed is commonly explained as reflecting an internal verbal monitoring. One can also find in the literature other arguments in favour of the monitoring or verification impairment hypothesis. However, none are persuasive. The first argument is the presence of the confabulatory symptom itself! Briefly summarised, the cause of confabulation is held to be faulty monitoring or verification, and the argument supporting this interpretation is the fact that patients produce confabulations and do not correct themselves. For example, DeLuca (1993, p. 641), argued "During a verbal list, learning task [...] patient BJ emitted numerous intrusive errors indicative of poor self-monitoring." This is obviously circular. The second type of argument often encountered in the literature for the monitoring or verification impairment is the presence of frontal lobe dysfunction (e.g. Conway & Tacchi, 1996, p. 336: "OP can access autobiographical knowledge but [...] she cannot evaluate accessed knowledge, due to executive impairments". This hypothesis is reminiscent of the idea of a "central deficit", which is now challenged by empirical data (Burgess & Shallice, 1994). Some confabulators had good performance in several tests assumed to be sensitive to frontal lesions, although these patients were not tested using modern batteries (e.g. Delbecq-Derouesné et al., 1990; Kapur & Coughlan, 1980). More critically, some patients with severe deficits in executive functions do not confabulate (e.g. Burgess & Alderman, 1990, cited by Burgess & Shallice, 1994). Then, there is a dissociation between what can be called frontal dysfunction and confabulation.

To sum up, although it can seem surprising that PAD confabulated and still had preserved memory verification and checking processes, this is both theoretically possible and empirically supported.

Consequences for Accounts of Confabulation

The present findings have several consequences. They suggest that a descriptor process or memory search process impairment can be sufficient to induce confabulation. In the framework of the memory control processes models, it supports the idea that different aspects of retrieval are mediated by different processes, namely that the search and memory monitoring processes can be dissociated one from the other. This is in agreement with Burgess and Shallice's (1996a) and Moscovitch and Melo's (1997) models. It is also consistent with the previously described patient showing such a deficit (ROB, reported by Hanley et al., 1994). On the other hand, our findings are inconsistent with the notion that search and monitoring are two aspects of the same processes or computational machinery (e.g. Moscovitch, 1989).

Differences between Amnesic with and without Confabulation

Two different hypotheses have been proposed to account for the difference between amnesics who do and who do not confabulate. According to Hanley et al. (1994), whereas confabulators have a monitoring or verification impairment, amnesic patients without confabulation have a search deficit. In contrast, Moscovitch and Melo (1997) proposed that confabulatory amnesic patients have both a search and monitoring impairment whereas non-confabulatory amnesics only exhibit a search deficiency. Indeed, previously reported patients who show both intact recognition and impaired recall do not confabulate (e.g. Hanley et al., 1994). Conversely, patients who confabulate, generally do not show intact recognition (e.g. Baddeley & Wilson, 1988; Dalla Barba et al., 1990; Delbecq-Derouesné et al., 1990). However, our findings challenge both ideas proposed in the literature because PAD exhibited confabulations and yet had preserved memory verification abilities, as described earlier.

Other findings in the neuropsychological literature challenge Moscovitch and Melo's (1997) hypothesis. Recently, Schacter et al. (1996), described a patient, BG, who exhibited a considerable number of false alarm errors in recognition tests after an infarction of the right frontal lobe, suggesting a deficit in monitoring or verification processes. In addition, BG was impaired in free recall and had normal recognition in the California Test, a finding that can be seen as a search deficiency. However, BG did not produce confabulations in two batteries often used to assess whether a patient is a confabulator: a questionnaire (Dalla Barba, 1993a) and a version of the Crovitz's test (Moscovitch, 1995).

What are the alternative hypotheses one can propose to differentiate patients with memory deficit who do and do not make confabulations? One possibility concerns the memory processes impairment: Patients with memory deficits could have an encoding and/or consolidation impairment whereas confabulatory patients would suffer from a retrieval deficit. As is well known, memory behavioural deficit can result from different types of cognitive impairments. However, this hypothesis cannot account for all patients in the literature: For instance, ROB (Hanley et al., 1994) is a nonconfabulatory amnesic patient with a selective search impairment. She displayed normal recognition despite very impoverished recall, even when the difficulty between the two tests was matched. The patient did not confabulate at the time of investigation. Although PAD and ROB had similar results in the Recognition Memory Words and Faces (Warrington, 1984), their performances in recall are very different: ROB's impairment is more severe. An ad hoc hypothesis could be that ROB had a more severe descriptor process impairment in the sense that she had problems in initiating memory search, i.e. in setting up retrieval strategies, whereas PAD had difficulty in setting up appropriate and subtle descriptors, but was able to initiate memory search.

The following hypothesis could therefore be added to the Burgess and Shallice model (1996a). Patients whose memory deficit were at retrieval but who do not confabulate would mostly have a difficulty in spontaneously elaborating description, whereas confabulatory patients would mostly elaborate inaccurate descriptions. In Schacter and colleagues' terms (Norman & Schacter, 1996; Schacter, et al., 1998), amnesic patients would suffer from a loss of the ability to apply focusing, whereas confabulators would use blurred focusing. A related theoretical distinction can be found in the original proposal of Norman and Bobrow (1979), later adapted by Burgess and Shallice (1996a), about the descriptor processes. Norman and Bobrow postulated two aspects that a description should have to be efficient: the *constructability*—likelihood that an appropriate description can be formed when the need for a memory trace is manifest—and the *discriminability*—the ability of the description to discriminate among all the possible records within memory. Using this approach, PAD would suffer from an inability to produce sufficiently discriminable descriptions.

REFERENCES

Bachy-Languedoc, N. (1989). *Batterie d'examen des troubles en dénomination*. Bruxelles: Editest.

Baddeley, A., Lewis, V., Eldridge, M., & Thompson, N. (1984). Attention and retrieval from long-term memory. *Journal of Experimental Psychology: General, 13*, 518–540.

Baddeley, A., & Wilson, B. (1986). Amnesia, autobiographical memory, and confabulation. In D.C. Rubin (Ed.), *Autobiographical memory* (pp. 225–252). Cambridge: Cambridge University Press.

Baddeley, A., & Wilson, B . (1988). Frontal amnesia and the dysexecutive syndrome. Special Issue: Single-case studies in amnesia: Theoretical advances. *Brain and Cognition, 7*, 212–230.

Battig, W.F., & Montague, W. E. (1969). Category norms for verbal items in 56 categories: A replication and extension of the Connecticut category norms. *Journal of Experimental Psychology Monograph, 80*, 1–43.

Berlyne, N. (1972). Confabulation. *British Journal of Psychiatry, 120*, 31–39.

Burgess, P.W., & Shallice, T. (1994). Fractionnement du syndrome frontal. *Revue de Neuropsychologie, 4*, 345–370.

Burgess, P.W., & Shallice, T. (1996a). Confabulation and the control of recollection. *Memory, 4*, 359–411.

Burgess, P.W., & Shallice, T. (1996b). Response suppression, initiation and strategy use following frontal lobe lesions. *Neuropsychologia, 34*, 263–273.

Buschke, H., & Fuld, P.A. (1974). Evaluating storage, retention, and retrieval in disordered memory and learning. *Neurology, 24*, 1019–1025.

Cardebat, D., Doyon, B., Puel, M., Goulet, P., & Joanette, Y. (1990). Evocation lexicale formelle et sémantique chez des sujets normaux. Performances et dynamiques de production en fonction du sexe, de l'âge et du niveau d'étude. *Acta Neurologica Belgica, 90*, 207–217.

Cinan, & Shallice, T. (1999). *Dual task interference in recall.* Manuscript in preparation.

Conway, M.A. (1990). *Autobiographical memory: An introduction.* Buckingham, UK: Open University Press.

Conway, M.A., & Tacchi, P.C. (1996). Motivated confabulation. *Neurocase, 2,* 325–339.

Coyette, F., & Van der Linden, M. (1999). *Adaptation française du Test de Mémoire Autobiographique de Kopelman.* Manuscript in preparation.

Coyette, F., Van der Linden, M., Calicis, F., & Wijn, C. (1998). *Adapatation en langue française de la procédure indicée de Grober et Buschke.* Manuscript in preparation.

Craik, F.I.M. (1979). Human memory. *Annual Review of Psychology, 30,* 63–102.

Craik, F.I.M. (1982). Selective changes in encoding as a function of reduced processing capacity. In F. Klix, J. Hoffman, & E. van Der Meer (Eds.), *Cognitive research in psychology,* (pp. 152–161). Berlin: Deutscher Verlag der Wissenschaft.

Craik, F.I.M., Govoni, R., Naveh-Benjamin, M., & Anderson, N.D. (1996). The effect of divided attention on encoding and retrieval processes in human memory. *Journal of Experimental Psychology: General, 125,* 159–180.

Craik, F.I.M., & Tulving, E. (1975). Depth of processing and the retention of words in episodic memory. *Journal of Experimental Psychology: General, 104,* 268–294.

Dalla Barba, G. (1993a). Confabulation: Knowledge and recollective experience. *Cognitive Neuropsychology, 10,* 1–20.

Dalla Barba, G. (1993b). Different patterns of confabulation. *Cortex, 29,* 567–581.

Dalla Barba, G., Cappelletti, J.Y., Signorini, M., & Denes, G. (1997). Confabulation: Remembering 'another' past, planning 'another' future. *Neurocase, 3,* 425–436.

Dalla Barba, G., Cipolotti, L., & Denes, G. (1990). Autobiographical memory loss and confabulation in Korsakoff's syndrome: A case report. *Cortex, 26,* 525–534.

Delbecq-Derouesné, J., Beauvois, M.F., & Shallice, T. (1990). Preserved recall versus impaired recognition. A case study. *Brain, 113,* 1045–1074.

Delis, D.C., Kramer, J.H., Kaplan, E., & Ober, B.A. (1987). *The California Verbal Learning Test.* San Antonio, TX: Psychological Corporation.

DeLuca, J. (1993). Predicting neurobehavioral patterns following anterior communicating artery aneurysm. *Cortex, 29,* 639–647.

DeLuca, J., & Cicerone, K.D. (1991). Confabulation following aneurysm of the anterior communicating artery. *Cortex, 27,* 417–423.

De Renzi, E., & Faglioni, P. (1978). Normative data and screening power of a shortened version of the Token Test. *Cortex, 14,* 41–49.

Deweer, B., Benoît, N., Ergis, A.M., Eustache, F., Pillon, B., & Van der Linden, M. (1999). *Le California Verbal Learning Test: Adaptation française et normalisation.* Manuscript in preparation.

Feinberg, J.F. (1980). The Wernicke-Korsakoff Syndrome. *American Family Physicians, 22,* 129–133.

Fischer, R.S., Alexander, M.P., D'Esposito, M., & Otto, R. (1995). Neuropsychological and neuroanatomical correlates of confabulation. *Journal of Clinical and Experimental Neuropsychology, 17,* 20–28.

Grober, E., & Buschke, H. (1987). Genuine memory deficit in dementia. *Developmental Neuropsychologia, 3,* 13–36.

Hanley, J.R., Davies, A.D.M., Downes, J.J., & Mayes, A.R. (1994). Impaired recall of verbal material following rupture and repair of an anterior communicating artery aneurysm. *Cognitive Neuropsychology, 11,* 543–578.

Hodges, J.R., & McCarthy, R.A. (1993). Autobiographical amnesia resulting from bilateral paramedian thalamic infarction. *Brain, 116,* 921–940.

Janowsky, J.S., Shimamura, A.P., & Squire, L.R. (1989). Source memory impairment in patients with frontal lobe lesions. *Neuropsychologia, 27,* 1043–1056.

Johnson, M.K. (1991). Reality monitoring: Evidence from confabulation in organic brain disease patients. In G. Prigatano & D. Schacter (Eds.), *Awareness of deficit after brain injury,* (pp. 176–197). New York: Oxford University Press.

Johnson, M.K. (1997). Source monitoring and memory distorsion. *Philosophical Transactions of the Royal Society of London, 352,* 1733–1745.

Johnson, M.K., Hashtroudi, S., & Lindsay, D.S. (1993). Source monitoring. *Psychological Bulletin, 114,* 3–28.

Johnson, M.K., Kounios, J., Nolde, S.F. (1996). Electropsysiological brain activity and memory source monitoring. *NeuroReport, 7,* 2929–2932.

Johnson, M.K., O'Connor, M., & Cantor, J. (1997). Confabulation, memory deficits and frontal dysfunction. *Brain and Cognition, 34,* 189–206.

Joslyn, D., Grundvig, J.L., & Chamberlain, C.J. (1978). Predicting confabulation from the Graham-Kendall Memory-For-Designs Test. *Journal of Consulting and Clinical Psychology, 46,* 181–182.

Kapur, N., & Coughlan, A.K. (1980). Confabulation and the frontal lobe dysfunction. *Journal of Neurology, Neurosurgery and Psychiatry*, *43*, 461–463.

Kennedy, K.J. (1981). Age effects on Trail Making Test performance. *Perceptual and Motor Skills*, *52*, 671–775.

Kern, R.S., Van Gorp, W.G., Cummings, J.L., Brown, W.S., & Osato, S.S. (1992). Confabulation in Alzheimer's disease. *Brain and Cognition*, *19*, 172–182.

Kinsbourne, M., & Winocur, G. (1980). Response competition and interference effects in paired associate learning by Korsakoff amnesics. *Neuropsychologia*, *18*, 541–548.

Kopelman, M.D. (1987). Two types of confabulation. *Journal of Neurology, Neurosurgery and Psychiatry*, *50*, 1482–1487.

Kopelman, M.D., Guinan, E.M., & Lewis, P.D.R. (1995). Delusional memory, confabulation, and frontal lobe dysfunction: A case study in De Clérambault's syndrome. *Neurocase*, *1*, 71–77.

Kopelman, M.D., Ng, N., & Van Den Brouke, O. (1997). Confabulation extending across episodic, personal and general semantic memory. *Cognitive Neuropsychology*, *14*, 683–712.

Kopelman, M.D., Wilson, B.A., & Baddeley, A.D. (1990). *The autobiographical Memory Interview*. Bury St. Edmunds, UK: Thames Valley Test Company.

Mercer, B., Wapner, W., Gardner, H., & Benson, F. (1977). A study of confabulation. *Archives of Neurology*, *34*, 429–433.

Meulemans, T., Vincent, E., Andres, P., & Van der Linden, M. (1999). *Adaptation française du test de Hayling*. Manuscript in preparation.

Morton, J., Hammersley, R.H., & Bekerian, D.A. (1985). Headed records: A model for memory and its failure. *Cognition*, *20*, 1–23.

Moscovitch, M. (1989). Confabulation and the frontal systems: Strategic versus associative retrieval in neuropsychological theories of memory. In H.L. Roediger, III & F.I.M. Craik (Eds.), *Varieties of memory and consciousness: Essays in honour of Endel Tulving* (pp. 133–160). Hillsdale, NJ: Lawrence Erlbaum Associates Inc.

Moscovitch, M. (1995). Confabulation. In D.L. Schacter (Ed.), Memory distortion, (pp. 226–251). Cambridge, MA: Harvard University Press.

Moscovitch, M., & Melo , B. (1997). Strategic retrieval and the frontal lobes: Evidence from confabulation and amnesia. *Neuropsychologia*, *35*, 1017–1034.

Norman, K.A., & Bobrow, D.G. (1979). Descriptions: An intermediate stage in memory retrieval. *Cognitive Psychology*, *11*, 107–123.

Norman K.A., & Schacter, D.L. (1996). Implicit memory, explicit memory and false recollection: A cognitive neuroscience perspective. In L.M. Reder (Ed.) *Implicit memory and metacognition* (pp. 229–259). Hillsdale, NJ: Lawrence Erlbaum Associates Inc.

Papagno, C., & Muggia, S. (1996). Confabulation: Dissociation between everyday life and neuropsychological performance. *Neurocase*, *2*, 111–118.

Parkin, A.J., Yeomans, J., & Bindschaedler, C. (1994). Further characterisation of the executive memory impairment following frontal lobes lesions. *Brain and Cognition*, *26*, 23–42.

Raven, J.C. (1982). *Revised manual for Raven's progressive matrices and vocabulary scale*. Windsor, UK: NFER-Nelson.

Sandson, J., Albert, M.L., & Alexander, M.P. (1986). Confabulation in aphasia. *Cortex*, *22*, 621–626.

Schacter, D.L. (1987). Memory, amnesia and frontal lobe dysfunction. *Psychobiology*, *5*, 21–36.

Schacter, D.L., Curran, T., Galluccio, L., Milberg, W.P., & Bates, J.F. (1996). False recognition and the right frontal lobe: A case study. *Neuropsychologia*, *34*, 793–808.

Schacter, D.L., Harbluk, J.L., & McLachlan, D.R. (1984). Retrieval without recollection an experimental analysis of source amnesia. *Journal of Verbal Learning and Verbal Behaviour*, *23*, 593–611.

Schacter, D.L., Norman, K.A., & Koutstaal, W. (1998). The cognitive neuroscience of constructive memory. *Annual Review of Psychology*, *49*, 289–318.

Schnider, A., Gutbrod, K., Hess, C.W., & Schroth, G. (1996). Memory without context: amnesia with confabulations after infarction of the right capsular genu. *Journal of Neurology, Neurosurgery and Psychiatry*, *61*, 186–195.

Schnider, A., von Däniken, C., & Gutbrod, K. (1996). The mechanisms of spontaneous and provoked confabulation. *Brain*, *119*, 1365–1375.

Shallice, T. (1982). Specific impairments of planning. *Philosophical Transaction of the Royal Society of London*, *B298*, 199–209.

Shallice, T. (1988). *From neuropsychology to mental structure*. Cambridge: Cambridge University Press.

Shallice, T., & Burgess, P.W. (1991). Deficit in strategy application following frontal lobe damage in man. *Brain*, *114*, 727–741.

Shapiro, B.E., Alexander, M.P., Gardner, H., & Mercer, B. (1981). Mechanisms of confabulation. *Neurology, 31*, 1070–1076.

Shimamura, A.P. (1995) Memory and frontal lobe function. In M.S. Gazzaniga (Ed.), *The cognitive neurosciences* (pp. 803–813). Cambridge, MA: MIT Press.

Shimamura, A.P., Janowsky, J.S., & Squire, L.R. (1990). Memory for the temporal order of events in patients with frontal lobe lesions and amnesic patients. *Neuropsychologia, 28*, 803–813.

Shimamura, A.P., Janowsky, J.S., & Squire, L.R. (1991). What is the role of frontal lobe damage in memory disorder? In H.S. Levin, H.M. Eisenberg, & A.L. Benton (Eds.), *Frontal lobe function and dysfunction* (pp. 171–195). Oxford: Oxford University Press.

Stuss, D.T., Alexander, M.P., Lieberman, A., & Levine, H. (1978). An extraordinary form of confabulation. *Neurology, 28*, 1166–1172.

Talland, G.A. (1965). *Deranged memory: A psychonomic study of the amnesic syndrome.* New York: Academic Press.

Vanier, M., & Lemyse, C. (1994). *Le Rivermead Behavioural Memory Test (French version).* Bury St Edmunds, UK: Thames Valley Test Company.

Volpe, B.T., & Hirst, W. (1983). Amnesia following the rupture and repair of an anterior communicating artery aneurysm. *Journal of Neurology, Neurosurgery and Psychiatry, 46*, 704–709.

Warrington, E.K. (1984). *Recognition Memory Test.* Windsor, UK: NFER-Nelson.

Watkins, O.C., & Watkins, M.J. (1975). Buildup of proactive inhibition as a cue-overload effect. *Journal of Experimental Psychology: Human Learning and Memory, 104*, 442–452.

Wechsler; D. (1970). *Echelle d'Intelligence de Wechsler pour Adultes, WAIS.* Paris: Centre de Psychologie Appliquée.

Wechsler D. (1991). *Echelle Clinique de Mémoire de Wechsler-Révisée, WMS-R.* Paris: Centre de Psychologie Appliquée.

Wickens, D.D. (1970). Encoding categories of words: An empirical approach to word meaning. *Psychological Review, 77*, 1–15.

Wickens, D.D., Moody, M.L, & Dow, R. (1981). The nature and timing of the retrieval process and of interference effect. *Journal of Experimental Psychology: General, 110*, 1–20.

Winocur, G., & Weiskrantz, L. (1976). An investigation of paired-associate learning in amnesic patients. *Neuropsychologia, 14*, 97–110.

COGNITIVE NEUROPSYCHOLOGY, 1999, 16 (3/4/5), 243–265

FALSE RECOGNITION FOLLOWING FRONTAL LOBE DAMAGE: THE ROLE OF ENCODING FACTORS

Alan J. Parkin and Jamie Ward
University of Sussex, Brighton, UK

Claire Bindschaedler
CHUV, Lausanne, Switzerland

Ella J. Squires and Georgia Powell
University of Sussex, Brighton, UK

This paper reports a series of experiments on patient JB, a man with memory difficulties following damage to the left frontal lobe. The primary characteristic of JB's recognition memory impairment is a high level of false recognition together with a normal hit rate. The hypothesis that JB's false recognition reflects an over-reliance on familiarity is considered, but discounted on the basis that the false alarm rate is not affected by increasing the similarity between distractors and targets, and remains high when nonword stimuli are used. It is suggested, instead, that JB relies on a poorly focused memory description, which lacks item-specific detail but contains more general, low-level properties of the target items—these properties being held by many distractor items as well. This deficit is considered to arise because of damage to frontally mediated control processes involved in the selection of elements for memory encoding. An encoding deficit is supported by the fact that JB's false recognition is significantly reduced by orienting instructions, and is eliminated when his remote memory is subjected to recognition testing. In contrast, it is shown that manipulations at the level of retrieval (e.g. restricting the number of "old" responses) have little effect on his false recognition.

INTRODUCTION

Recent studies of certain patients with frontal lobe damage have indicated that their recognition memory exhibits a very characteristic impairment that differs markedly from that found in patients who have become amnesic due to lesions of the medial temporal cortex or the diencephalon (Parkin, 1997). Delbecq-Derouesné, Beauvois, and Shallice (1990) report RW, who developed memory problems following a ruptured aneurysm of the anterior communicating artery (ACoA)—this form of aneurysm is reliably associated with frontal lesions in addition to lesions of the basal forebrain (e.g. Parkin & Leng, 1993). On tests of recognition RW performed very poorly and made many false alarms. However, he was always confident about the "accuracy" of his responses. In contrast, RW's performance on tests of recall was relatively spared (excluding confabulations). Parkin, Bindschaedler,

Requests for reprints should be addressed to Alan J. Parkin, Laboratory of Experimental Psychology, University of Sussex, Falmer, Brighton, BN1 9QG, UK (E-mail: alp@biols.susx.ac.uk).

This research was funded by a Human Frontiers grant (RG–126/97). We are grateful to Tim Shallice and Gordon Winocur for comments on an earlier draft and to Rebecca Poz and Claudia Metzler for assistance in collecting some of the data, and to JB for his cheerful co-operation with testing.

Harsent, and Metzler (1996) examined the recognition memory of JB, another patient who suffered a ruptured ACoA aneurysm. Over a range of recognition tests, involving both verbal and nonverbal materials, JB's hit rate was within normal range but his false alarm rate varied between 39% and 52%. Like RW, his responses were associated with a high degree of certainty. Thus, when asked if he was "sure" or "not sure" about any given response, he produced the same proportion of "sure" responses for hits and false alarms. Finally, Schacter, Curran, Galluccio, Milberg, and Bates (1996; see also Curran, Schacter, Norman, & Galluccio, 1997) describe the memory performance of BG, who suffered frontal damage following a stroke. Seven experiments showed that BG produced normal hit rates but pathologically high false alarm rates on recognition tests involving words, nonwords, environmental sounds, and pictures.

Although the phenomenon of high false alarm rates following frontal damage is well established, the underlying cause of this deficit remains to be explained. Recently, Schacter et al. (1996) have suggested that high false alarms may arise because the patient sets up, at retrieval, a poorly focused event description. Norman and Schacter (1996) defined a focused memory description as containing a maximal number of features associated with the sought-after trace but that are not characteristic of competing traces[1]. An unfocused description therefore contains information that is common to all the target traces and lacks information pertaining to individual targets within the sequence (cf. "gist" or "general event" memory; Brainerd, Reyna, & Kneer, 1995; Conway & Rubin, 1993). In the case of word stimuli, for example, it is argued that patient BG's event description amounts to little more than "I saw a bunch of words" and, as a result, BG is willing to accept most word stimuli as plausible targets with, presumably, only his general awareness that not all the items can be targets preventing him from responding "yes" to every item. A number of lines of evidence support this interpretation of BG's false alarm errors. First, it was shown that BG's false alarm rate is not affected by the degree of associative relationship between real-word targets and their distractors on a recognition test. If BG's impaired recognition memory were due to a simple over-reliance on item familiarity, then one would expect greater susceptibility to associated distractors. It is possible, however, that with verbal memory, high false alarms could be uninfluenced by target-distractor association because prior experience of words per se is sufficient to make distractors seem familiar. Crucial to dismissing this argument is the fact that BG also makes high levels of false alarms when nonword stimuli are used. By definition these items cannot have pre-experimental levels of familiarity and their lack of meaning greatly reduces their scope for generating inter-item familiarity effects at recognition. Finally, Schacter et al. (1996) demonstrated that BG's false alarms could be reduced by presenting him with targets and distractors drawn from different taxonomic categories. The event description in this instance is more focused because features that are consistently present in the target sequence are not present at all in the distractors.

The aim of the present study was to extend investigations of JB in the light of the recent study of Schacter et al. (1996) with the aim of discovering more about the nature and underlying basis of JB's recognition memory impairment. On a priori grounds there is some reason to suspect that JB's impairment, despite its superficial similarity to that of BG, might have a different origin. A number of functional neuroimaging studies have implicated the right frontal region in retrieval operations (Shallice et al., 1994; Tulving, Kapur, Craik, Moscovitch, & Houle, 1994). BG's lesion, although not in exactly the same place as that identified via functional neuroimaging, is also right frontal and thus supports a retrieval-based explanation of his deficit. JB, in contrast, has a left-sided lesion and, with reference to the same body of functional neuroimaging data, we might expect a deficit in encoding.

[1] Other studies have referred to this as a process of "pattern separation" (e.g. McClelland, McNaughton, & O'Reilly, 1995).

CASE BACKGROUND

JB's case history has been described elsewhere (Parkin et al., 1996; Parkin, Leng, Stanhope, & Smith, 1988) so will only be briefly recounted here. JB, now aged 54, suffered a ruptured ACoA aneurysm in October 1984. Following repair a large left frontal horn lesion with an adjacent low density area was detected by CAT scan. Unfortunately the extent of aneurysmal clipping (three clips used) prevented detailed neuroradiological assessment but, minimally, JB was considered to have damage to the left frontal cortex and the left caudate. Initially there was a severe confusional state characterised by fantastic confabulation but this ameliorated and by 1987 JB's primary deficit was a marked disturbance of anterograde memory and significant personality change. He is excessively prone to repeating himself and, despite numerous visits to the laboratory, he still has to ask directions once he has arrived at the University. Despite his psychometric profile JB does not give the impression of being amnesic. He has got to know the research team well and is able to recognise them outside the department without difficulty. In addition he can, if appropriately prompted, give quite detailed accounts of events in his life, both before and after his illness. Such observations have been confirmed by formal comparisons between JB and "classical" amnesic patients, suggesting that JB's remote memory for faces from previous decades is normal and markedly superior to that of Korsakoff's patients and that his ability to learn paired associates is markedly improved by supplying him with learning strategies (e.g. mediational sentences, imagery), unlike Korsakoff and bitemporal amnesics (Parkin et al., 1988).

Table 1 shows JB's performance on the Wechsler Adult Intelligence Scale-Revised (WAIS-R; Wechsler, 1981) and it can be seen that there has been no significant decline in intelligence relative to his estimated premorbid IQ (NART; Nelson, 1985). He also performs extremely well on the Standard Progressive Matrices (Raven, 1960). On the Wechsler Memory Scale Revised (WMS-R; Wechsler, 1984) JB shows marked impairments on both tests of logical memory, paired associates, and the delayed visual reproduction test.

Further testing confirmed indications from WMS-R that JB's deficit is worse for verbal than for non/verbal material—a finding consistent with his left-sided lesion. On the Warrington Recognition Memory Test (Warrington, 1984) he scored 30/50 for words (percentile < 5) but on faces he scored 39/50 (percentile 10). On "frontal" tests, JB was normal on the modified Wisconsin Card Sorting Test (Nelson, 1976)—6 categories, 0 perseverative errors; FAS word fluency (Benton & Hamsher, 1976)—52; cognitive estimation (Shallice & Evans, 1978)—3; Stroop (Trenerry, Crosson, DeBoe, & Leber, 1989)—78th percentile; and within normal limits on the Ruff figural fluency test (Ruff, Light, & Evans, 1987)—45 correct reproductions and no perseverations. However, JB did perform poorly on the Alternate Uses Test (Guildford, Christensen, Merrifield, & Wilson, 1978).

In summary, JB presents with a frontally associated memory impairment, although this does not appear to be part of a wider "dysexecutive syndrome" (cf. Baddeley, 1996). This is consistent with the notion that different frontal functions have different neurological substrates, which may be differentially affected by brain damage (e.g. Allport, 1993; Monsell, 1995; Parkin, 1998). The focus of this investigation, however, is JB's poor recognition memory and, specifically, his tendency to recognise falsely nonpresented items.

EXPERIMENTAL INVESTIGATION

The experimental investigation will be divided broadly into two parts. The first set of experiments will attempt to characterise JB's false recognition disorder in more detail, with particular reference to the question of whether false recognition is influenced by target distractor similarity (contrasting associative relationship) or pre-experimental familiarity with the target material (using nonword stimuli). The second set of experiments will attempt to identify the functional locus of JB's false recognition disorder by investigating the influence of encoding and retrieval manipulations on his false alarm rate.

Table 1. *JB's Profile on WAIS-R and WMS-R*

WAIS-R				*WMS-R*			
Verbal		*Performance*		*Percentiles*		*Indices*	
Information	10	Picture complete	9	Digits Forward	28	Verbal Memory	68 (70)
Digit span	10	Picture arrangement	8	Digits Backward	29	Visual Memory	88 (77)
Vocabulary	12	Block design	11	Visual Span Forward	99	General Memory	68 (68)
Arithmetic	15	Object assembly	10	Visual Span Backward	71	Delayed Recall	55 (57)
Comprehension	11	Digit symbol	9	Logical Memory	9	Attention/Conc.	105 (91)
Similarities	12			Logical Memory Delay	< 1		
				Visual Reproduction	54		
Verbal IQ	113	Performance IQ	107	Visual Reproduction Delay	5		
Full Scale IQ	110						
National Adult Reading Test estimated pre-morbid IQ	117						

Figures in parentheses indicate mean performance of eight Korsakoff patients (Wechsler, 1984).

Effects of Target-distractor Similarity and Target Familiarity

Previous investigations of JB's false recognition have provided at least some support for the notion that JB's recognition memory may be based on an over-reliance upon familiarity. Recognition judgements based on familiarity rely upon a unidimensional signal, which does not take account of the specific content of the memory or the context in which it was acquired. Familiarity-based recognition is often defined as lacking "conscious awareness" of the study episode (e.g. Gardiner, 1988; Rajaram, 1993) and may be based, at least in part, upon the ease/fluency with which the stimulus is processed (e.g. Gardiner & Java, 1993; C.M. Kelley & Jacoby, 1990). Parkin et al. (1996) gave JB a recognition and conscious awareness (RCA) task in which he was required to classify his "yes" responses subjectively as being based upon an episodic recollection of an encounter ("remember"), or a feeling of familiarity ("know"). His performance was remarkable in two ways. First he produced high levels of false alarms along with a normal hit rate and, second, he classified all his "yes" responses, correct or not, as "know," suggesting reliance on familiarity[2]. In contrast, a matched group of control subjects tended to produce "remember" classifications.

A further study suggesting that JB is unable to rely upon contextual detail of the encoding episode to support recognition memory was described briefly by Parkin, Yeomans, and Bindshaedler (1994). In the first block, subjects were first shown a list a target words to remember (e.g. "sky") and were later required to recognise the target from a non-presented unrelated distractor in a forced/choice recognition test (e.g. "sky" or "cave"). In the critical second block, subjects were shown a new list of targets to remember (e.g "mile") but the forced-choice recognition test contained distractors that had appeared as targets in the previous list (e.g. "mile" or "sky"). Under these conditions all items can be assumed to have high levels of familiarity and correct identification depends on the ability to recollect the correct context of an item. To check that any deficit observed in the second test was not simply a general proactive interference effect, two additional blocks were the given in which no items were repeated. The most important finding was that JB was at chance on the second block but within normal limits on the subsequent tests. Thus JB again

[2] It should be noted that this pattern could arise out of a failure to appropriately apply theory-of-mind type words rather than deficient memory. However, other lines of evidence suggest that a memory-based explanation is more likely. Parkin et al. (1988) have shown that JB has poor source and temporal context memory—indicative of a lack of a specific recollection and consistent with "know" responding.

seems most impaired when he is required to rely on context to respond.

Although it can be argued that over-reliance on familiarity could be the basis of JB's poor recognition memory, an alternative explanation can be offered. As we saw earlier, Schacter et al. (1996) have argued that high false alarms rates arise because a patient might rely on poorly focused event descriptions, which set up an inappropriately liberal response bias that is uninfluenced by target-distractor similarities unless these are extremely obvious. In JB's case it could be argued that evidence suggesting over-reliance on familiarity could be re-interpreted in terms of a poorly focused event description. Thus the high false alarms in the RCA task and predominance of "know" responses could easily reflect a vague event description such that he is able to use his memory for the features of the whole list to guide recognition, but unable to use the features associated with individual items in the list. Furthermore, good performance on a forced/choice task could arise because the procedure precludes the influence of a liberal response bias, requiring as it does selection of only one item per trial. Thus, on the assumption that the target has some minimal memorial advantage over the distractor, the target will be reliably accepted even though, under single probe conditions, both might well be accepted as targets.

The first experiment was conducted in order to assess whether JB's recognition memory is influenced by the semantic similarity between individual target and distractor items. If recognition is determined by familiarity then distractors that are more similar to targets should be processed more fluently and appear more familiar, resulting in higher false alarms. If JB relies on a poorly focused event description, then this type of item-specific detail should not influence his false alarm rate.

Experiment 1: Synonym Distractors

JB undertook a series of recognition tests in which the associative relationship between targets and distractors was varied systematically. In one series each target was matched with a distractor that was a strong synonym. In a second series each target was matched with a weakly related synonym, and in a final series there was no associative relationship between targets and distractors.

Method

Subjects. JB and seven control subjects participated (mean age 48.8; range 45–54). In this experiment, and all subsequent ones, control subjects were approximately matched to JB in terms of NART IQ.

Materials. Six lists of 48 items were devised using the synonym norms produced by Whitten, Suter, and Frank (1979). Two lists (H1; H2) comprised 24 pairs of items that had a strong synonym relationship (e.g. purchase–buy), two lists (L1; L2) comprised 24 pairs with a weak synonym relationship (e.g. novel–book) and in the remaining two lists (N1; N2) there was no synonym relationship—these latter two lists comprised individual items from synonym pairs in the norms. Items in the target sequence were presented in a random order and items in the recognition sequence were presented in a pseudorandom order such that members of a pair were never adjacent in the sequence.

Procedure. In this experiment and subsequent experiments in this section, subjects were instructed to try to remember the items for a later test and items were presented centrally, one at a time, on an Apple Macintosh computer using a standard font. Targets were presented for 2000msec each with an inter-trial interval of 1000msec. Immediately following the target sequence, subjects were shown the recognition sequence, in which items were presented singularly and subjects were required to make a "yes/no" response according to whether the item had been presented previously. The experiment was conducted in two sessions separated by at least a day with lists presented in the order H1–L1–N1–N2–L2–H2.

Results and Discussion

Initial inspection of the data indicated that the order in which conditions were run did not affect performance, so the data were collapsed across sessions. The mean number of hits and false alarms were calculated for each subject and these data are illustrated in Table 2. In this, and all following

Table 2. *Hit Rate and False Alarm (FA) Rate (%) for JB and Controls as a Function of Distractor Type (High, Low, or No Synonym Relationship)*

Distractor Type	*JB*			*Controls (SD)*		
	Hits	*FA*	*d'*	*Hits*	*FA*	*d'*
High	77.1	45.8	0.8	69.1 (10.4)	12.9 (8.3)	1.8 (0.9)
Low	85.4	33.3	1.5	73.8 (12.5)	5.8 (5.8)	2.5 (0.8)
None	75.0	43.8	0.8	75.0 (14.6)	5.0 (6.7)	2.6 (0.9)

analyses, JB's performance is considered abnormal if his scores are greater than 2 SDs away from the mean of the control group. Examination of Table 2 shows that JB's hit rate is well within normal limits but that his false alarm rate is abnormally high in all three conditions. Moreover, although there is a slight depression of his false alarm rate in the L condition it is notable that there is no difference in his error rates for H and N conditions. In order to ensure that the lists could produce a semantic distraction effect, the control data were converted to d' values, which yielded means of 1.8, 2.5, and 2.6 for the H, L and N lists respectively (corresponding values for JB were 0.8, 1.5, and 0.8). The control data were then analysed in a one-way repeated measures ANOVA and this indicated that performance was poorer in the H condition than in either L or N conditions [$F(1, 7) = 4.56$, $P < .05$].

Experiment 1 showed, as expected, that JB made far more false alarms than control subjects. More importantly, there was no difference in his false alarm rate to highly related distractors compared with unrelated distractors, although this had a substantial effect on control subjects' performance. As discussed earlier, this type of finding argues against an explanation that attributes a high false alarm rate to an over-reliance on familiarity of individual items in the list.

Experiment 2: Semantic, Visual, and Rhyming Distractors

This experiment was designed to replicate and extend the finding of the previous experiment, that JB does not produce more false alarms with synonymously related distractors, by taking into consideration rhyming and visual distractors as well as semantically related ones.

Method

Subjects. JB and 14 control subjects participated (mean age = 53.6, SD = 3.0).

Materials. Forty pairs of rhyming words (e.g. node–toad), 40 pairs of visually related words (e.g. glean–gleam), 40 pairs of semantically related words (e.g. stench–stink), and 120 unrelated words were selected. Rhyming (R), visual (V), and semantic pairs (S) were assigned to one of six lists (R1, R2, S1, S2, V1, V2) and one item from each pair was randomly assigned to appear as either a target or distractor. The recognition sequences consisted of the 20 targets, the 20 related distractors, and 20 unrelated distractors.

Procedure. Words in both target and recognition sequences were presented in a random order. Words in the target sequence were presented for 3000msec followed by an interval of 1000msec. The recognition sequence was presented immediately after the target sequence. Words in the recognition sequence were presented for the same duration, during which time subjects were required to give an oral "yes/no" response according to whether the word had been presented in the target sequence or not. Blocks were presented in a single session in the order R1–R2–S1–S2–V1–V2.

Results and Discussion

The results are summarised in Table 3. Control subjects produced significantly more false alarms for semantically related distractors [$t(13) = 2.78$, $p < .05$] and visually related distractors [$t(13) = 2.85$, $p < .05$], relative to unrelated distractors. There was a nonsignificant trend for the rhyming distractors [$t(13) = 1.50$, n.s.). In contrast,

Table 3. *Effect of Semantic, Rhyming, and Visually Related Distractors on JB's Hit and False Alarm Rates (%) Compared to Control Subjects Mean (SD)*

Distractors	*JB*	*Controls*
Rhyming		
Hits	87.5	82.3 (16.7)
FA (R)	50.0	6.8 (9.7)
FA (U)	55.0	3.6 (3.2)
Semantic		
Hits	85.0	85.7 (14.8)
FA (S)	55.0	7.5 (8.2)
FA (U)	52.5	4.3 (6.0)
Visual		
Hits	92.5	83.8 (14.1)
FA (V)	52.5	9.8 (8.9)
FA (U)	57.5	3.0 (6.7)

R: rhyming; S: semantic; V: visual; U: unrelated.

JB's false alarm rate was uninfluenced by any of these manipulations and remained pathologically high.

These results support the previous conclusion that an over-reliance on item-specific familiarity cannot account for JB's elevated false alarm rate. If familiarity was important then distractors that share more features with target items should be processed more fluently and should therefore seem more familiar, resulting in greater false recognition; but this was not found.

Experiment 3: Nonword Targets and Distractors

It is possible that the high false alarm rates in Experiments 1–2 could be uninfluenced by experimentally defined target-distractor association because prior experience of words per se may be sufficient to make distractors seem familiar. The counter to this is to examine how JB performs when given a recognition memory test involving nonwords. The argument is that these are inherently unfamiliar and thus a false alarm could not be attributed to pre-experimental familiarity with the stimulus materials.

JB's recognition memory using nonwords as both targets and distractors was assessed. Two types of nonword list were used; one in which nonwords were highly "word-like" and one where the nonwords did not resemble known words. This manipulation allowed for the possibility that a high false alarm rate to nonword distractors might arise because the subject notes the similarity between nonwords and real words and thus inadvertently uses global information about word familiarity to influence responding. If a process of this kind is operating then one would expect to see far less evidence of high false alarm rates when using nonwords that do not resemble known words.

Method

Subjects. JB and seven controls participated (mean age 48, range 44–52).

Materials. A total of 160 nonwords were devised. Of these 80 were word-like (WL), in that a real word could be formed by substituting just one letter (e.g. duture, munnel), the remaining 80 did not resemble words (NWL) in that no real word could be formed by substituting just one letter (e.g. balvit, borrut), but were nevertheless pronounceable. The WL and NWL lists were each randomly divided into 2 sets of 40 and randomly divided again into 20 targets and 20 distractors.

Procedure. In the target sequence, nonwords were presented for 2000msec. Immediately after, subjects were shown the recognition sequence and asked to give a "yes/no" response according to whether it had been present in the target sequence. Four blocks were given in the order WL(1)–NWL(1)–NWL(2)–WL(2).

Results and Discussion

Preliminary analysis indicated that list order did not affect the results and so data from the two lists comprising each nonword type were pooled. The number of hits and false alarms as a function of nonword type (NWL, WL) were calculated for both JB and controls and these data are summarised in Table 4. Again, it can be seen that the main difference between JB and controls is JB's excessively high false alarm rate. Importantly, his false alarm rate was uninfluenced by the type of nonword and his hit rate was within the normal limits.

Table 4. *Hit Rate and False Alarm Rate (%) for JB and Controls, Experiment 3, as a Function of Nonword Type*

Nonword Type	*JB*			*Controls (SD)*		
	Hits	*FA*	*d'*	*Hits*	*FA*	*d'*
Not word-like	85.0	30.0	1.5	65.5 (13.5)	8.0 (5.5)	1.9 (0.6)
Word-like	75.0	35.0	1.0	74.0 (7.0)	7.0 (4.0)	2.2 (0.5)

In conclusion, Experiment 3 showed that JB generated high levels of false alarms when nonwords were used as stimuli. This cannot easily be explained in terms of overlaps in familiarity between targets and distractors because the scope for generating familiarity cues is greatly reduced in stimuli devoid of meaning. Furthermore, the presence of high false alarm rates even when nonwords do not resemble real words argues against any pre-experimental exposure to words per se as being significant in the generation of these false alarm rates. By implication, therefore, one can also argue that the high false alarm rates found with real-word stimuli (e.g. Experiments 1–2) do not have their origin in pre-experimental familiarity. One further test of the familiarity hypothesis was conducted in Experiment 4.

Experiment 4: No targets in the Recognition Sequence

If JB's recognition memory does not depend on familiarity information then it is possible to predict that his recognition memory would not be affected if there were no overlap at all between targets and distractors—for instance, if none of the targets are presented in the recognition sequence. In contrast, if individual item familiarity is important then one would minimally expect lower false alarm rates when targets are present in the recognition sequence because no immediate familiarity information would be available.

Method

Only JB took part in this experiment. The materials consisted of 200 words that were allocated, randomly, to appear as targets (4 sets of 20) or distractors (2 sets of 20 and 2 sets of 40). Words were not systematically related to each other (e.g. synonyms) in any way. In the targets-absent condition, the 20 target words were shown one at a time for 1500msec followed by a 200msec gap. The recognition sequence, containing only the 40 distractor words, was given immediately afterwards. The targets-present condition was identical, except that the recognition sequence contained 20 previously shown target words and 20 distractors. The conditions were presented in an AB–BA design over 2 sessions separated by 4 months (A = present condition, B = absent condition).

Results and Discussion

JB's performance did not differ across testing sessions, so results are collapsed across this dimension. Under conditions where the targets did appear in the recognition sequence, JB made 57 "yes" responses of which 33 were hits and 24 were false alarms, and when no targets were present he made 54 "yes" responses and 26 "no" responses (false alarm rates of 60% and 68% respectively). Thus, JB is at least as willing to produce false alarms when targets are absent from the recognition sequences as when they are present. An explanation based upon an over-reliance on familiarity would predict that false alarm rates should be lowered in the targets-absent condition. Interestingly, JB was unaware of the fact that no targets had been presented for recognition, even when prompted.

Summary of Experiments 1–4

Experiments 1–4 have ruled out a familiarity-based explanation of JB's false recognition deficit. In contrast, the results are consistent with the notion that JB relies on poorly focused event descriptions in recognition. This poorly focused description contains features that are shared by many other items, including those not presented as targets, resulting in high levels of false recognition.

The findings presented so far are similar to those reported by Schacter et al. (1996) for BG. However, whereas Schacter et al. have argued that a failure to set up a focused description at retrieval reflects a failure of a retrieval mechanism, another possibility remains. Namely, that the retrieval description is unfocused because a deficit at encoding has failed to select an appropriate set of features from which to base future recognition judgements. For instance, if JB only encodes the general characteristics of the items (i.e. real words, similar length, composed of the same letters) then these properties will also tend to be present in the distractor items, including the case in which no targets are present at recognition. The next set of experiments will address the question of whether this pattern can best be accounted for by an encoding or retrieval deficit.

Effect of Encoding and Retrieval Manipulations on False Recognition

Attempts to locate deficits at levels of either encoding or retrieval have had a chequered history in memory research (e.g. see Mayes & Downes, 1997). This is because there may well be some overlap between these processes. Thus, laying down new memories may activate previous memories of a similar nature and retrieving a memory is necessarily contingent upon the information being appropriately laid down in the first place. Nevertheless, there is reason to believe that there will be at least some divergence between processes involved in encoding and those at retrieval. For instance, retrieval may involve the use of certain decision heuristics that are of little relevance at encoding (e.g. Johnson, Raye, Foley, & Foley, 1981; Schacter, Israel, & Racine, 1999) and encoding may involve more attention-based processes that select certain input streams for further processing. Furthermore, on purely empirical grounds, the encoding-retrieval distinction would appear to be supported by neuroimaging studies suggesting the involvement of different brain regions (Shallice et al., 1994; Tulving, Kapur, Craik, et al., 1994.

First of all, we will consider how JB's false recognition is affected by manipulations at the retrieval stage. We will then go on to consider how JB's false recognition can be accounted for by a deficit at the level of encoding.

Experiment 5: Targets and Distractors Drawn from Different Taxonomic Categories

As noted earlier, Schacter et al. (1996) demonstrated that BG showed a very marked reduction in false alarms using a recognition test in which targets and distractors were drawn from different taxonomic categories. They argued that a manipulation of this kind enabled BG's deficient retrieval mechanism to operate efficiently because a very obvious cue enabled targets and distractors to be discriminated from one another (e.g. "I saw items from categories A, B, C but not D, E, F"). This hypothesis was examined in JB.

Method

Subjects. JB and 11 control subjects participated (mean age = 55.1, SD = 5.2).

Materials. The materials comprised 2 target lists of 20 words. Each of these lists in turn comprised five words from four different categories. Each target list was pseudorandomised to ensure that no two items from the same category were in adjacent positions. List A involved fish, spices, sports, and parts of the body. List B comprised spirits, flowers, vehicles, and fruits. For List A, a recognition test was constructed involving a random sequence of the 20 targets and 20 distractors derived from 4 additional taxonomic categories (5 in each): furniture, insects, buildings, precious stones. For List B a similar recognition test was constructed except that the 20 distractors were 5 more items from each of the taxonomic categories used to construct the target list.

Procedure. There were some procedural differences between test administration for JB and controls. For JB the target items were presented individually on index cards for 2 seconds each. Immediately following this the recognition test was given. Each stimulus was presented for 3 seconds and JB had to indicate "yes" if a word had occurred in the previous list and "no" if it had not. It was anticipated that the conditions under which JB was tested would prove too easy for controls so the procedure was modified in that target exposure was reduced to 1 second per item and recognition involved presentation of each item for 3 seconds with a 1-second inter-trial interval. For controls the items were presented on a MacIntosh powerbook. In addition, a 10-minute distractor period involving subjects crossing out Es and Rs from a random array of letters was interpolated between study and test. All subjects received List A followed by List B a few minutes later.

Results and Discussion

The results of Experiment 5 are illustrated in Table 5. JB's hit rate is virtually identical to that of controls. Of more interest, however, is JB's pattern of false alarms compared with controls. JB makes the same number of false alarms in both lists whereas for controls significantly more false alarms are made in List B [$t(10) = 3.96$, $P < .005$]. Furthermore, while JB's false alarm rate on list B lies within 2SDs of the control mean his false alarm rate on List A is over 10 times greater than that of controls.

In summary, JB is unable to attenuate his false alarms if targets and distractors are drawn from different taxonomic categories, even though this manipulation produced a strong result in BG (Schacter et al., 1996). This result could be interpreted as evidence for different functional impairments in the two patients. JB may have an encoding deficit in that he tends to encode only more superficial detail and therefore cannot take advantage of taxonomic category information. BG may have a retrieval deficit in that all types of information are encoded well (including higher-level detail), but he is unable to utilise this information at retrieval unless there is an obvious organising principle.

One potential difficulty with this experiment is that good performance may depend on the subjects' ability to formulate deliberate strategies as much as it depends on the content of their memory. In the next experiment, the retrieval strategy to be adopted was directly controlled in an attempt to reduce JB's tendency to produce false alarms.

Experiment 6: Restricting the Number of "Yes" Responses

JB's response pattern is typically characterised by an excessive number of affirmative responses. This experiment examined whether restricting the number of "yes" responses at retrieval can be used as a basis for more accurate discrimination between targets and distractors. JB saw lists of 25 words followed by a recognition test in which he was urged to be as accurate as possible and only allowed to make 25 responses. In addition he numbered his responses as he worked through the recognition test. This enabled a measure of confidence in that it established whether or not those items he identified earlier were ones that he knew to be targets. This was contrasted with conditions in which he was free to use his normal retrieval criteria.

Method

Subjects. JB and nine control subjects participated (mean age = 56.2, SD = 3.5).

Materials. Eight sets of 50 words were selected mainly from the Toronto Word Pool. These were randomly assigned to appear as either targets or distractors in one of eight lists (four restricted, four unrestricted), with equal numbers in each.

Procedure. Target items were displayed individually for 2000msec. In the restricted condition subjects

Table 5. *Hit Rate and False Alarm Rate (%) for JB and Controls as a Function of Whether Targets and Distractors are Drawn from the Same Taxonomic Categories*

Taxonomic Category	*JB* Hits	*JB* FA	*JB* d'	*Controls (SD)* Hits	*Controls (SD)* FA	*Controls (SD)* d'
Different	70.0	35.0	0.9	74.0 (18.0)	1.5 (3.0)	3.1 (0.8)
Same	80.0	35.0	1.2	80.0 (14.5)	19.0 (16.5)	2.0 (1.1)

were presented with a sheet of paper containing 2 columns of 25 items. In addition there was a sheet of labels each with a number from 1 to 25. They were instructed to be as accurate as possible and could only make 25 responses. This was done by placing a label next to each word that was recognised. They were instructed to use the labels in numerical order but they did not have to work through the list systematically. The unrestricted condition was similar except that no constraint was placed on how subjects should respond. The experiment was conducted over two sessions, separated by at least a day, and blocks were presented in the order UURR–RRUU (R = restricted, U = unrestricted).

Results and Discussion

Preliminary analysis of the data indicated that there were no differences between the two experimental sessions, so the data were collapsed across this factor for further analysis. The results are summarised in Table 6. JB's false alarm rate was not reduced by restricting the number of "yes" responses at retrieval. If anything, this manipulation reduced his hit rate. In contrast, the hit rate of control subjects was uninfluenced by this manipulation [$t(8) = 1.77$, n.s.]. Since the control subjects generally produced fewer than 25 "yes" responses in the unrestricted condition, applying the response restriction actually increased their false alarm rate [$t(8) = 5.43$, $p < .001$]—presumably because they were being forced to guess. Indeed, control subjects gave false alarms significantly higher ranks than hits [$t(7) = 11.60$, $p < .001$], suggesting that they were less confident about their false alarms[3]. JB, however, was just as confident about his false alarms (in terms of rankings) as he was about his hits.

Experiment 6 showed that an emphasis on accuracy at retrieval had no beneficial effect on false alarm rates. It was also notable that JB did not choose to identify distractors any later than targets. This suggests that JB is unable to change his retrieval criteria on the basis of relative familiarity of individual items, consistent with previous findings. Patient RW (Delbecq-Derouesné et al., 1990) also

Table 6. *Performance When Subjects Must Make a Restricted Number of "Yes" Responses Compared To When There Is No Restrictions. Mean (SD)*

	Unrestricted (Score /25)		*Restricted (Score /25)*		*Restricted (Rank)*	
	Hits	*FA*	*Hits*	*FA*	*Hits*	*FA*
JB	19.8	8.5	16.5	8.5	13.0	13.2
Controls	19.8	1.4	20.7	4.3	11.3	20.1
	(2.7)	(1.1)	(2.2)	(2.2)	(0.5)	(2.1)

showed a similar pattern, in that requiring an exact number of "yes" responses did not improve performance, although this patient, unlike JB, was at chance. Given that encouraging JB to adopt a different strategy at retrieval has no effect on false alarm rates, the next set of experiments were designed to assess whether encouraging him to use a different strategy at encoding may produce a beneficial effect.

Experiment 7: Orienting at Encoding with Concrete and Abstract Words

Encoding manipulations directly affects the processing of targets but not that of distractors. If false recognition arises simply out of a failure to process distractors properly (e.g. over-confident responding), then encoding manipulations should have no effect on false alarm rates. Similarly, if targets are processed adequately in the first place then the scope for improving performance by using encoding manipulations would be limited. On the other hand, if targets are not encoded adequately and false recognition of distractors is dependent on the quality of memories for target items then orienting manipulations should have a beneficial effect.

Experiment 7 compared JB's recognition memory for unrelated words under semantic orienting conditions versus conditions where he was free to use his normal learning strategy. Visual imagery was also manipulated in that half the target lists comprised concrete words and the other half comprised abstract words. The reasoning behind this was that if JB had an encoding problem, it might be

[3] One subject was excluded from the analysis of ranks because he failed to produce any false alarms in the restricted condition.

more pronounced for abstract words because of the lesser opportunity for encoding that these stimuli provide (e.g. Craik & Lockhart, 1972; Craik & Tulving, 1975).

Method

Subjects. The subjects were JB and eight control subjects (mean age = 49, SD = 2.8).

Materials. Three hundred and twenty words were selected from the Toronto Word Pool, of which 160 were concrete and 160 abstract in nature. Each set of 160 was further subdivided into 4 lists of 40 words designated C1, C2, C3, C4 and A1, A2, A3, A4 for concrete and abstract words respectively, and each list was randomly divided again into equal numbers of targets and distractors. Lists Cl, C4, and A1, A4 were allocated to the free study condition and lists C2, C3, A2, A3 were allocated to the semantic orienting condition.

Procedure. The experiment was conducted in two sessions separated by at least a day. In the free study condition they were told to try and learn the words but no further instruction was given. In the semantic orienting condition subjects were told to study each word and decide whether it was pleasant or unpleasant; under these conditions subjects were also aware that they would have to remember the words later. The lists and conditions were given in the following order—Session 1: C1, A1 (free study), C2, A2 (orienting task); Session 2: A3, C3 (orienting task), A4, C4 (free study). For each condition target words were presented for 2000msec with an inter-trial interval of 1000msec.

Results and Discussion

Preliminary analyses of the data indicated that session did not affect JB's results [$\chi^2(1) = 0.23$, *n.s.*, with session as a factor], and so equivalent conditions across sessions were pooled. Table 7 summarises the results of the study. It can be seen that, in every condition, JB's false alarm rate is well in excess of the controls but that, with the exception of concrete words in the no-orientation condition, his hit rate is within normal limits. The table also indicates that false alarms are reduced in the condition where JB was asked to carry out an orienting task. In particular his ability to identify concrete words is greatly enhanced by the imposition of orienting tasks. The effect of orientation is also emphasised when considering the d' scores generated by this experiment (see Table 6). Thus for concrete words JB's performance improves from 0.74 without orientation to 2.79 with orientation. For abstract words the improvement is, however, quite modest: 1.28 without orientation, 1.69 with orientation. This improvement was further assessed using a chi-squared analysis and this showed that JB's frequency of false alarms was significantly reduced following orienting instructions [$\chi^2 = 3.47$, $P < .05$ (1-tailed)]. A 2 × 2 ANOVA of the control data indicated a main effect of word type [$F(1, 7) = 61.89$, $P < .001$] with concrete words producing higher d' scores, but no effect of orienting task.

This experiment showed that conditions designed to improve encoding led to a marked improvement in JB's recognition memory, including his false alarm rate. The demonstration that this effect was most pronounced in the concrete word conditions is most likely to stem from the greater opportunities that these types of stimuli provide for encoding via the potential generation of both verbal and imaginal codes. The lack of an effect of orienting task in controls is most likely to reflect a ceiling effect.

Experiment 8: Further Orienting Measures at Encoding

This experiment was designed to replicate the previous finding, that orientation at encoding significantly reduces false recognition. The experiment does, however, differ in a number of ways. A variety of different orienting manipulations were used on JB rather than just pleasantness judgements since it is expected that different "levels of processing" might influence subsequent recognition (e.g. Craik & Lockhart, 1972). Also, the control subjects did not perform the orienting tasks. This was done to determine whether orienting effects in JB can produce equivalent levels of performance to that found in subjects who are free to adopt their own strategy.

Table 7. *Percentage Hit Rate and False Alarm Rates for JB and Controls as a Function of Word Type and Acquisition Conditions*

	JB			*Controls (SD)*		
	Hits	*FA*	*d'*	*Hits*	*FA*	*d'*
No-orientation						
Concrete	72.5	45.0	0.74	93.0 (8.0)	0.0 (0.0)	4.05 (0.61)
Abstract	80.0	32.5	1.28	79.5 (13.5)	2.0 (2.0)	3.05 (0.65)
Orientation						
Concrete	97.5	22.5	2.80	95.5 (5.5)	1.0 (1.5)	4.10 (0.60
Abstract	82.5	22.5	1.70	85.0 (10.0)	2.5 (1.0)	3.26 (0.71)

Method

Subjects. JB and 10 control subjects participated (mean age = 56.1, range = 52–59).

Materials. Two hundred and eighty concrete nouns were selected and randomly assigned to appear as targets or distractors in one of 7 blocks (20 of each in every block).

Procedure. Words in the target sequence were displayed for 4000msec each, followed by a gap of 1000msec. Immediately after each target sequence, the recognition sequence was given in which items were displayed for 2000msec and subjects were required to make a "yes/no" response. The procedure was identical for both JB and controls except for the instructions given at encoding. In four of the blocks JB was given instructions to memorise and an orienting task: pleasantness judgements, sentence construction, read the spelling of the word, or visual imagery. In the remaining blocks he was just given instructions to memorise. The order of the orientation and no-orientation blocks were alternated. Control subjects did not perform orienting tasks in any of the blocks.

Results and Discussion

Table 8 shows that JB shows a substantial benefit of orienting instructions at encoding, particularly in the visual imagery condition. Collapsing data across the no-orientation condition with the various orientation conditions shows that JB's false alarm rates are significantly lower in the orientation conditions [$\chi^2(1) = 25.23$, $P < .001$] and his hit rates are significantly higher [$\chi^2(1) = 8.78$, $P < .001$]. However, his false alarm rates remain outside the 2SD range of control subjects.

Thus, the results of this experiment are consistent with the previous one and suggest that JB has an encoding deficit that, at least in part, can be circumvented by giving him orienting instructions. The reason why JB's false alarm rate remains higher than that of control subjects in these conditions is not entirely clear. One possibility, is that the encoding manipulations used were not potent enough to abolish his deficit completely. Another possibility is that the control subjects, despite being given only instructions to memorise, were in fact using some encoding strategy themselves. Finally, the suggestion that JB may have some additional difficulty (e.g. with retrieval mechanisms) cannot be completely ruled out. However, this latter account is not favoured on the basis of previous results suggesting no benefit of retrieval manipulations. We will return to this in the General Discussion.

Experiment 9: Recognition Memory for Items Encoded Premorbidly

If JB suffers only from an encoding deficit then it follows that memory for information acquired prior to his brain injury should be unaffected, i.e. it should not be prone to false alarms. It was therefore decided to devise a famous names test, tapping remote memory.

Method

Subjects. JB and six control subjects participated (mean age, 49, SD 2.8).

Table 8. *Effects of Orientation on JB's Hit and False Alarm Rates (%)*

	JB		*Controls*		
	Hits	*FA*	*Hits*	*FA*	*Example*
Nice/Nasty	100	30	93 (9)	3 (4)	"nasty"
No orientation	75	45	93 (9)	2 (2)	—
Spelling	95	25	95 (8)	1 (2)	"S,P,I,D,E,R"
No orientation	100	55	93 (10)	2 (2)	—
Sentence	100	40	97 (5)	2 (5)	"the spider crawled down the pipe"
No orientation	75	55	93 (12)	4 (5)	—
Imagery	95	20	95 (7)	4 (4)	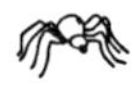

Materials and Procedure. The first test involved a list of 40 famous people (e.g. Sarah Ferguson, Rupert Murdoch), which was randomly interspersed with the names of 40 people with fictitious names that nonetheless sounded plausible (e.g. Alex Langer, Conrad Nash). The second test was designed to be more difficult, and revolved around the names of people involved in popular music in the 1960s and 1970s (a particular interest of JB). The names of 40 singers or groups (e.g. Bobby Vee, Ventures) were randomly interspersed with the names of unknown singers and groups (e.g. Sharon Sugar, Delta Cats). These latter names were not truly fictitious but selected from a record catalogue on the grounds that they had never become famous. In this way it was hoped that the distractor names would be plausible. In each test, targets and distractors were printed on a single page and subjects were instructed to place a circle around any name they thought was famous.

Results and Discussion

JB performed the famous name task faultlessly (100% hits, 0% false alarms). Control subjects produced average hit and false alarm rates of 93% (SD = 3.8) and 2.1% (SD = 4.0) respectively. In the more difficult test, JB had a hit rate of 75% and a false alarm rate of 2.5%. This compared favourably with the control group's score of 51% hits (SD = 10.6) with a false alarm rate of 2.9% (SD = 4.0). Thus, JB's tendency to produce false alarms does not extend to premorbidly acquired information.

The results so far have shown that JB does not benefit substantially from manipulations designed to improve accuracy at retrieval but that he does benefit from such manipulations when they are applied at encoding; this is consistent with the notion that he has an encoding deficit. The remaining experiments aim to elucidate further the nature of this deficit. In particular, we will examine the hypothesis that JB may benefit from orienting instructions at encoding simply because this allows for greater engagement in the task. If this is so, then we would expect to find a similar beneficial effect if he was given orienting instructions at retrieval. Also it is possible that JB has a difficulty in encoding because of a deficit in extracting higher-level relationships (such as taxonomic categories) per se, even in non-memory tasks[4].

Experiment 10: Orientation Effects at Retrieval

In order to determine that the beneficial effect of orienting observed in the previous experiment is due to processes specific to encoding (as opposed to, say, greater engagement in the task per se), a similar experiment was conducted in which JB was required to orient towards certain properties at retrieval. The orienting task chosen was visual imagery, since previous experiments have shown this to be particularly effective during encoding.

[4] For instance, it has been suggested that some frontal patients have difficulties in understanding proverbs and jokes, despite performing well on more traditional tests of language/semantics (e.g. Stuss, 1991).

Method

Subjects. JB and 10 controls participated (mean age = 54.2, range = 46–60).

Materials. One hundred and sixty concrete nouns were selected and randomly assigned to appear in 1 of 4 blocks as either a target or distractor (making 4 sets of 20 targets and 20 distractors). Two of the lists were assigned to the orienting condition (O) and the remaining two to the no-orienting (N) condition.

Procedure. Subjects were given general memory instructions for all target sequences. Items in the target sequence were displayed for 200msec each followed by an interval of 2000msec. The recognition sequence was given immediately afterwards and items were presented for 4000msec followed by a 1000msec interval. The procedure was identical in both orienting and no-orienting conditions except in terms of the instructions given to the subject. In the orienting condition, subjects were told that during the recognition sequence they should try to imagine a picture of the item for 4000msec before giving a "yes/no" response. In the no-orienting condition, they were simply told to give a "yes/no" response before presentation of the next item. Blocks were presented in a single session in the order N–O–O–N.

Results and Discussion

Table 9 shows that JB showed no benefit of orientation at retrieval. The effect did, however, reach significance for control subjects in terms of false alarms [hits: $t(9) = 0.18$, n.s. false alarms $t(9) = 1.91$, $P < .05$, 1-tailed]. This suggests that previous studies showing that JB benefits from orientation instructions at encoding cannot be attributable to a greater level of engagement in the memory task per se. The results also suggest that JB's poorly focused event description is not arising from a damaged retrieval mechanism since attempts to get him to focus on item-specific features at retrieval have little benefit, presumably because such information was not encoded in the first place.

Experiment 11: Attending to Different Features in a Non-memory Task

It has been found that JB does not always encode taxonomic categories (Experiment 5) and, although he shows a significant improvement when given orienting instructions, his performance is still somewhat worse than controls. It is therefore important to assess the hypothesis that JB's encoding deficit might stem from a more basic conceptual deficit in attending to certain properties of items. The procedure that was used was to give JB lists of words (as in the memory experiments) but to ask him to try and spot the common feature between them. The feature could either be a low-level property (e.g. ambulance, earth, art ... [all contain an "A"]) or a higher-level property (e.g. cabbage, jade, envy ... [green things]). The dependent measure was the number of words shown before the common feature was correctly spotted.

Method

Subjects. JB and seven control subjects participated (mean age = 54.4, range = 50–59).

Materials. There were 14 sequences of 20 words. Half of the sequences had a low-level property in common (compound words, seven-letter words, "A" words, double letters, three syllables, -er endings, "B" words) and the remainder had a high-level property in common (green things, islands, metal things, alphabet names, pop groups, politicians,

Table 9. *Effect of Orientation at Retrieval on Hit and False Alarm Rates (%)*

	JB			*Controls (SD)*		
	Hits	*FA*	*d'*	*Hits*	*FA*	*d'*
No orientation	87.5	67.5	0.74	91.5 (9.2)	3.3 (4.4)	3.8 (1.0)
Orientation	90.0	60.0	1.02	92.3 (8.2)	1.5 (2.7)	3.8 (0.9)

brand names). Items were printed on individual cards.

Procedure. Subjects were shown a sequence of words one at a time, for 2 seconds, and instructed to try to find the similarity or common factor. Subjects could take as many guesses as they liked and the experimenter informed them if they were right or wrong, stopping if they had correctly guessed. Only a single word was visible at any one time and subjects could not look back to previous items. If the subject failed after 20 words the sequence was stopped and the subject was informed of the common factor.

Results and Discussion

JB performed the task as well as controls for high-level features and was marginally worse for the low-level features. He failed to guess correctly, after all 20 words, 1 of the high-level features and 4 of the low-level features (control mean 1.1 (SD 0.7) and 2.6 (SD 1.3) respectively). Of those that he did get correct he needed to be shown, on average, 5.7 words for the high-level features and 13.3 words for the low-level features (controls: 8.4 (SD 2.9) and 7.4 (SD 2.5) respectively). Thus, JB is unimpaired at attending to higher-level features of items when the task explicitly requires him to do so, but he apparently does not always extract such information when given instructions to memorise. This occurs even though the experimental procedure is essentially the same in both instances, i.e. lists of words given one at a time.

Having established the locus of JB's deficit, it is important to consider in more detail what type of information JB does and does not encode. There is already some evidence to suggest that JB fails to encode certain higher/level properties, since he shows no benefit of having target and distractors drawn from nonoverlapping semantic categories. The final experiment investigates whether this holds true for other types of information.

Experiment 12: Orthograhic Overlap between Targets and Distractors

There is already some evidence to suggest that JB is able to attenuate false alarms when targets and distractors are composed of non-overlapping pools of low-level features. Parkin et al. (1996) presented JB with two tests involving memory for abstract designs constructed out of various shapes, lines, colours, and patterns. In one version, the distractors were composed out of an entirely different set of features to that used to construct the targets (non-overlapping feature condition). In another version, the targets and distractors were identical except for one feature (overlapping feature condition). JB produced no false alarms in the non-overlapping version. However, he was severely impaired on the overlapping version, producing an excessive level of false alarms along with a normal hit rate.

Although the results of the abstract designs test are encouraging, it is still possible that control subjects may strategically adopt a more conservative criteria for responding in the overlapping condition if they are aware that targets and distractors are very similar to each other. The experiment described below was designed to rule out this possibility.

Method

Subjects. JB and 10 control subjects participated (mean = 54.9, range = 50–58).

Materials. The experiment used 160 four-letter words. Half of the words were used in the no-overlap (N) condition, and the remainder in the overlap (O) condition. In the no-overlap condition, target words were created using only 13 letters of the alphabet (i, a, u, f, r, m, b, d, l, w, p, q, h), and the distractors were composed entirely of the remaining 13 letters (o, e, y, s, t, g, n, z, c, j, v, k, x). In the overlap condition, both targets and distractors were created using all 26 letters, taking at least 1 letter from each of the target and distractor letter pools that had been used in the no-overlap condition (e.g. goal, yarn), thus maximising the difference between the conditions.

Procedure. The target sequence consisted of 20 words presented for 1500msec followed by a gap of 200msec. In between each target and recognition sequence there was an interval of 9–10 min to prevent ceiling effects, during which time the subject was given nonverbal puzzles. In the recognition sequence, 40 words (20 targets and 20 distractors) were presented 1 at a time in randomised order and the subject was required to make a "yes/no" recognition response. The lists were presented in the order NO–ON, over two sessions separated by 1 week. At the end of the second session subjects were asked to report whether they had noticed any differences/similarities between the words used in the experiment.

Results and Discussion

Preliminary analysis of the data indicated that there were no differences between the two experimental sessions so the data were collapsed across this factor for further analysis. Table 10 shows that control subjects performed better in the no-overlap condition relative to the overlap condition. This difference was statistically significant for false alarm rates [paired $t(9) = 3.68$, $P < .005$], but failed to reach significance for hit rates [paired $t(9) = 0.76$, n.s.]. JB's false alarm rates remained pathologically high in both overlap and no-overlap conditions. However, as with the control subjects, his false alarm rate was nevertheless attenuated in the no-overlap condition. One measure of attenuation is the ratio of false alarms in the overlap condition relative to the no-overlap condition. JB's ratio of 1.36 is well within the range of controls (mean = 2.47, SD = 1.71; z = − .65). In the debriefing, subjects often reported that words looked similar or had similar meanings but no subject was aware of the fact that targets and distractors were composed of different letters in some blocks. Thus, the reduction of false recognition in the no-overlap condition in both JB and controls is unlikely to reflect an overt change in retrieval strategy or a shift in bias. Indeed, signal detection analyses of the control subjects data revealed that the difference in performance between the conditions is entirely attributable to greater discriminability in the no-overlap condition [$t(9) = 2.20$, $P < .05$] with no change in bias [$t(9) = 1.54$, n.s.] (measures based on the nonparametric method described by Donaldson, 1992).

Given that control subjects also show a benefit from this manipulation, one might wonder whether JB's ability to benefit from encoding really does differ in any qualitative way from controls, with the difference between JB and controls in other orienting experiments arising from a ceiling level of performance from controls. However, the most important point is to contrast JB's performance in the encoding manipulation tasks with his performance in other experiments. Thus, control subjects show a significant effect of semantic distraction whereas JB shows none (Experiment 1) and, in contrast, JB shows a substantial benefit of encoding manipulations whereas controls show little/none (Experiment 7). This cross-over between manipulations that affect controls and manipulations that affect JB suggests that the difference between controls and JB does not lie in the fact that JB's memory is simply worse.

In summary, JB is unable to alter his retrieval criteria in order to attenuate his false alarm rate on the basis of item familiarity or taxonomic category organisation at retrieval. However, he is able to attenuate his false alarm rate if targets and distractors are composed of different pools of low-level elements, even without awareness of this manipulation. This is consistent with an encoding deficit that results in only superficial aspects of the items being retained. The results of this experiment also go some way to explaining why JB may be willing to make false alarms to distractors when no targets are present

Table 10. *Hit and False Alarm Rates (%) When Targets and Distractors Are Made Up of Words Composed of Either Overlapping or Non-overlapping Pools of Letters*

	JB			*Controls (SD)*		
	Hits	*FA*	*d'*	*Hits*	*FA*	*d'*
Overlap	73.0	75.0	0.47	78.0 (18.9)	13.4 (9.2)	0.88 (0.10)
No overlap	78.0	55.0	0.70	81.0 (14.1)	5.9 (4.4)	0.93 (0.04)

(Experiment 4), since the distractors in that experiment were made up of the same letters as the targets.

GENERAL DISCUSSION

This study has investigated a patient with damage to the left frontal lobe, JB, who generally produces a high level of false alarms in single probe recognition memory tasks, together with a normal level of true recognition. The deficit can be explained by reliance on a poorly focused event description but cannot readily be accounted for by an over-reliance on familiarity. If JB were relying on familiarity cues then distractors that are more similar to targets should be processed more fluently, appear more familiar, and therefore produce more false alarms. This was not the case (Experiments 1 and 2). Furthermore, JB produces high false alarm rates to nonword targets that have no intrinsic familiarity (Experiment 3), and continues to produce false alarms even if none of the target words are presented in the recognition sequence (Experiment 4).

Following Schacter et al. (1996), we assume that JB relies on a poorly focused event description, which contains features that are shared by many items (including those not presented) but has impoverished item-specific detail. However, we postulate that this pattern reflects a failure at encoding rather than retrieval. In support of this, we demonstrated that JB's false alarms are reduced by encoding manipulations but not retrieval manipulations. One important retrieval manipulation, according to Schacter et al. (1996), is to take targets and distractors from different taxonomic categories. Their patient, BG, was able to suppress his false alarm rates significantly after this manipulation; the argument being that this manipulation provides a focused memory description since targets and distractors are composed from nonoverlapping features. However, it would only lead to a focused memory description if such features were encoded in the first place. Indeed, JB showed no effect of this manipulation (Experiment 5), suggesting that he may not spontaneously encode higher-level category features. Furthermore, he showed no tendency to reduce his false alarms following another retrieval manipulation; that is, requiring him to restrict the number of affirmative responses at retrieval (Experiment 6).

Evidence for an encoding deficit in JB comes from the fact that he benefits significantly from orienting instructions at encoding (Experiments 7 and 8). Our hypothesis is that JB fails to select an appropriate set of features to encode when given instructions to memorise, and that providing an orienting instruction (e.g. pleasantness judgements) enables him to overcome this difficulty. Parkin et al. (1988) report a similar finding for paired associate recall in which JB was able to achieve a normal level of performance following imagery instruction but was significantly impaired otherwise (see also Signoret & Lhermitte, 1976). Further evidence for an encoding deficit comes from the fact that JB does not produce false alarms to items that were encoded pre-morbidly (Experiment 9). The effect of orienting appears to be specific to encoding, since he shows no benefit of this manipulation at retrieval (Experiment 10), and the encoding deficit is not due to a difficulty in extracting higher-level properties from words per se, since he is unimpaired at finding common features amongst words in a non-memory task (Experiment 11). Finally, we considered what types of feature JB does and does not encode. It was suggested that JB encodes only the more superficial, low-level properties of stimuli, since he *is* able to utilise nonoverlapping features between targets and distractors as a basis for attenuating false alarms when these features correspond to letters or perceptual elements (Experiment 12, and the Abstract Designs test; Parkin et al., 1996). Given that these types of low-level features are, in most recognition tasks, present in distractors as well as targets, this would lead JB to accept distractors as if they were targets. However, because it is highly unlikely that a given set of targets and distractors, would share exactly the same elements in equal proportions, JB is able to discriminate some distractors while maintaining a high hit rate (i.e. his performance is not at chance).

It is important to mention that although the results that we have presented are more consistent with an encoding deficit than with a retrieval deficit, the suggestion that JB has no retrieval difficulty whatsoever (perhaps as the result of a separate impairment) is hard to rule out completely. This difficulty stems, at least in part, from a lack of consensus in the literature as to what the characteristics of a retrieval deficit should be, and disagreement over which manipulations are sensitive to retrieval. Nevertheless, we can consider a number of alternatives. One possibility is that retrieval difficulties should be characterised by the setting of an inappropriate response criterion at retrieval. However, we have shown that forcing an appropriate criterion by requiring a set number of "yes" responses does not improve JB's performance. Furthermore, we would predict that if JB simply had a liberal response criterion then this would lead to a consistently higher hit rate than controls as well as a higher false alarm rate. A meta-analysis of 30 experimental conditions, however, reveals that whereas 29/30 conditions show an increase in false alarms (all significant), in 14/30 conditions his hit rate is higher (not significant in any), in 14/30 conditions his hit rate is lower (significant in one instance) and in 2/30 it is identical to that of controls. One might also expect that a retrieval deficit should be characterised, at least in some patients, by a tendency to confabulate, either because the retrieval description is too broad or the retrieved memory is not properly evaluated (e.g. Burgess & Shallice, 1996). JB, however, no longer shows any tendency to confabulate and does not produce an excessive amount of intrusions in list recall. Thus, in the absence of a sufficiently explicit theoretical framework for understanding retrieval and in the interests of parsimony, it seems reasonable to conclude that JB's deficit is primarily at the level of encoding.

Having established the locus of JB's deficit, we will now go on to consider in more detail the relationship to other patients that have been reported in the literature and how it may relate to more general theories of frontal function and memory.

Relationship to Other Patients

A primary objective of this study was to contrast the performance of JB with that of BG (Schacter et al., 1996). Although both patients have similar presenting characteristics (i.e. pathological false alarm rates) and may base their recognition judgements on qualitatively similar memory descriptions (i.e. poorly focused), the functional locus of their deficits may differ. Thus, JB may fail to encode item-specific information in sufficient detail and BG may fail to set up a detailed event description at retrieval. The present conclusions fit well with data from functional neuroimaging studies, which have consistently attributed retrieval processes to right frontal involvement and encoding to left frontal activity (Fletcher et al., 1995; Kapur et al., 1994; Tulvin, Kapur, Markowitsch, et al., 1994)—BG and JB having right and left frontal lobe damage respectively. This convergence of neuropsychological data with those from functional neuroimaging is further supported by a recent study by Ward, Parkin, and Squires (1998) who report patient MR—a man suffering from a demyelinating illness centred on the left frontal lobe whose false alarm rates exceeded even those made by JB. As one might predict from his left-sided lesion, the provision of encoding instructions at test significantly reduced his false alarm rate. In contrast, RW (Delbecq-Derouesné et al., 1990), who had a bilateral frontal lesion more extensive on the right, did not benefit from semantic orienting at encoding in a single probe recognition test (performance was at chance). However, the patient did show signs of an "overactive" retrieval mechanism in that the patient produced a large amount of intrusions in recall tasks and confabulatory-type responses in a number of other tests.

There are also some reasons for caution in postulating a simple left–right dichotomy for encoding and retrieval. More recent neuroimaging studies have suggested a role of the left prefrontal cortex in retrieval (Nolde, Johnson, & D'Esposito, in press; Nolde, Johnson, & Raye, in press) and of the right prefrontal cortex in encoding (Kelley et al., 1998; Wagner et al., 1998). With regards to encoding, the left hemisphere appears to be involved in the encoding of words, the right hemisphere is involved in the encoding of nonverbal material (faces, W.M. Kelley et al., 1998; abstract images, Wagner et al., 1998), and there is evidence of bilateral encoding for pictures of familiar objects (W.M.

Kelley et al., 1998). With regards to retrieval, Nolde, Johnson, and Raye (in press) have suggested that the right hemisphere plays a dominant role in more automatic aspects of retrieval (e.g. yes/no recognition) whereas the left hemisphere is involved in more strategic aspects of retrieval (e.g. source memory). Leaving aside the issue of neuroanatomical correlates, it is still possible to describe the lesion in terms of *functional* damage and this should be able to provide constraints upon normal models of memory and executive function.

An important finding in JB is that he does not take advantage of semantic categories in memory tasks. Similar findings have also been reported in group studies of frontal patients. For example, Gershberg and Shimamura (1991) report that in free recall, frontal lobe patients often do not perform any better on lists containing semantically related words and do not group similar words at retrieval (e.g. reporting "lion, dog, zebra" consecutively), unlike controls. However, this study is neutral with regards to the question of whether the failure to take advantage of semantic similarity is arising because of a failure to encode the information adequately or a failure of retrieval strategies.

One effect that is dependent on subjects' ability to encode relevant stimulus dimensions is "release from proactive interference" (e.g. Wickens, 1970). When subjects are given a free recall test in which successive lists contain semantically similar words (e.g. canary, robin, sparrow), performance deteriorates from proactive interference (PI), but when the categories are changed performance increases to its original level (e.g. Loess, 1968). Moscovitch (1982) studied release from PI in several groups of memory-impaired subjects and found that the only group who failed to show this effect had left frontal lesions (right frontal, left and right temporal, and temporal+hippocampal groups all showed normal release). This is consistent with the idea that left frontal patients are encoding at a more superficial level, such that they do not always take account of taxonomic category. Indeed, a previous study of JB has shown that he shows very little release from PI, and no benefit in recalling semantically related lists of words relative to unrelated lists of words, unlike controls (Parkin et al., 1988).

Relationship to Models of Normal Memory

Traditionally, models of memory assume that episodic memories are encoded via medial temporal lobe structures, which act as a consolidator and/or provide a temporary "index" to the memory trace, which is ultimately distributed throughout the neocortex (e.g. Damasio, 1989; Squire, Cohen, & Nadel, 1984). However, there is also a theoretical motivation to suppose that frontally associated control processes might play an important role in encoding. Attempting to encode every aspect of every event would impose a substantial computational burden on the memory system. Even in a task such as remembering lists of words, the range of possible parameters to encode is large (e.g. font, text size, phonology, temporal order, word associations) and presumably requires some form of selection mechanism in order to prioritise which features to encode and (perhaps) to deprioritise or inhibit other features. Selection may be based upon goals and task demands, meta-memory assumptions (e.g. use of imagery as a mnestic strategy), or properties of the stimulus items themselves. A failure of these mechanisms may result in a tendency to encode only lower-level features and/or those features that are shared by many other items, including items that were not presented. This would then give rise to a pathological false alarm rate. This deficit may be compensated for, at least partially, by external selection of features to encode (i.e. by giving orienting instructions). Alternatively, the deficit may be reduced by using targets and distractors made up of nonoverlapping sets of features (particularly low-level features) so that the differentiating features can act as cues at retrieval, even implicitly.

This account of the role of the frontal lobes in encoding resembles several existing theories. The encoding manipulations that we carried out on JB draw on the levels of processing assumption that semantic encoding enhances later retrieval (e.g. Craik & Lockhart, 1972; Craik & Tulving, 1975). Indeed, neuroimaging studies have shown that left frontal regions are activated by level of processing manipulations (Kapur et al., 1994). This region may be involved in producing a focused event description at encoding by selecting appropriate features and reducing the influence of irrelevant features, at least for verbal material. This account is also similar to Shimamura's (1995) notion of the frontal lobes acting as a gating mechanism by filtering extraneous activity using inhibitory mechanisms. However, it is not clear whether it is possible at the present time to distinguish between the hypothesis that JB fails to inhibit inappropriate features at encoding from the hypothesis that he fails to select appropriate features in the first place.

McClelland (1995) found that in his connectionist model, a failure to encode a proportion of features was essential to the model's later ability to produce memory distortions at retrieval. Without this assumption, it was found there is little scope for constructive processes at retrieval to intrude new features erroneously into the pattern. Our hypothesis is similar to this, with the further assumption that a failure to select certain features for encoding is not arbitrary (a simplifying assumption made by McClelland) but is mediated by frontally associated control processes.

Brainerd, Reyna, and colleagues (e.g. Brainerd & Reyna, 1998; Brainerd et al., 1995) have recently proposed that memories consist of two different types of trace: a "verbatim" trace which contains the perceptual/contextual detail associated with an event, and a "gist" trace, which contains the general meaning of the event. Furthermore, they make the claim that hits and false alarms draw upon these traces to different extents, with false alarms more associated with the gist trace and hits with the verbatim trace. In order to explain JB's deficit within this framework we would need to assume that his ability to encode verbatim traces has been compromised such that this trace would be unable to reject distractors on the basis of item-specific properties and so recognition relies on more general gist characteristics of the studied items. However, this account generates a number of predictions not borne out by our data. Brainerd et al. (1995) claim that the gist trace consists of information at a conceptual/semantic level, whereas we know that this type of information is often not encoded by JB. Furthermore, they make the claim that distractors that share more features with targets are more likely to be accepted by a gist trace. Again, the lack of effect of target-distractor similarity in both JB and BG suggests that they are not relying on this gist trace, at least as currently defined by Brainerd et al.

The extent to which JB's encoding deficit can be considered to be memory-specific or part of a more general deficit (e.g. to an attentional mechanism) requires further investigation. As we have already noted, encoding may involve the interplay of many cognitive components some of which may be primarily memory-based and others that may be related to more general cognitive mechanisms. The findings so far, however, suggest that JB does not have general difficulties in setting up a "task set" in non-memory tasks (e.g. Stroop, WCST) or attending to higher-level properties of stimuli in non-memory tasks (e.g. when asked to find the similarities between items). Thus, the hypothesis that JB's deficit reflects damage to memory-specific processes remains viable.

REFERENCES

Allport, A. (1993). Attention and control: Have we been asking the wrong questions? A critical review of 25 years. In D.E. Meyer & S. Kornblum (Eds.), *Attention and performance XIV*. Cambridge, MA: MIT Press.

Baddeley, A. (1996). Exploring the central executive. *Quarterly Journal of Experimental Psychology, 49A*, 5–28.

Benton, A.L., & Hamsher, K.D. (1976). *Multilingual Aphasia Examination*. Iowa City: University of Iowa.

Brainerd, C.J., & Reyna, V.F. (1998). When things that were not experienced are easier to "remember" than things that were. *Psychological Science, 9*, 484–489.

Brainerd, C.J., Reyna, V.F., & Kneer, R. (1995). False-recognition reversal: When similarity is distinctive. *Journal of Memory and Language, 34*, 157–185.

Burgess, P.W., & Shallice, T. (1996). Confabulation and the control of recollection. *Memory, 4*, 359–411.

Conway, M.A., & Rubin, D.C. (1993). The structure of autobiographical memory. In A.F. Collins, S.E. Gathercole, M.A. Conway, & P.E. Morris (Eds.), *Theories of Memory*. Hove, UK: Lawrence Erlbaum Associates Ltd.

Craik, F.I.M., & Lockhart, R.S. (1972). Levels of processing: A framework for memory research. *Journal of Verbal Learning and Verbal Behaviour, 11,* 671–684.

Craik, F.I.M., & Tulving, E. (1975). Depth of processing and the retention of words in episodic memory. *Journal of Experimental Psychology: General, 104,* 268–294.

Curran, T., Schacter, D.L., Norman, K.A., & Galluccio, L. (1997). False recognition after a right frontal lobe infarction: Memory for general and specific information. *Neuropsychologia,* 35, 1035–1049.

Damasio, A.R. (1981). The brain binds entities and events by multiregional activation from convergence zones. *Neural Computation,* 1, 123–32.

Delbecq-Derouesné, J., Beauvois, M.F., & Shallice, T. (1990). Preserved recall versus impaired recognition. *Brain, 113,* 1045–1074.

Donaldson, W. (1992). Measuring recognition memory. *Journal of Experimental Psychology,* 121, 275–277.

Fletcher, P.C., Frith, C.D., Grasby, P.M., Shallice, T., Frackowiak, R.S.J., & Dolan, R.J. (1995). Brain systems for encoding and retrieval of auditory-verbal memory: An in vivo study in humans. *Brain, 118,* 401–416.

Gardiner, J.M. (1988). Functional aspects of recollective experience. *Memory and Cognition, 16,* 309–313.

Gardiner, J.M., & Java, R.I. (1993). Recognising and remembering. In A.F. Collins, S.E. Gathercole, M.A. Conway, & P.E. Morris (Eds.), *Theories of Memory.* Hove, UK: Lawrence Erlbaum Associates Ltd.

Gershberg, F.B., & Shimamura, A.P. (1991). The role of the frontal lobes in free recall: Interference, organisation and serial position effects. *Society for Neuroscience Abstracts, 17,* 136.

Guildford, J.P., Christensen, P.R., Merrifield, P.R., & Wilson. R.C. (1978). *Alternate Uses: Manual of instructions and interpretation.* Orange, CA: Sheridan Psychological Services.

Johnson, M.K., Raye, C.L., Foley, H.J., & Foley, M.A. (1981). Cognitive operations and decision bias in reality monitoring. *American Journal of Psychology,* 94, 37–64.

Kapur, S., Craik, F.I.M., Tulving, E., Wilson, A.A., Houle, S., & Brown, G.M. (1994). Neuroanatomical correlates of encoding in episodic memory: Levels of processing effect. *Proceedings of the National Academy of Science, USA, 91,* 2008–2011.

Kelley, C.M., & Jacoby, L.L. (1990). The construction of subjective experience: Memory attributions. *Mind and Language, 5,* 49–68.

Kelley, W.M., Miezin, F.M., McDermott, K.B., Buckner, R.L., Raichle, M.E., Cohen, N.J., Ollinger, J.M., Akbudak, E., Conturo, T.E., Snyder, A.Z., & Petersen, S.E. (1998). Hemispheric specialisation in human dorsal frontal cortex and medial temporal lobe for verbal and nonverbal memory encoding. *Neuron,* 20, 927–936.

Loess, H. (1968). Short-term memory and item similarity. *Journal of Verbal Learning and Verbal Behaviour, 7,* 87–92.

Mayes, A.R., & Downes, J.J. (1997). What do theories of the functional deficit(s) underlying amnesia have to explain? *Memory, 5,* 3–36.

McClelland, J.L. (1995). Constructive memory and memory distortions: A parallel distributed processing approach. In D.L. Schacter (Ed.), *Memory distortion.* Cambridge, MA: Harvard Press.

McClelland, J.L., McNaughton, B.L., & O'Reilly, R.C. (1995). Why there are complementary learning systems in the hippocampus and neocortex: Insights from the successes and failures of connectionist models of learning and memory. *Psychological Review, 102,* 419–457.

Monsell, S. (1995). Control of mental processes. In V. Bruce (Ed.), *Unsolved mysteries of the mind.* Hove, UK: Erlbaum Associates Ltd.

Moscovitch, M. (1982). Multiple dissociations of function in amnesia. In L.S. Cermak (Ed.), *Human memory and amnesia.* Hillsdale, NJ: Lawrence Erlbaum Associates Ltd.

Nelson, H.E. (1976). A modified card sorting test sensitive to frontal lobe deficits. *Cortex, 12,* 313–324.

Nelson, H.E. (1985). *National Adult Reading Test.* London: NFER-Nelson.

Nolde, S.F., Johnson, M.K., & D'Esposito, M.D. (in press). Left prefrontal activation during episodic remembering: An event-related fMRI study. *NeuroReport.*

Nolde, S.F., Johnson, M.K., & Raye, C.L. (in press). The role of prefrontal cortex during tests of episodic memory. *Trends in Cognitive Sciences.*

Norman. K.A.. & Schacter, D. (1996) Implicit memory, explicit memory, and false recollection: A cognitive neuroscience perspective. In L.M. Reder (Ed.), *Implicit Memory and Metacognition.* Hillsdale, NJ: Lawrence Erlbaum Associates Inc.

Parkin, A.J. (1997). The neuropsychology of false memory. *Learning and Individual Differences, 9,* 341–357.

Parkin, A.J. (1998). The central executive does not exist. *Journal of the International Neuropsychology Society, 4,* 518–522.

Parkin, A.J., Bindschaedler, C., Harsent, L., & Metzler, C. (1996). Pathological false alarm rates following damage to the left frontal cortex. *Brain and Cognition,* 32, 14–27.

Parkin, A.J., & Leng, N.R.C. (1993). *Neuropsychology of the amnesic syndrome.* Hove, UK: Lawrence Erlbaum Associates Ltd.

Parkin, A.J, Leng, N.R.C., Stanhope, N., & Smith, A.P. (1988). Memory impairment following ruptured aneurysm of the anterior communicating artery. *Brain and Cognition, 7,* 231–243.

Parkin. A.J., Yeomans, J., & Bindschaedler, C. (1994). Further characterisation of the executive memory impairment following frontal lobe lesions. *Brain and Cognition, 26,* 23–42.

Rajaram, S. (1993). Remembering and knowing: Two means of access to the personal past. *Memory and Cognition, 21,* 89–102.

Raven, J.C. (1960) *Guide to the Standard Progressive Matrices.* London: H.K. Lewis.

Ruff, M., Light, R.H. & Evans, R.W. (1987). Ruff figural fluency test: A normative study with adults. *Developmental Neuropsychology, 3,* 37–51.

Schacter, D.L., Curran, T., Galluccio, L., Milberg, W.P., & Bates, J.F. (1996). False recognition and the right frontal lobe: A case study. *Neuropsychologia, 34,* 793–808.

Schacter, D.L., Israel, L., & Racine, C. (1999). Suppressing false recognition in younger and older adults: The distinctiveness heuristic. *Journal of Memory and Language, 40,* 1–24.

Shallice, T., & Evans, M.E. (1978). The involvement of the frontal lobes in cognitive estimation. *Cortex, 14,* 294–303.

Shallice, T., Fletcher, P., Frith, C.D., Grasby, P., Frackowiak, R.S.J., & Dolan, R.J. (1994). Brain regions associated with acquisition and retrieval of verbal episodic memory. *Nature, 368,* 633–635.

Shimamura, A.P. (1995). Memory and frontal lobe function. In M.S. Gazzaniga (Ed.), *The cognitive neurosciences.* Cambridge, MA: MIT Press.

Signoret, J.L., & Lhermitte, F. (1976). The amnesic syndromes and the encoding process. In M.R. Rosenzweig & E.L. Bennett (Ed.), *Neural mechanisms of learning and memory.* Cambridge, MA: MIT Press.

Squire, L.P., Cohen, N.J., & Nadel, L. (1984). The medial temporal region and memory consolidation: A new hypothesis. In H. Weingartner & E. Parker (Eds.), *Memory consolidation.* Hillsdale, NJ: Lawrence Erlbaum Associates Inc

Stuss, D.T. (1991). Self-awareness and the frontal lobes: A neuropsychological perspective. In J. Strauss & G.R. Goethals (Eds.), *The self: Interdisciplinary approaches.* New York: Springer-Verlag.

Trenerry, M.R., Crosson, B., DeBoe, J., & Leber, W.R. (1989). *Stroop Neuropsychological Screening Test.* Odessa, FL: Psychological Assessment Resources.

Tulving, E., Kapur, S., Craik, F.I.M., Moscovitch, M., & Houle, S. (1994). Hemispheric encoding/retrieval asymmetry in episodic memory: Positron emission tomography findings. *Proceedings of the National Academy of Science, USA, 91,* 2016–2020.

Tulving, E., Kapur, S., Markowitsch, H.J., Craik, F.I.M., Habib, R., & Houle, S. (1994). Neuroanatomical correlates of retrieval in episodic memory: Auditory sentence recognition. *Proceedings of the National Academy of Science, USA, 91,* 2012–2015.

Wagner, A.D., Poldrack, R.A., Eldridge, L.L., Desmond, J.E., Glover, G.H., & Gabrieli, J.D.E. (1998). Material-specific lateralisation of prefrontal activation during episodic encoding and retrieval. *Neuroreport, 9,* 3711–3717.

Ward, J., Parkin, A.J., & Squires, E. (1998). *Phenomenal misidentification due to left frontal lobe disease.* Manuscript in preparation.

Warrington, E.K. (1984). *Recognition Memory Test.* London: NFER-Nelson.

Wechsler, D. (1981). *Wechsler Adult Intelligence Scale-Revised.* New York: Psychological Corporation.

Wechsler, D. (1984). *Wechsler Memory Scale-Revised.* New York: Psychological Corporation.

Whitten, W.B, Suter, W.N, & Frank, M.L. (1979). Bidirectional synonym ratings of 464 noun pairs. *Journal of Verbal Learning and Verbal Behaviour, 18,* 109–127.

Wickens, D.D. (1970). Encoding categories of words: An empirical approach to meaning. *Psychological Review, 77,* 1–15.

COGNITIVE NEUROPSYCHOLOGY, 1999, 16 (3/4/5), 267–292

NEUROPSYCHOLOGICAL MECHANISMS OF FALSE FACIAL RECOGNITION FOLLOWING FRONTAL LOBE DAMAGE

Steven Z. Rapcsak
VA Medical Center and University of Arizona, Tucson, USA

Sheryl L. Reminger, Elizabeth L. Glisky, and Alfred W. Kaszniak
University of Arizona, Tucson, USA

James F. Comer
VA Medical Center, Tucson, USA

Previous neuropsychological studies have demonstrated an association between false recognition and frontal lobe dysfunction. In the experiments reported here we explore the contribution of memory impairment and executive dysfunction to the pathogenesis of false facial recognition in patients with focal frontal lobe damage. Memory illusions in response to novel faces were observed in both anterograde and retrograde tests of face recognition memory. However, in neither memory domain could false recognition be accounted for by face memory loss. Instead, our findings suggest that false facial recognition in frontal patients reflects the breakdown of strategic memory retrieval, monitoring, and decision functions critical for attributing the experience of familiarity to a specific source. Frontal executive memory functions are primarily recruited under conditions of uncertainty when the face cue does not automatically elicit relevant contextual information, leaving the source of familiarity unspecified. Our results indicate that frontal patients do not spontaneously engage in effortful recollection of specific contexts that can normally be used to oppose and inhibit recognition decisions based on general or context-free familiarity. However, frontal patients can use context recollection to suppress false recognition once this strategy is pointed out to them. In some frontal patients false recognition may be material-specific.

INTRODUCTION

Face memory impairment in neurological patients is typically associated with right hemisphere damage and may take different clinical forms. The most extensively studied face recognition disorder is prosopagnosia—a condition characterised by the loss of memory for familiar faces. Prosopagnosics do not experience a sense of familiarity with the faces of people they knew prior to their illness and are unable to identify these individuals from facial cues. In fact, patients usually report that all faces look completely unfamiliar. The retrograde face recognition deficit is regularly accompanied by severe anterograde face memory impairment. The critical lesion site in prosopagnosia involves the right ventromedial occipito-temporal region, including extrastriate and inferotemporal (IT) visual association cortex and adjacent medial temporal lobe limbic/paralimbic areas (hippocampus and related structures) (Damasio, Tranel, & Damasio, 1990; De Renzi, Perani, Carlesimo,

Requests for reprints should be addressed to Steven Z. Rapcsak, M.D., Neurology Section (1-127), VA Medical Center, Tucson, Arizona 85723, USA (Fax: (520) 629-4783; E-mail: szr@u.arizona.edu).

Silveri, & Fazio, 1994; Sergent & Signoret, 1992; Tovée & Cohen-Tovée, 1993).

The absence of conscious facial recognition that is the hallmark of prosopagnosia stands in striking contrast with another type of face memory disorder, in which patients mistakenly believe that unfamiliar faces are familiar (A.W. Ellis, Hillam, Cardno, & Kay, 1991; Rapcsak et al., 1998; Rapcsak, Polster, Comer, & Rubens, 1994; Rapcsak, Polster, Glisky, & Comer, 1996; Young, De Haan, & Newcombe, 1990; Young, Flude, Hay, & Ellis 1993). The spurious sense of familiarity evoked by novel faces that characterises false facial recognition is sometimes accompanied by the retrieval of false identity-specific biographic information, resulting in frank misidentification, which in certain patients can approach delusional proportions (Rapcsak et al., 1994, 1996).

Although the clinical phenomenon is well documented, false facial recognition has received considerably less attention from cognitive neuroscientists than prosopagnosia. Consequently, our knowledge of the psychological mechanisms and neural substrates underlying this type of face memory impairment is much more limited. It seems to us, however, that a complete understanding of face recognition disorders requires that we develop neuropsychological models capable of accounting for both memory loss and memory distortion. Furthermore, by studying false facial recognition in neurological patients we can gain important insights into the cognitive processes and brain systems that normally safeguard against memory illusions and thereby help maintain the high accuracy of face recognition memory. Such efforts are also likely to improve our understanding of the neurocognitive changes responsible for the age-related increase in false facial recognition errors in normal individuals (Bartlett & Fulton, 1991; Bartlett, Leslie, Tubbs, & Fulton, 1989; Bartlett, Strater, & Fulton, 1991), and may ultimately lead to the discovery of a possible organic basis for the delusional misidentification syndromes (e.g. Capgras delusion, Frégoli syndrome, intermetamorphosis), which until recently have been discussed primarily in the psychiatric literature (Christodoulou, 1986; H.D. Ellis & Young, 1990; Rapcsak et al., 1994, Young et al., 1990). Finally, false facial recognition has obvious applied implications for eyewitness testimony (Searcy, Bartlett, & Memon, in press).

In this paper we explore further the relationship between frontal lobe damage and false facial recognition—an association we documented in previous neuropsychological studies of face memory (Rapcsak et al., 1994, 1996, 1998). Specifically, we examine the contribution of memory impairment and executive dysfunction to the pathogenesis of false facial recognition both within the anterograde and the retrograde domains of face memory. We also present evidence that experimental manipulations designed to encourage the use of stringent decision criteria can virtually eliminate false facial recognition in patients with frontal lobe damage—a finding that may have practical implications for rehabilitation. Finally, we provide data consistent with the notion that false recognition following frontal lobe damage may be material-specific. We conclude with a discussion of the role of prefrontal cortex in face recognition memory.

METHODS

Subjects

Frontal Patients. Two patients with frontal lobe damage participated in the experiments. JS is a 67-year-old right-handed man with 16 years of formal education who developed severe memory impairment following surgical repair of an anterior communicating artery aneurysm (Rapcsak et al., 1998). CT scan revealed bilateral infarction of the basal forebrain/septal area and the ventromedial frontal region, including orbitofrontal cortex and anterior cingulate gyrus. Frontal lobe involvement was more extensive on the right side, where the lesion extended into anterior (frontopolar) and inferior dorsolateral prefrontal areas (Fig. 1a). BW is a 51-year-old right-handed man with 12 years of formal education. BW underwent surgical removal of a right frontal lobe tumour in 1988, which was followed by radiation therapy. MRI scan showed extensive right frontal lobe damage, involving orbitofrontal, dorsolateral, anterior (frontopolar), and superior medial prefrontal cortex (Fig. 1b). Areas of abnormal signal intensity were also seen in the right anterior temporal lobe and the basal ganglia region, consistent with radiation necrosis or residual tumour. Detailed neuropsychological profiles of the two frontal patients are presented in Table 1.

Temporal Patients. Five patients (age range: 41–72) with evidence of right medial temporal lobe damage were also recruited to serve as controls for the frontal patients in the anterograde face memory experiments. Three patients had undergone temporal lobectomy for the control of epilepsy that proved refractory to medical management, while in the remaining two patients the lesion aetiology was infarction in the distribution of the posterior cerebral artery. As expected, the right temporal group showed evidence of face memory impairment on the Warrington Recognition Memory Test (WRMT; mean = 35.0, SD = 6.78), whereas verbal memory was generally well preserved (mean = 44.2, SD = 6.38).

Controls. The normal control group included six subjects (age range: 53–76) without a history of neurological or psychiatric illness.

Anterograde Face Recognition Memory Experiments

Experiment 1

The paradigms used in our previous studies of false facial recognition required subjects to make decisions about familiarity within the context of autobiographical memory (i.e. they had to decide whether they had ever seen a particular face before) (Rapcsak et al., 1994, 1996, 1998). By contrast, most investigations of false facial recognition in normal subjects have used anterograde episodic memory tests, where old/new recognition judgements were made with respect to the study phase of the experiment (e.g. Bartlett & Fulton, 1991; Bartlett et al., 1989, 1991). Previous case studies of false recognition in frontal patients have also relied primarily on anterograde tests of episodic memory (Curran, Schacter, Norman, & Gallucio, 1997; Delbecq-Derouesné, Beauvois, & Shallice, 1990; Parkin, Bindschaedler, Harsent, & Metzler, 1996; Schacter, Curran, Gallucio, Milberg, & Bates,

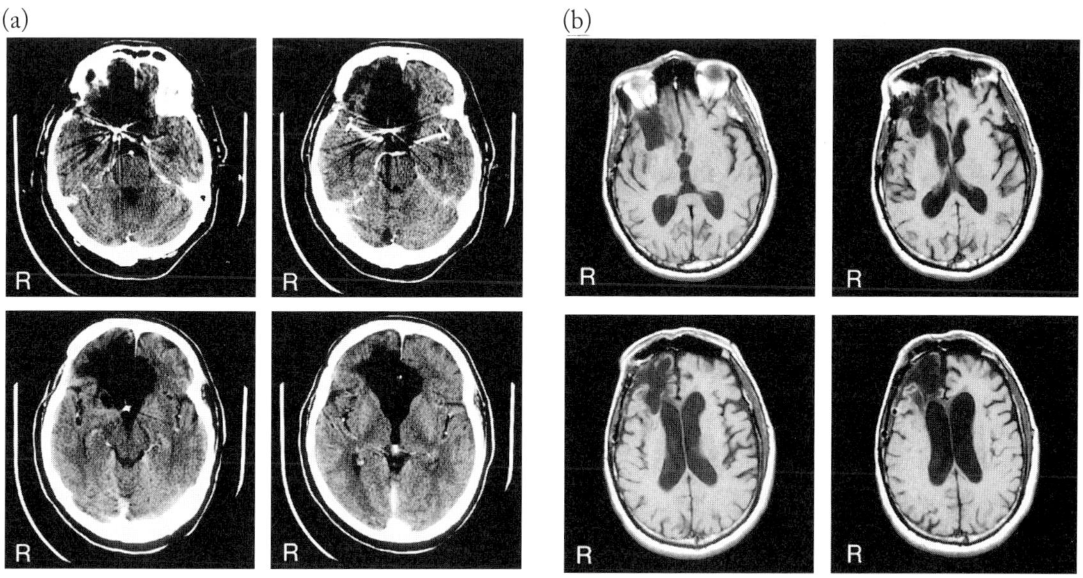

Fig. 1. *CT and MRI scans in (a) JS and (b) BW showing extent of frontal lobe damage.*

Table 1. *Neuropsychological Profiles of the Two Patients with Frontal Lobe Damage*

	Patient JS	*Patient BW*
Age	67	51
Education (yrs)	16	12
WAIS[a]		
Full Scale IQ	100	126
Verbal IQ	102	133
Performance IQ	99	113
WMS[a]		
General Memory	78	100
Verbal Auditory	83	138
Visual	78	75
Delay	60	114[b] 78[c]
CVLT		
Trial 1	5	8
Trial 5	6	13
Long Delay FR	2	12
Long Delay CR	3	14
Hits	16	15
False positives	21	0
Bias	.90	0
WRMT		
Words	23	49
Faces	32	37
WCST		
Categories	2	6
Pers. Errors	64	0
FAS	12	30
Trails B	420" 7 errors	160" 0 errors

[a] JS received the WAIS-R and WMS-R; BW received the WAIS-III and WMS-III.
[b] Auditory
[c] Visual
WAIS: Wechsler Adult Intelligence Scale; WMS: Wechsler Memory Scale; CVLT: California Verbal Learning Test; FR: Free Recall; CR: Cued Recall; WRMT: Warrington Recognition Memory Test; WCST: Wisconsin Card Sorting Test; FAS: Verbal Fluency Test.

1996b). Therefore, in Experiment 1 we examined false facial recognition within the context of standard old/new tests of recognition memory.

Procedure. Stimuli were presented on a Macintosh IIci computer using SuperLab software. In the Study Phase, pictures of faces taken from a college yearbook were presented to subjects one at a time on the computer screen. Each face was presented for 5 seconds. The pictures of faces were cropped so that minimal amounts of clothing and other extraneous information could be seen in each picture. There were four different versions of this test, varying by the number of faces to be remembered: 32 faces, 24 faces, 16 faces, and 8 faces. An equal number of male and female faces were used in each set. In the Test Phase, which immediately followed the completion of the Study Phase, pictures of faces were again presented one at a time on the computer screen. Subjects were instructed to press either a "yes" key, if the picture was of a face that they had seen in the Study Phase, or a "no" key, if the picture was of a face not presented before. Each test version included an equal number of randomly distributed targets and distractors. Distractor items were pictures of male and female college students taken from the same yearbook as the target faces. Before each picture appeared on the screen, a fixation point appeared for 250msec to signal subjects that a picture was about to be displayed. After a 250msec pause, a picture of a face appeared. The face remained on the screen until subjects responded with a key press.

Results. Hit and false alarm rates for the four sets of faces are presented in Fig. 2. All groups showed a tendency toward improved recognition memory performance as a function of decreasing set size, manifested generally as an increase in hits and a corresponding decrease in false alarms. Statistical analyses on the collapsed hit and false alarm data from the four face memory experiments were conducted using the Kruskal-Wallis test to detect significant differences among the subjects groups, followed by the Mann-Whitney U test for pairwise comparisons. Kruskal-Wallis tests indicated significant group differences for both hits ($H = 8.6$, $P = .01$) and false alarms ($H = 7.9$, $P = .02$). Mann-Whitney U tests revealed no significant differences between hit rates for frontal patients and normal controls ($U = 5$, $P = .74$), whereas temporal lobe

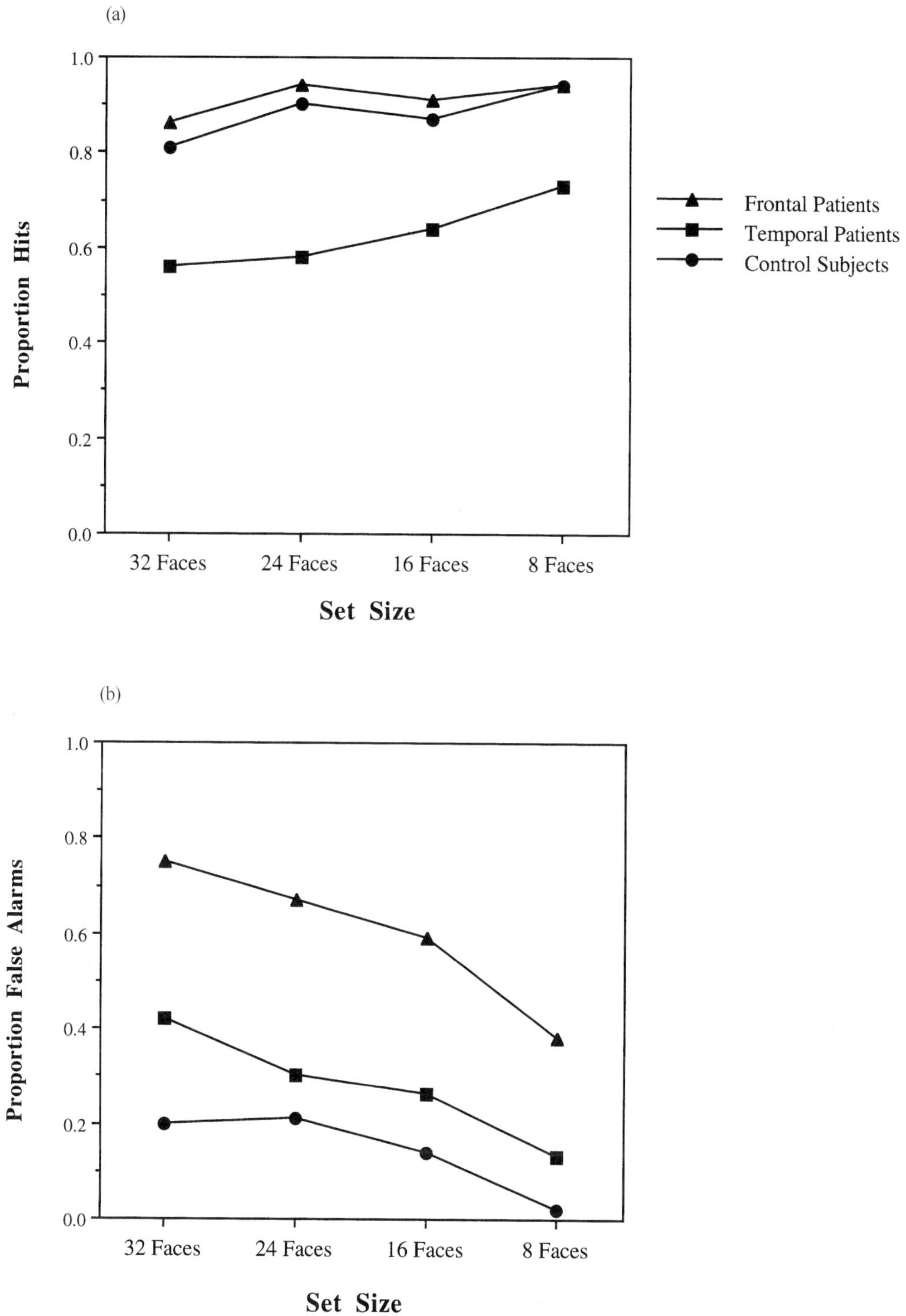

Fig. 2. *Hit (a) and false alarm (b) rates in Experiment 1.*

patients were impaired relative to both groups (temporals vs. controls $U = 0$, $P = .006$; temporals vs. frontals $U = 0$, $P = .05$). Frontal patients had higher false alarm rates than both temporal patients ($U = 0$, $P = .05$) and controls ($U = 0$, $P = .05$). Temporal patients also had higher false alarm rates than control subjects ($U = 3.5$, $P = .04$)

To obtain a more precise index of memory accuracy and examine possible differences in response bias, we computed the discrimination and bias measures derived from the two-high-threshold model of recognition memory (Snodgrass & Corwin, 1988). In brief, the two-high-threshold model assumes that in making recognition decisions the subject enters into one of three possible memory states: old recognition, new recognition, and uncertainty. Old items crossing the old recognition threshold are identified as old, whereas new items crossing the new threshold are classified as new. When the subject is in the uncertain state, items will be classified as old or new depending on the subject's response bias. The measure of recognition accuracy derived from the model is the Discrimination Index (Pr), computed by the formula H–FA where H = hit rate and FA = false alarm rate. The Bias Index (Br), which reflects the probability of the subject saying "yes" to an item when in the uncertain state, is computed as FA/1–Pr. A Br value of .5 indicates neutral response bias (i.e. equal number of "yes" and "no" responses when uncertain), values greater than .5 are indicative of a liberal bias, whereas values less than .5 are consistent with a conservative bias. In all calculations of hit and false alarm rates we applied the correction recommended by Snodgrass & Corwin (1988).

Pr and Br scores for the three subject groups are presented in Fig. 3. All three groups showed improved memory accuracy as a function of decreasing set size, indicated by a progressive increase in discrimination (Pr) scores. Kruskal-Wallis tests on the collapsed data from the four face memory experiments indicated significant group differences for both the Pr ($H = 8.17$, $P = .02$) and the Br ($H = 5.9$, $P = .05$) measures. Mann-Whitney U tests revealed that both frontal and temporal groups were impaired relative to controls on the Pr measure (frontals vs. controls, $U = 0$, $P = .05$; temporals vs. controls, $U = 1$, $P = .01$), but the two patient groups were not significantly different from each other ($U = 5$, $P = 1.0$). By contrast, Br scores were higher in the frontal group than in both the temporal ($U = 0$, $P = .05$) and control groups ($U = 0$, $P = .05$), indicating a liberal response bias in frontal patients. Br scores were not significantly different for controls and temporal lobe patients ($U = 8$, $P = .20$), and were generally indicative of a neutral or slightly conservative response bias[1].

Discussion. The results of Experiment 1 are consistent with previous case studies documenting relatively normal hit rates but pathologically elevated false alarm rates in frontal patients on old/new recognition tests of episodic memory (Curran, Schacter, Norman, & Gallucio, 1997; Parkin et al., 1996; Schacter et al., 1996b). False alarms to new faces in our frontal subjects exceeded not only the rates observed in normal controls but also the rate of false alarms produced by patients with right temporal lobe damage.

Temporal patients produced more false recognition responses than normal controls, but their hit rates were also significantly lower. Taken together, these findings suggest that their defective performance was most likely related to poor memory for the study faces. Frontal patients also showed evidence of face memory impairment, since their corrected recognition accuracy scores reflected by the discrimination index (Pr) were substantially lower than those obtained by controls. However, discrimination scores for temporal and frontal patients were not significantly different, suggesting that face memory impairment alone cannot explain the high false recognition rates observed in subjects with frontal lobe damage. This hypothesis receives further support from the response bias data which revealed that, despite equivalent levels of memory discrimination, frontal patients showed evidence of

[1] Essentially identical results were obtained when the data were analysed using discrimination (d_L) and bias (C_L) measures derived from signal detection theory (for details, see Snodgrass & Corwin, 1988).

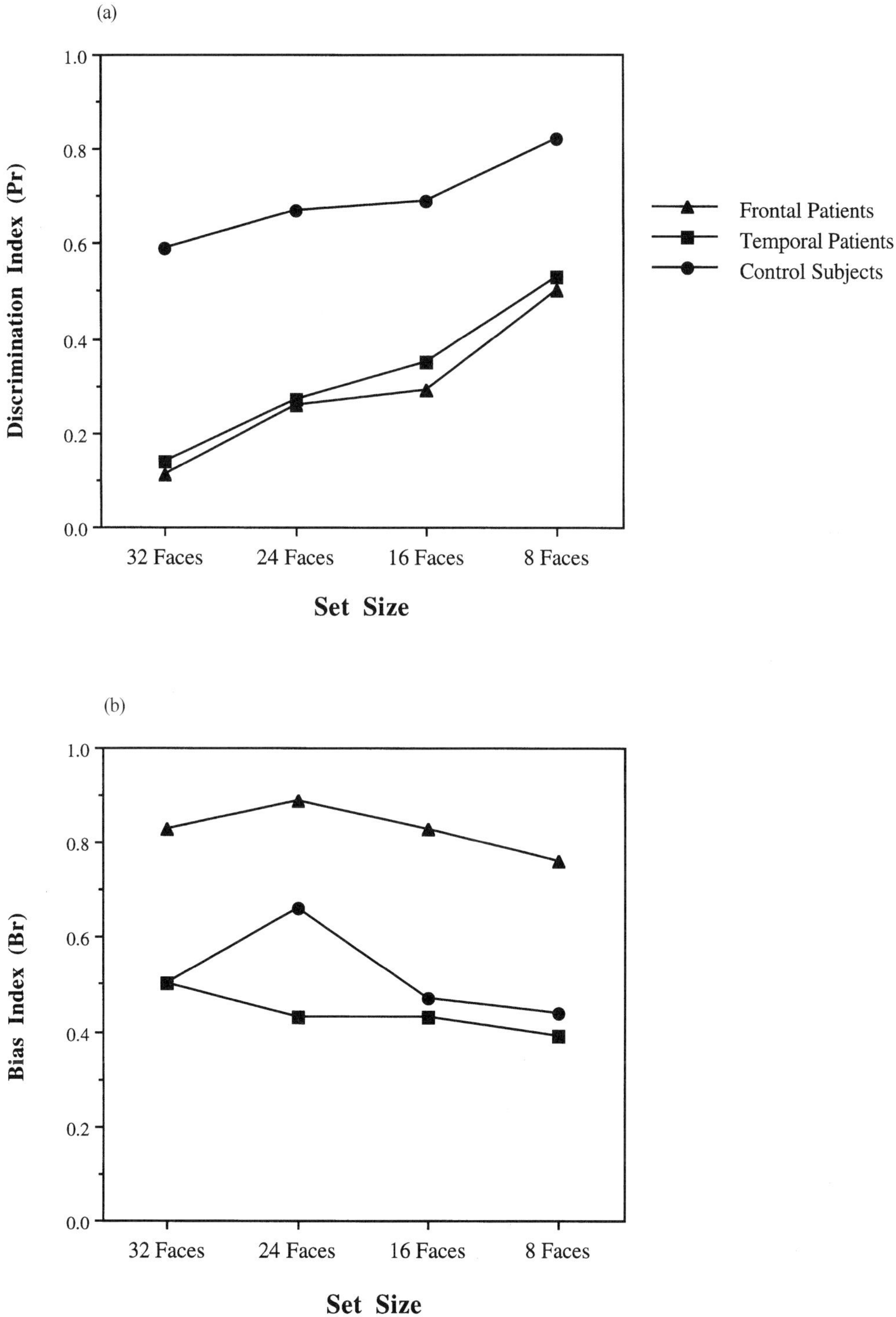

Fig. 3. *(a) Discrimination (Pr) and (b) Bias (Br) scores in Experiment 1.*

a liberal response bias whereas temporal patients, as a group, showed no significant bias relative to normal controls. That a liberal response bias is not simply the result of poor memory is also suggested by the observation that the patient in the temporal group who obtained the lowest discrimination scores of all participants tested was actually also the experimental subject who showed the most conservative bias.

It seems reasonable to assume that both temporal and frontal patients had difficulty encoding distinctive memory representations for the faces presented at study—a conclusion that is also supported by the poor performance of both groups on the faces subtest of the Warrington Recognition Memory Test. Due to this encoding deficit, patients did not have access to high-quality item-specific information critical for reliably distinguishing target faces from distractors. Impoverished item-specific memory is expected to have devastating consequences for face recognition. Faces represent a visual category where the structural similarity between category members is normally very high (i.e. all faces share the same basic components and general configuration). To recognise a particular face, the recognition system must be able to perform fine within-category discriminations based on subtle differences in global or configurational characteristics (Sergent, 1984). The accuracy of face recognition memory, therefore, depends on the ability to assign distinct and nonoverlapping memory codes to each individual face. Consistent with this hypothesis, a number of studies have demonstrated that distinctive faces are better discriminated in recognition memory experiments than are typical faces (e.g. Bartlett, Hurry, & Thorley, 1984; Light, Kayra-Stuart, & Hollander, 1979; Vokey & Read, 1992). The advantage of distinctive faces over typical ones is presumably due to the fact that the latter are harder to assign unique item-specific memory codes because of the larger number of structurally similar representations in memory. The greater encoding specificity of distinctive faces translates into higher hit rates in recognition experiments, whereas false alarms occur more frequently to typical faces.

Assuming that item-specific face memory was compromised to a similar degree in both frontal and temporal patients, as reflected by their near identical discrimination (Pr) scores, we need to explain why frontal patients showed and exceedingly liberal response bias while temporal patients performed similarly to normal controls on the bias (Br) measure. Response bias reflects the decision strategy adopted under conditions of uncertainty (i.e. when discrimination is less than optimal because the information immediately available in memory is insufficient to determine conclusively whether an item is old or new). An explanation of the liberal response bias in frontal patients, therefore, requires that we identify the abnormal criterion setting and judgement processes responsible for the production of false alarms in excess of what would be expected on the basis of random guessing.

It has been proposed that recognition decisions reflect the outcome of two distinct but closely related and highly interactive psychological processes (Atkinson & Juola, 1973; Hintzman & Curran, 1994; Jacoby & Dallas, 1981; Mandler, 1980). The first component is relatively automatic and involves the detection and assessment of stimulus familiarity. The second component is more effortful and involves strategic memory search to retrieve possible contexts in order to attribute familiarity to a specific source. Under normal circumstances these cognitive operations take place conjointly and judgements about prior occurrence reflect the additive effects of recognition by familiarity and context retrieval or identification (Mandler, 1980). Specifically, we assume that in making recognition decisions subjects monitor both the strength of the familiarity signal and the output of the context retrieval process and set criteria with respect to the amount and quality of information required for producing a particular response. However, since positive identification of an event is not possible on the basis of familiarity alone, context retrieval normally provides a more reliable basis for recognition judgements (Jacoby & Dallas, 1981; Mandler, 1980). As a result, subjects can optimise performance in recognition memory experiments by endorsing items only when they can retrieve detailed contextual information that uniquely specifies the study episode as the appropriate source for the experience of familiarity (i.e. requiring that test items exceed both a familiarity criterion and an "identification" criterion based on a mental representation of the study context). Responses based on context retrieval play an important role in rejecting related distractor items that have features in common with targets and, therefore, also give rise to a feeling of familiarity (i.e. items that exceed the familiarity criterion but do not meet the contextually based criterion for identification). By adopting stringent response criteria and relying consistently on context recollection or identification, subjects can oppose and suppress the potentially misleading influence of undifferentiated or context-free familiarity on recognition decisions (Jacoby & Kelly, 1992; Johnson, Hashtroudi, & Lindsay, 1993).

In situations where item-specific contextual information is unavailable, however, subjects may resort to less analytical approaches to decision making. For instance, in the absence of detailed item-specific memory subjects may rely on general or "gist" information about the study episode (Brainerd, Reyna, & Kneer, 1995). Gist memory reflects general stimulus characteristics (i.e. what the study items had in common), but this type of memory trace is not sufficient to distinguish between targets and related distractors since both types of items are consistent with the gist representation. According to "fuzzy-trace" theory (Brainerd et al., 1995), hits in recognition memory tests are driven by item-specific information whereas gist memory is the primary source of false alarms. In our face recognition experiment a gist representation may have corresponded to a generic description of the study episode (e.g. "pictures of young students"). Over-reliance on this type of gist memory trace could have accounted for the high false alarm rates (as well as the inflated hit rates) in our frontal patients, who may have uncritically endorsed items that matched this general description. In short, without access to detailed item-specific memory representations (either because of impoverished encoding or because of a failure to engage in effortful and strategic memory search to retrieve critical contextual information), frontal patients may have adopted lenient decision criteria and accepted gist-based or general familiarity as diagnostic of the item having been presented in the Study Phase.

It is also possible that some false alarm responses in our frontal patients were triggered by face familiarity signals from sources other than the study episode. For example, some distractor faces may have had general similarity to faces encountered in everyday life. As noted earlier, this type of structurally induced familiarity is generally held responsible for the higher false alarm rates to typical faces in recognition memory experiments (Bartlett et al., 1984; Light et al., 1979; Vokey & Read, 1992). False recognition errors in frontal patients thus may have reflected defective source monitoring (Johnson et al., 1993), manifested by an inability to distinguish between facial familiarity from an extra-experimental source and familiarity based on a specific prior exposure to the face (i.e. the Study Phase).

Patients with right temporal lobe damage also produced more false alarms than normal controls. Considering their reduced hit rates, this finding probably reflects the fact that temporal patients were less able to rely on item-specific memory in discriminating between target faces and distractors. Indeed, the pattern observed in temporal patients is similar to the "mirror effect" in normal subjects, where lower hit rates in recognition memory tasks are generally accompanied by an increase in false alarms (Glanzer & Adams, 1985). However, temporal patients made fewer false recognition errors than patients with frontal lobe damage despite the fact that both groups showed similar levels of item-specific face memory impairment. This relative paucity of false alarms in the temporal group suggests that monitoring and decision functions in these patients were largely preserved. That is, temporal patients produced fewer false alarm responses than frontal patients because they were more likely to realise that the absence of detailed item-specific memory is inconsistent with a positive judgement of prior occurrence. In fact, response strategies in temporal patients may not have been all that different from the strategy adopted by normal controls under conditions of uncertainty, as suggested by their similar bias (Br) scores in Experiment 1. It is possible, however, that in addition to item-specific memory impairment, temporal patients also retained a less robust gist representation of the study episode. Consequently, temporal patients may have experienced lower levels of gist-based or general familiarity with test items, reducing their susceptibility to false recognition.

Theoretically, the influence of gist memory on false alarms can be evaluated by designing a recognition experiment using both within-category (gist-consistent) and out-of-category (gist-inconsistent) distractors (e.g. Koutstaal & Schacter, 1997). If false alarms are driven primarily by gist information, then such errors should predominantly occur in response to within-category distractors. In the next experiment we examine the contribution of gist memory to false facial recognition.

Experiment 2

Procedure. In the Study Phase, 32 pictures of novel faces were presented to subjects one at a time on the computer screen. The target faces were all pictures of white males. As in Experiment 1, exposure duration was set at 5 seconds. In the Test Phase, which immediately followed the completion of the Study Phase, pictures of faces were again presented one at a time on the computer screen. Subjects were instructed to press either a "yes" key, if the picture was of a face that they had seen previously, or a "no" key, if the picture was of a face not seen before. The Test Phase included an equal number of randomly distributed targets and distractors. Three different types of distractor items were used: 16 pictures of other white males (within-category or gist-consistent distractors), 8 pictures of white females, and 8 pictures of non white males. The latter two categories of distractors were considered out-of-category or gist-inconsistent with respect to the items presented in the Study Phase. Before each picture, a fixation point appeared for 250msec to signal subjects that a picture was about to appear. After a 250msec pause, a picture of a face appeared. The face remained on the screen until subjects responded with a key press.

Results. Hit and false alarm rates for Experiment 2 are presented in Table 2. For comparison, we also included similar data from the 32-item face recognition memory test in Experiment 1, where no obvious category differences existed between targets and distractors. As can be seen from the Table, hit rates for the different subject groups were similar in the two experimental conditions, with temporal patients obtaining the lowest scores in both. By contrast, false alarm rates were lower for all three groups in Experiment 2, consistent with a general effect of distractor category on recognition memory performance.

The proportions of gist-consistent versus gist-inconsistent false alarms (computed as #gist-consistent FA/#gist-consistent distractors and #gist-inconsistent FA/#gist-inconsistent distractors) for the three subject groups are shown in Fig. 4. Additional analyses revealed that in normal controls virtually all false alarms (94%) occurred in response to gist-consistent distractor items. Gist-consistent false alarms also accounted for the majority of false recognition errors in frontal patients (81%). However, the difference between gist-consistent (63%) and gist-inconsistent (37%) false alarms appeared to be reduced in patients with right temporal lobe damage. These findings suggest that gist memory made a relatively smaller contribution to false alarm responses in temporal patients than in controls and frontal patients.

Discussion. The results of Experiment 2 demonstrate the powerful influence of gist memory on false recognition errors in normal subjects. However, controls produced relatively few false alarm responses overall, presumably because they could use

Table 2. *Hit and False Alarm Rates for the 32-item Face Memory Tests in Experiments 1 and 2*

	Experiment 1 (Noncategorised Distractors)		*Experiment 2 (Categorised Distractors)*	
	Hits	*False Alarms*	*Hits*	*False Alarms*
Frontal patients	.86	.75	.94	.42
Temporal patients	.56	.42	.51	.27
Control subjects	.81	.20	.81	.11

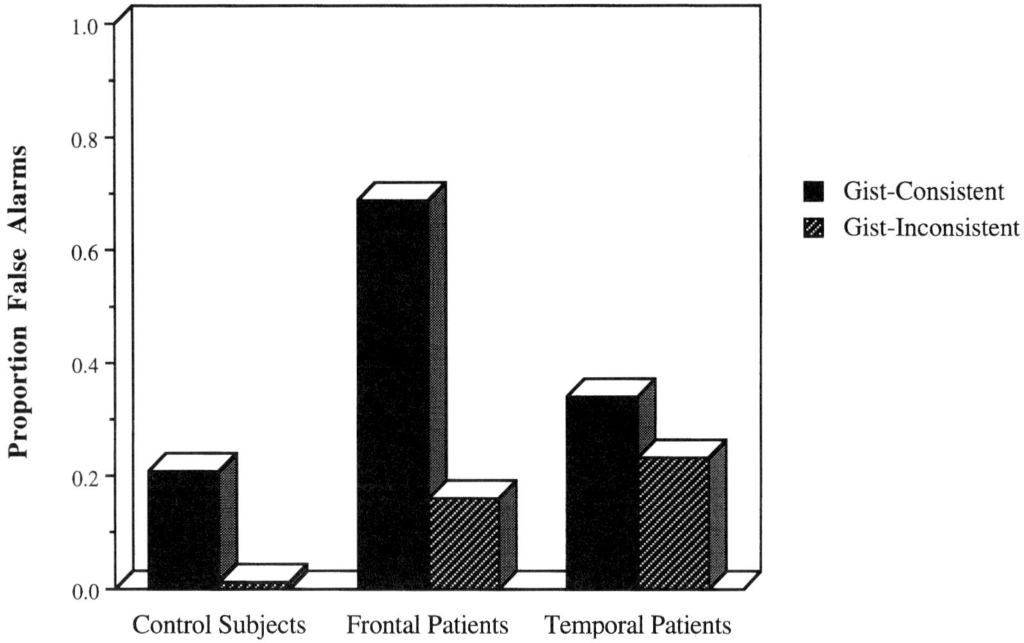

Fig. 4. *False alarm rates in Experiment 2.*

item-specific memory to oppose the effect of gist memory on recognition decisions. Gist memory also made a large contribution to the false alarms produced by frontal patients. This finding is in agreement with previous reports that false recognition errors in frontal patients are more frequent to within-category distractor items (Parkin et al., 1996; Schacter et al., 1996b). On the other hand, in patients with right temporal lobe damage the influence of gist memory seemed to be attenuated, providing support for the hypothesis that in addition to item-specific memory impairment these patients also experienced difficulty encoding general or categorical information about what study items had in common. This latter finding is consistent with the results of Schacter et al. (Schacter, Verfaellie, & Anes, 1997; Schacter, Verfaellie, Anes, & Racine, 1998; Schacter, Verfaellie, & Pradere, 1996c), who found that amnesic subjects exhibited reduced levels of false recognition for semantically or perceptually related distractor items in verbal memory paradigms. Similar results were recently obtained within the nonverbal memory domain by Koutstaal, Schacter, Verfaellie, Brenner, and Jackson (this issue), who demonstrated reduced gist-based false recognition in amnesic patients using pictures of novel abstract objects as stimuli. Taken together, these observations suggest that the medial temporal regions of the brain play an important role in encoding not only the item-specific information that supports veridical recognition but also the general or gist memory representation that is the major source of false recognition errors (cf. Schacter et al., 1996c, 1997, 1998). Based on these results, we predict that recognition memory performance in individual patients with temporal lobe damage may vary depending on the degree to which these two different components of memory are compromised. For instance, the potential for false alarms would be higher in temporal patients who could no longer rely on item-specific memory to suppress false recognition but in whom gist memory representations were still relatively preserved. By contrast, the likelihood of false recognition would be minimal in temporal patients in whom item-specific and gist memory were both significantly reduced. For additional discussion on the relationship between item-specific and gist memory with respect to the issue of false recognition in amnesia see Schacter et al. (1998).

Retrograde Face Recognition Memory Experiments

In these experiments we examined the question whether the false recognition effects observed in frontal patients in anterograde face memory tests also extended into the retrograde domain of face memory. In contrast to anterograde tests, where old/new recognition decisions are made with reference to information learned in the study phase, in retrograde memory experiments facial familiarity is judged within a larger autobiographical context. We reasoned that retrograde recognition memory tests may prove particularly useful for assessing the dysfunctional decision making and monitoring operations implicated in false recognition, since in these paradigms the performance of frontal patients is not expected to be significantly contaminated by retrograde face memory impairment (i.e. prosopagnosia).

The retrograde face memory tests included two related experiments that used different sets of unfamiliar faces. The order of presentation was counterbalanced, so that half the subjects were exposed to Unfamiliar Faces Set 1 in Experiment 3 and Unfamiliar Faces Set 2 in Experiment 4, whereas for the rest of the subjects the order was reversed.

Experiment 3

Procedure. The stimulus set consisted of 32 Famous Faces (i.e. entertainers, politicians) and 32 Unfamiliar Faces. An attempt was made to include unfamiliar faces that had a "celebrity-type" appearance (e.g. actor/actress portraits from an out-of-town talent agency, faces from ads in low circulation magazines, etc.). Pictures of faces were presented one at a time on the computer screen in random order. Subjects were instructed to press either a "yes" key, if the picture was the face of a familiar person, or a "no" key if the face was unfamiliar. Prior to testing, subjects were explicitly told to call a face familiar only if they thought that they had seen that particular individual before, either in person or through the media. After completing the test, subjects were shown the Famous Faces again and were asked to identify these individuals. Responses were considered correct if subjects produced either the appropriate name or other identity-specific biographic information (e.g. "One of the Beatles, he was killed in New York City a few years ago").

Results. Hit and false alarm rates for Experiment 3 are shown in Figure 5. Mann-Whitney U tests revealed that hit rates were not significantly different for frontal patients (.94) and normal controls (.85) ($U = 4$, $P = .51$). Similar results were obtained when we compared the proportion of Famous Faces that frontal patients and controls could identify correctly (.78 vs. .81). By contrast, false alarm rates were significantly higher in frontal patients (.52) than in control subjects (.06) ($U = 0, P = .05$).

Discussion. The results of Experiment 3 demonstrate pathologically high false alarm rates in frontal patients in retrograde tests of face recognition memory. False recognition in our frontal subjects cannot be attributed to retrograde face memory impairment, since both BW and JS were able to identify Famous Faces as well as controls. These results are consistent with our previous observation that false facial recognition and prosopagnosia are dissociable (Rapcsak et al., 1994, 1996).

We propose that the high false alarm rates observed in frontal patients in both anterograde and retrograde face memory tests may have similar underlying mechanisms. In particular, we suggest that recognition decisions in the retrograde domain also involve a *specific* and a *general* or "gist" memory component, which work in opposition in determining overall recognition accuracy. The specific memory component in the retrograde domain is mediated by face recognition units (FRUs) (Bruce & Young, 1986), which contain stored memory representations for familiar faces. The activation of a specific FRU by a familiar face is normally followed by the retrieval of identity-specific biographic information, providing the appropriate context for the experience of familiarity and resulting in person identification. Although novel faces by definition have no pre-existing representations in memory, they can nonetheless give rise to a feeling of familiarity. In fact, such misattributions of familiarity are not uncommon in everyday life (Young, Hay, & Ellis, 1985). An example of this

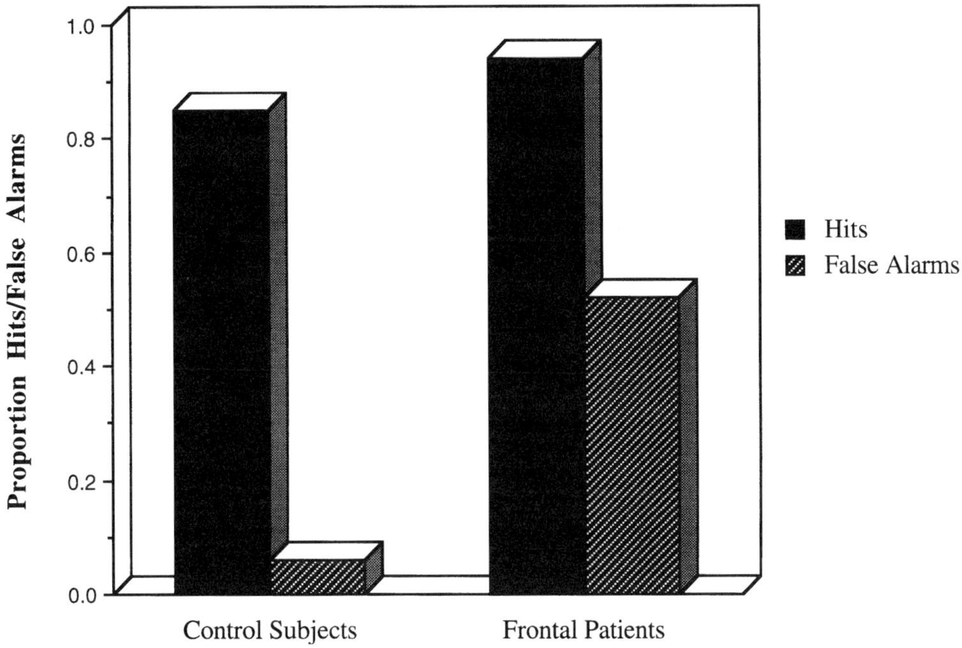

Fig. 5. *Hit and false alarm rates in Experiment 3.*

kind of recognition error is when an unfamiliar face has strong physical resemblance to the face of a person we know (i.e. look-alike effect). False recognition in this situation is presumably mediated by the spurious activation of a specific FRU, followed by the retrieval of false semantic information resulting in misidentification. Frequently, however, the subjective experience of familiarity evoked by a novel face is context-free. This type of familiarity, we suggest, is mediated by the general or gist component of face recognition memory. General memory effects arise from the intrinsic properties of memory systems to store information not only about specific exemplars but also about what category members have in common (McClelland & Rumelhart, 1985). In the case of face recognition, the strength of this general memory signal may reflect the global similarity between a novel face stimulus and all individual faces represented in memory, or it may be determined by the amount of structural overlap between the target item and abstract facial prototypes extracted from faces encountered in everyday life (Bruce, 1988; Light et al., 1979; Valentine & Bruce, 1986; Valentine & Ferrara, 1991). Facial prototypes are generalisations based on the accumulated effects of prior experience with faces and do not correspond to any particular FRU. Novel faces that closely resemble stored facial prototypes or have a large number of structurally similar exemplars represented in memory may give rise to a spurious but nonetheless compelling sense of familiarity. The hypothesis that this type of general or context-free familiarity may contribute to incorrect recognition decisions is supported by the finding that typical faces or faces that bear a categorical resemblance to certain occupational stereotypes (e.g. "actress type") are associated with high false alarm rates in normal subjects (Bartlett et al., 1984; Klatzky, Martin, & Kane, 1982; Light et al., 1979; Vokey & Read, 1992),

As noted earlier, however, the process of identification that involves the conscious recollection of specific contexts can oppose recognition judgements based on undifferentiated or context-free familiarity. Strategic context retrieval is not usually necessary when dealing with highly familiar faces where identity-specific contextual information is readily available, but it assumes a more critical role when operating under conditions of uncertainty. Consider the example of encountering a face that looks familiar but there is no other information immediately available in memory. This type of ambiguity can be resolved by attempting to retrieve possible contexts in order to attribute familiarity to a specific source. By engaging in context retrieval, we may ultimately discover that the person is indeed somebody we know. In this situation, a positive recognition judgement is made by determining not only that the face exceeded the criterion for familiarity but also that the contextual information retrieved from memory in response to the face cue met the criterion for identification. On the contrary, if we are unable to generate likely contexts for the experience of facial familiarity we may decide that the person is in fact unfamiliar. Here we use context recollection to reject a novel face that exceeded the familiarity criterion but failed to meet the contextually based criterion for identification. In short, we can improve recognition accuracy (and avoid potentially embarrassing social situations) by relying primarily on context recollection in face recognition judgements.

Normal subjects produced few false recognition errors in the retrograde face memory paradigm, suggesting that they primarily endorsed faces when they had access to appropriate identity-specific contextual information via the activation of specific FRUs. By relying consistently on the specific component of face recognition memory, normals were successful in opposing the influence of general or context-free familiarity on recognition decisions. Frontal patients also had relatively preserved retrograde memory for specific faces, as indicated by the fact that they were able to recognise famous faces as well as controls. As noted earlier, however, contextual information is readily available for these well-known individuals and identification does not require strategic memory search. Despite their good performance in recognising highly familiar faces, frontal patients experienced significant difficulty in situations where there was uncertainty about the origin of familiarity (i.e. when a face stimulus exceeded the familiarity criterion but identity-specific contextual information was not directly available). Under conditions of uncertainty, frontal patients demonstrated a tendency to respond on the basis of general or context-free familiarity without attempting to engage in strategic recollection of likely contexts and use this information as the basis for recognition judgements. Although the failure to use context recollection to oppose judgements based on context-free familiarity may have been the primary abnormality, it is possible that frontal patients also used inappropriate decision criteria with respect to the dimension of familiarity itself, accepting lower levels of general familiarity as diagnostic of previous encounter. This dual-deficit account is consistent with the notion that the frontal lobes play an important role not only in memory for context (Moscovitch, 1994; Schacter, 1987) but also in cognitive judgements of familiarity/novelty (Metcalfe, 1993, 1994). As discussed earlier, false recognition errors in frontal patients may have reflected defective source monitoring (Johnson et al., 1993), manifested as an inability to distinguish between familiarity based on memory for specific faces and familiarity based on memory for faces in general.

If the hypothesis that recollection of specific contexts can be used to suppress false recognition is correct, then it might be possible to reduce false alarms in frontal patients by requiring that they adopt stringent decision criteria and respond primarily on the basis of context retrieval or identification. This prediction was tested in Experiment 4, where we placed recognition by familiarity and identification in opposition.

Experiment 4

Procedure. Subjects were shown the same 32 Famous Faces as in Experiment 3, but these were now mixed randomly with a different set of 32 Unfamiliar Faces. Again, an effort was made to include unfamiliar faces with a "celebrity-type" appearance. As in Experiment 3, subject were asked to press the "yes" key if the face was that of a familiar person and the "no" key if the face was unfamiliar. However, in Experiment 4 subjects were explicitly instructed to call faces familiar only if they could remember the occupation and name of the person. The face remained on the screen until subjects responded with a key press.

Results. As can be seen from Fig. 6, false recognition errors were dramatically reduced in frontal patients when they were encouraged to use stringent response criteria that emphasised identification rather than familiarity as the basis for face recognition judgements. In fact, false alarm rates for frontal patients (.06) and controls (.01) were not significantly different under these conditions ($U = 1$, $P = .12$). Hit rates for both groups were slightly lower than in Experiment 3, reflecting the use of stricter criteria for identifying Famous Faces.

Discussion. The results of Experiment 4 are consistent with previous demonstrations in normal subjects that context retrieval or source recollection can oppose the influence of general familiarity on memory decisions (e.g. Dodson & Johnson, 1993; Jacoby, Kelley, Brown, & Jasechko, 1989; Lindsay & Johnson, 1989; Multhaup, 1995). Most importantly, our findings suggest that although patients with frontal lobe damage do not spontaneously engage in effortful context recollection, they can use identification to inhibit responses based on undifferentiated familiarity once this strategy is pointed out to them. In fact, both JS and BW commented during the test that although some of the unfamiliar faces looked very familiar, they were going to reject them because they could not come up with the profession and name of the person. These observations suggest that it might be possible to reduce false recognition in frontal patients by training them to rely consistently on the recollection of specific contexts in decision making. Such interventions could have important practical implications, since some frontal patients also demonstrate false facial recognition and misidentification in real-life situations (Rapcsak et al., 1994, 1996, 1998).

From a more general perspective, the results of Experiments 3 and 4 underscore further the critical importance of the decision criteria adopted by subjects in making recognition memory judgements. Decision criteria may vary both with respect to the quantity and the quality of information required, but the most stringent criteria will include multiple kinds of information rather than focusing on just one type (e.g. degree of familiarity) (Dodson & Johnson, 1993; Johnson et al., 1993; Multhaup, 1995). In Experiment 3, normal subjects seemed to

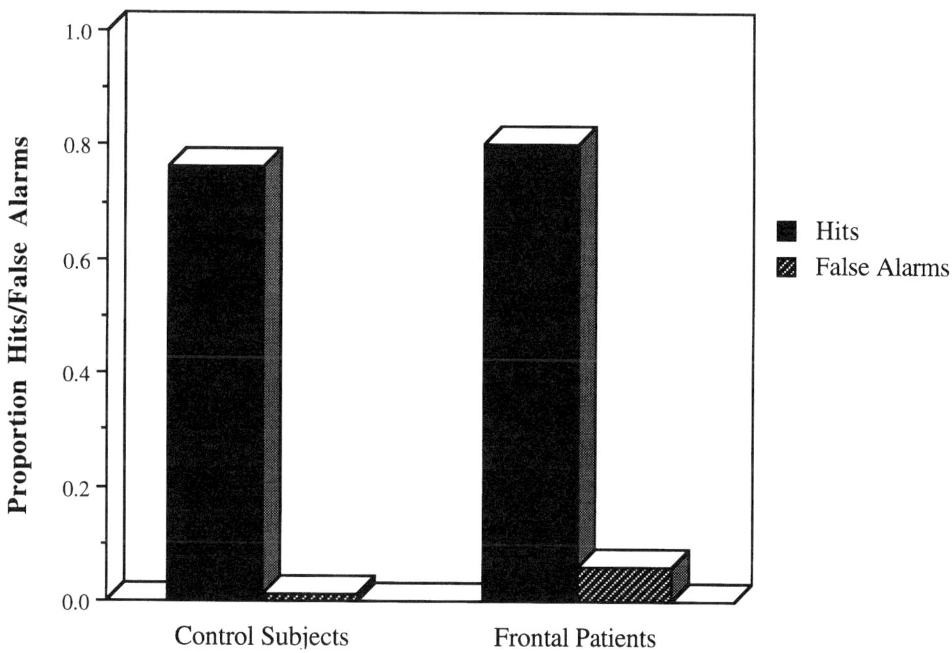

Fig. 6. *Hit and false alarm rates in Experiment 4.*

have discovered spontaneously the decision strategy most effective in reducing false recognition errors (i.e. context retrieval). To the extent that they required access to detailed contextual information to support a positive recognition decision, normal subjects may have adopted a mode of responding based on what has been referred to as the "distinctiveness heuristic" by Schacter, Israel, and Racine (1999). Using a distinctiveness heuristic in decision making involves setting criteria based on metamemory assumptions about the phenomenal characteristics of veridical recollection (e.g. expectations about the amount of perceptual and/or contextual detail the activated memory trace should contain in order to be accepted as genuine) (see also Dodson & Johnson, 1993; Johnson et al., 1993). When such metamemory expectations are not met, subjects are likely to produce a negative recognition decision. Consistent with this hypothesis, normal controls in Experiment 3 were generally able to interpret the *absence* of detailed contextual information as diagnostic that the face was probably novel, even though it may have seemed familiar at first. However, our findings suggest that frontal patients may not spontaneously employ a distinctiveness heuristic in decision making and consequently fail to regard the absence of specific recollection as inconsistent with a positive judgement of prior occurrence.

Material-specificity of False Recognition

Memory impairment following frontal lobe damage may be material-specific. For instance, Milner, Corsi, and Leonard (1991) found that patients with right frontal lesions performed worse on recency judgement tasks with nonverbal stimuli, whereas left frontal patients were more impaired when verbal materials were used. Material-specific false recognition, however, has not been demonstrated convincingly. In fact, most patients with frontal lobe damage show false recognition effects across a wide range of experimental stimuli (Parkin et al., 1996; Rapcsak et al., 1998; Schacter et al., 1996b). Nonetheless, in a previous report (Rapcsak et al., 1994) we noted that patients with false facial recognition following right hemisphere lesions that involved the frontal lobe did not produce false recognition errors in response to unfamiliar names or handwriting samples. In addition, Schacter et al. (1996b) provided some evidence that patient BG, whose lesion was confined to the right frontal lobe, produced more false alarms to pictures than to words. Patient BW in our study also had a unilateral right frontal lobe lesion, whereas JS had evidence of bilateral frontal lobe involvement. These differences in lesion laterality provided an opportunity to examine the issue of material-specificity in our patients by assessing their performance on verbal tests of recognition memory.

Experiment 5

Procedure. Verbal recognition memory was tested using three different types of stimuli: unrelated nouns (e.g. elbow, concept), animal names (e.g. turtle, lion), and pronounceable nonwords (e.g. tamal, fronge). In each version of the test, 32 study items from the same category were presented to subjects one at a time on the computer screen. Exposure duration was set at 5 seconds and subjects were instructed to read each word out loud. In the Test Phase, which immediately followed the completion of the Study Phase, words were again presented one at a time on the computer screen. Subjects were instructed to press either a "yes" key if the word was one that they had seen previously, or a "no" key if the word was one not seen before. Each test included an equal number of randomly distributed targets and distractors. Distractors were drawn from the same general category as targets (i.e. other unrelated nouns, animal names, nonwords). Before each word appeared on the screen, a fixation point appeared for 250msec to signal subjects that a word was about to be displayed. After a 250msec pause, a test item appeared. Words remained on the screen until subjects responded with a key press.

Results. Data from the three verbal recognition memory tests were combined since subjects performed similarly in all test conditions. Hit and false alarm rates are summarised in Table 3. Hit rates for both BW and JS were similar to those obtained by controls. However, JS produced significantly more false alarms than control subjects, whereas false alarm rates for BW were within normal limits. As can be seen from Table 3, Pr scores for BW were also within the range of controls, whereas JS's discrimination scores were significantly lower. In striking contrast to his performance on face memory tasks, bias (Br) scores for BW on the verbal tests were within normal range. On the other hand, Br scores for JS on the verbal tests were indicative of a liberal response bias, consistent with his performance in face recognition memory paradigms.

The results of the verbal recognition memory tests in Experiment 5 were generally consistent with the pattern noted on the CVLT, where BW showed preserved verbal learning and did not produce false alarms on the recognition trials, whereas JS showed poor verbal recall and produced numerous false recognition errors (see Table 1).

Discussion. Patient JS, who had bilateral frontal lobe damage, demonstrated false recognition in memory tests involving both words and faces. By contrast, false recognition in BW, who had a unilateral right frontal lobe lesion, was only apparent in face memory tests. A similar pattern was also observed on the Warrington Recognition Memory Test (WRMT), where JS performed poorly with both words and faces, whereas BW was only impaired on the faces subtest (see Table 1). We wish to emphasise that we do not claim that false recognition was necessarily face-specific in BW, only that it was specific to visual (pictorial) as opposed to verbal materials. In fact, BW did show evidence of general visual memory impairment on the WMS-III (see Table 1).

Although the results of Experiment 5 are consistent with material-specific false recognition in BW, there are some other possible interpretations. As noted earlier, frontal lobe involvement in episodic memory tests may only become critical under conditions where item-specific information is not readily available. For instance, in a PET study of verbal memory Schacter et al. (Schacter, Alpert, Savage, Rauch, & Albert, 1996a) observed greater prefrontal activation in conditions associated with low recall/high effort than in conditions characterised by high recall/low effort. Consistent with his good performance on verbal memory tasks in general (Table 1), BW probably had easy access to high-quality item-specific information in the recognition memory tests in Experiment 5 and may not have had to engage in the types of effortful memory retrieval, monitoring, and decision functions that normally depend on frontal lobe mechanisms. Therefore, in order to prove material-specificity, we need to demonstrate that BW also performs similar to controls under conditions of impoverished item-specific verbal memory.

Experiment 6

Procedure. In order to reduce memory accuracy, we tested recognition memory for verbal materials after a 48 hour delay. In the Study Phase, BW was asked to read a list of 32 high-frequency nouns (e.g. girl, tree) presented one at a time on the computer screen. Forty-eight hours later BW returned to the laboratory and was given an old/new recognition test using the items from the original study list mixed randomly with 32 high-frequency noun distractors. Five control subjects (age range = 43–53) were also tested under the same experimental conditions.

Results. The results of Experiment 6 are presented in Table 3. As can be seen from the Table, hit and false alarm rates for BW were both within normal range. Similarly, his Pr and Br scores were within the range of scores obtained by control subjects. These results indicate that in verbal memory tests the response strategy adopted by BW under conditions of poor discrimination was similar to the strategy used by normal controls.

Additional support for material-specificity comes from comparing BW's verbal memory performance in Experiment 6 to his performance on the eight-item face memory test in Experiment 1. Although his overall memory accuracy (Pr) was similar in the two experimental conditions (.48 vs. .44), he showed a more liberal response bias in the face memory test (.90) than in the verbal memory test (.62).

Table 3. *Hit (H) and False Alarm (FA) Rates and Discrimination (Pr) and Bias (Br) Scores in Experiments 5 and 6*

	Experiment 5				*Experiment 6*			
	H	*FA*	*Pr*	*Br*	*H*	*FA*	*Pr*	*Br*
Controls	.89	.09	.77	.45	.74	.38	.35	.59
(SD)	(.06)	(.09)	(.14)	(.09)	(.12)	(.14)	(.15)	(.16)
BW	.87	.02	.82	.27	.81	.31	.48	.62
JS	.88	.50	.36	.79	–	–	–	–

Discussion. Taken together, the results of Experiments 5 and 6 provide strong support for the hypothesis that false recognition in BW was specific to visual materials. These observations suggest that right prefrontal cortex plays a dominant role in memory retrieval, monitoring, and decision functions involving complex visual stimuli such as faces, whereas left prefrontal structures may perform similar cognitive operations for verbal materials. This interpretation of our data is of course perfectly consistent with classic notions of hemispheric functional specialisation (Bradshaw & Nettleton, 1981). However, our results seem to be at odds with recent PET studies, which demonstrated right prefrontal activation during memory retrieval for both verbal and visual stimuli in normal subjects (for reviews, see Cabeza & Nyberg, 1997; Nyberg, Cabeza, & Tulving, 1996). In order to reconcile the functional imaging data with the neuropsychological findings in patient BW, one might propose that right prefrontal cortex normally performs memory retrieval and monitoring operations for both verbal and visual materials. Left prefrontal areas, however, might be able to take over these functions for verbal (but apparently not for visual) stimuli following right frontal lobe damage. According to this view, the material-specificity observed in BW may be the result of functional compensation and neuronal plasticity.

Future studies of false recognition in patients with unilateral frontal lobe lesions should explore the issue of material-specificity in more detail. Such neuropsychological observations would provide a useful complement to the data from functional imaging studies in normal subjects and impose further constraints on theories about the neural basis of memory.

GENERAL DISCUSSION

Frontal lobe structures are not traditionally included in neuropsychological models of face recognition memory. This omission is probably due to the fact that damage to the frontal lobes does not result in the kind of pervasive face memory loss seen in prosopagnosia that has been the focus of intense neuropsychological investigation for over a century (Benton, 1990). It is well established, however, that in primates the temporal lobe visual areas implicated in face recognition (Desimone, 1991; Gross, 1992; Perrett, Hietanen, Oram, & Benson, 1992; Perrett et al., 1986) project to inferior convexity and ventromedial prefrontal cortex through both direct (via the uncinate fasciculus) and indirect limbo-thalamic pathways (via the amygdala, hippocampus, and the dorsomedian and anterior nuclei of the thalamus) (Mishkin, 1982; Tovée & Cohen-Tovée, 1993; Ungerleider, Gaffan, & Pelak, 1989). Furthermore, single cell recordings in monkeys have demonstrated that the inferior frontal convexity region, which receives input from temporal lobe visual areas, contains neurons that respond selectively to faces (Ó Scalaidhe, Wilson, & Goldman-Rakic, 1997; Wilson, Ó Scalaidhe, & Goldman-Rakic, 1993). Intracranial recordings of neural activity in humans have also documented differential responses in orbitofrontal and lateral prefrontal cortex to repeated versus nonrepeated faces in a continuous memory task (Seeck et al.,

1997a, b). Finally, prefrontal activation has been observed in a number of PET studies of face recognition memory (e.g. Courtney, Ungerleider, Keil, & Haxby, 1997; Grady et al., 1995; Haxby et al., 1996). However, the frontal lobe activations documented in the functional neuroimaging studies may not be face-specific, since the same cortical regions are also activated in memory tasks involving verbal materials and visual stimuli other than faces (Buckner, 1996; Cabeza & Nyberg, 1997; Nyberg et al., 1996).

Our findings suggest that the face memory disorder associated with right prefrontal damage is better characterised as memory distortion rather than memory loss. Memory illusions in response to novel faces were readily elicited in our frontal patients in both anterograde and retrograde tests of recognition memory. Although frontal subjects did demonstrate face memory impairment in the anterograde tests, it is noteworthy that patients with equivalent levels of item-specific face memory deficit following right temporal lobe damage produced fewer false recognition responses overall. Furthermore, frontal patients also produced numerous false recognition errors in the retrograde memory task, without evidence of significant retrograde face memory loss. Conversely, we have shown previously that patients with severe prosopagnosia following right temporal lobe damage do not produce false recognition errors in retrograde face memory paradigms (Rapcsak et al., 1994, 1996). Taken together, these observations suggest that face memory loss and false facial recognition are dissociable both at the behavioural and at the neuroanatomic level.

We propose that false facial recognition in frontal patients results from the breakdown of strategic memory retrieval, monitoring, and decision functions critical for attributing the experience of familiarity to its appropriate source. In particular, we suggest that right prefrontal cortex normally exerts executive control over face recognition by monitoring and verifying the various types of information retrieved from memory in response to the facial cue (Fig. 7). The putative frontal executive system receives information from two principal sources. The first of these corresponds to the signal generated by the face recognition module located within the right ventral occipito-temporal region (Allison et al., 1994; Kanwisher, McDermott, & Chun, 1997; McCarthy, Puce, Gore, & Allison, 1997; Puce, Allison, Asgari, Gore, & McCarthy, 1996; Sergent, Ohta, & McDonald, 1992). The face recognition module is a domain-specific perceptual recognition device that automatically compares current face percepts with representations of faces in memory. It is assumed that memory representations for previously encountered faces are stored within inferotemporal (IT) visual association cortex and that an interaction between IT cortex and the hippocampus is required for encoding new faces into memory. As noted earlier, damage to the face recognition module results in prosopagnosia, characterised by both retrograde and anterograde face memory loss.

Consistent with the characteristics of input modules in general (Fodor, 1983; Moscovitch, 1994), the face recognition module operates in a mandatory or "bottom-up" fashion and produces a shallow output that signals resemblance without specifying the source or providing the appropriate context for the sense of familiarity that accompanies the activation of memory representations. Thus, the module is not intrinsically capable of indicating whether the subjective experience of familiarity is due to the activation of a *specific* memory trace (e.g. the FRU for a particular familiar person, or the representation of a study face in a recognition memory experiment), or whether it reflects the *general* structural similarity between a novel face stimulus and representations in memory. In order to attribute facial familiarity to a specific source, additional contextual information must be retrieved. The product of the context retrieval process, therefore, provides the second major input to the frontal executive system (Fig. 7). In the case of familiar faces, context retrieval means gaining access to stored identity-specific biographic records (e.g. the person's occupation, name, etc.). In anterograde face memory tests context retrieval means activating information pertaining to the study episode. It is only when appropriate contextual information is recovered that we feel confident that the face had been successfully identified.

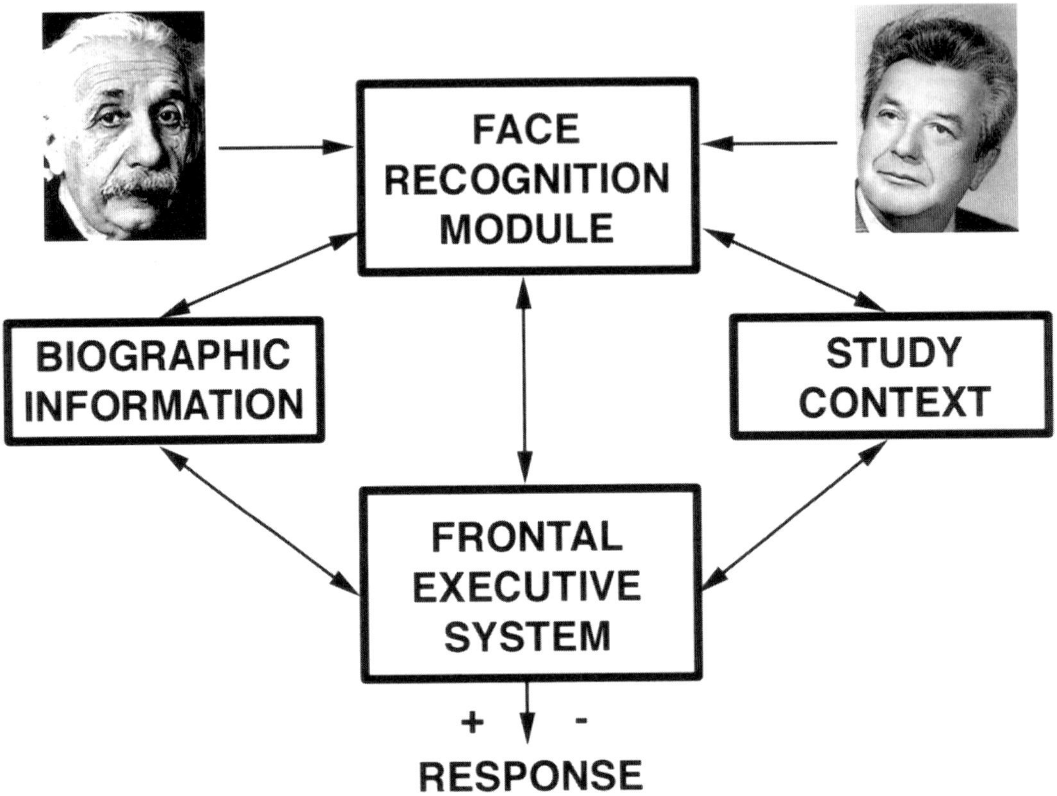

Fig. 7. *Simplified model of retrograde and anterograde face recognition memory.*

Although the frontal lobes normally have access to both the output of the face recognition module and the product of the context retrieval process, we do not wish to suggest that frontal lobe participation in face recognition is mandatory or that it occurs in an all-or-none fashion. As noted earlier, identity-specific biographic information is automatically available for most familiar faces under normal circumstances. Similarly, frontal lobe involvement is not essential when subjects have easy access to high-quality item-specific contextual information in episodic face memory tests. However, frontal lobe participation becomes critical under conditions of uncertainty when the face cue does not directly elicit relevant contextual information, leaving the source of familiarity unspecified (e.g. when we are not sure whether a familiar face is somebody we know, or when we can't decide whether or not a familiar looking face presented at test was on the original study list). In these situations the frontal executive system must initiate a strategic memory search (cf. Moscovitch, 1994) in order to reinstate the appropriate context for the feeling of familiarity evoked by the face. As we have seen, effortful recollection of specific contexts plays a critical role in opposing the influence of general facial familiarity on recognition judgements and provides the principal mechanism for suppressing false recognition. Patients with frontal lobe damage do not spontaneously engage in context recollection and tend to base recognition decisions on the shallow, context-free familiarity signal generated by the face recognition module, rendering them vulnerable to memory illusions. It remains an open question, however, whether frontal patients also have difficulty in evaluating the strength of the familiarity signal coming from the face recognition module. As noted earlier, it has been proposed that frontal lobe structures are involved in the monitoring and assessment of stimulus familiarity/novelty

(Metcalfe, 1993, 1994). Defective monitoring of the face familiarity signal may make it difficult to set appropriate decision criteria and may contribute to false recognition errors in patients with frontal lobe damage. Accurate monitoring of familiarity also plays an important role in metacognitive judgements of "feeling of knowing" (Metcalfe, 1993, 1994). Damage to prefrontal cortex is associated with impaired feeling of knowing judgements for information that is not immediately available in memory (Janowski, Shimamura, & Squire, 1989). It may be that impaired monitoring of facial familiarity creates a pathologically heightened feeling of knowing state in some frontal patients, promoting false recognition and reinforcing confidence in the reality of memory illusions.

False recognition of unfamiliar faces in patients with focal right frontal lobe damage has important implications for our understanding of the neuropsychological mechanisms underlying the age-related increase in false facial recognition errors in normal subjects (Bartlett & Fulton, 1991; Bartlett et al., 1989, 1991). To account for this phenomenon, Bartlett et al. (1991) proposed that elderly subjects may base face recognition judgements more on perceived familiarity and less on the recollection of contextual information. Our findings are consistent with the hypothesis that defective context recollection is a major factor in the pathogenesis of false facial recognition and suggest that face memory illusions in the elderly may be attributable to an age-related decline in right frontal lobe functioning.

Defective cognitive judgements of facial familiarity and personal identity also play a prominent role in the delusional misidentification syndromes (DMS) (e.g. Capgras delusion, Frégoli syndrome, intermetamorphosis). Patients with DMS frequently show neuropsychological evidence of face perception and memory impairment, consistent with right hemisphere dysfunction (H.D. Ellis & Young, 1990; Young, Ellis, Szulecka, & De Pauw, 1990). However, most patients with severe face perception and memory deficits following posterior right hemisphere damage are not delusional. Consequently, we believe that the bizarre memory distortions and reality monitoring failures that characterise DMS are primarily related to the breakdown of frontal supervisory and executive functions (cf. Benson & Stuss, 1990; Johnson, 1991; Johnson et al., 1993). In fact, neuroradiological evidence of right frontal lobe damage has been documented in a number of patients with DMS (Alexander, Stuss, & Benson, 1979; Forstl, Burns, Jacoby, & Levy, 1991; Malloy & Richardson, 1994; Rapcsak et al., 1994, 1996). In our experience, some patients with right frontal lobe damage only demonstrate false facial recognition (i.e. they claim that an unfamiliar face had been encountered before, but they cannot provide additional information or simply "guess" that it might be somebody from TV or the movies). Other patients, however, spontaneously confabulate in response to novel faces and produce false identity-specific biographic information resulting in frank misidentification. Misidentifications in some patients are also observed in real-life situations and in severe cases may reach delusional proportions (Rapcsak et al., 1994, 1996). In our view, false recognition, confabulation, and delusional misidentification represent a clinical continuum of increasingly severe memory distortions and reality monitoring failures attributable to right frontal lobe dysfunction.

Although we have focused primarily on false facial recognition in our discussion, we believe that the basic neuropsychological mechanisms of false recognition in frontal patients will be similar regardless of the stimulus category involved. A common theoretical interpretation of false recognition phenomena observed across a wide range of experimental stimuli seems plausible, given that the frontal lobes have the functional characteristics of "central systems" (Fodor, 1983) that perform strategic monitoring and control operations on the output generated by multiple domain-specific posterior cortical modules (Moscovitch, 1994; Stuss & Benson, 1986). This generic description of frontal lobe function, however, should not be taken to imply the existence of a single, general-purpose "executive faculty" that can be localised to a specific region within prefrontal cortex. In fact, the available neuropsychological evidence is more consistent with the view that there are several frontal supervisory and executive subsystems, each of which may be associated with a distinct neuroanatomic substrate (Parkin, 1998; Shallice & Burgess, 1996). In support of this hypothesis, studies in frontal patients have demonstrated low correlations between neuropsychological tests assumed to measure executive function, calling into question the usefulness of the concept of a general frontal "dysexecutive syndrome" (for reviews, see Parkin, 1998; Shallice & Burgess, 1996). Furthermore, individual case studies have shown that focal damage to prefrontal cortex may be associated with severe and pervasive impairments in strategic planning, problem solving, decision making, and social behaviour, even when performance on standard neuropsychological tests of frontal executive function is entirely within normal limits (e.g. Eslinger & Damasio, 1985; Shallice & Burgess, 1991).

Our cases provide additional empirical evidence that frontal executive functions are dissociable. We have shown that both JS and BW produced numerous memory distortions, consistent with the breakdown of putative frontal executive systems involved in the strategic control of conscious recollection. However, whereas JS was also severely impaired on standard tests of frontal executive function, BW obtained a perfect score on the WCST and performed within low normal range on the FAS (see Table 1). Similar dissociations are actually not all that uncommon in patients with false recognition and/or confabulation following prefrontal damage. For instance, BG (Schacter et al., 1996b) is described as showing moderate impairment on the WCST and the FAS, whereas JB (Parkin et al., 1996) performed within normal range on both of these tests, as well as on a number of other frontal lobe tests. RW (Delbecq-Derouesné et al., 1990) was impaired on the FAS, but he performed normally on the WCST and on several additional tests of frontal executive function. The opposite dissociation, normal FAS score but poor performance on the WCST, was reported by Moscovitch (1989) in the confabulating patient HW. These findings demonstrate that the breakdown of executive memory functions following prefrontal damage need not be part of a more general frontal "dysexecutive syndrome." Overall, the neuropsychological evidence reviewed here supports the view that prefrontal cortex comprises several functionally and anatomically distinct regions, each of which makes a unique contribution to the executive control of cognition and behaviour (Bechara, Damasio, Tranel, & Anderson, 1998; Goldman-Rakic, 1996; Parkin, 1998; Petrides, 1996; Shallice & Burgess, 1996). One of the major challenges facing contemporary cognitive neuroscience is to elucidate the functional role of the various prefrontal cortical subdivisions and determine how frontal executive systems interact with medical temporal lobe and posterior neocortical memory systems in providing strategic control over the constructive process of remembering past experiences.

REFERENCES

Alexander, M.P., Stuss, D.T., & Benson, D.F. (1979). Capgras syndrome: A reduplicative phenomenon. *Neurology*, *29*, 334–339.

Allison, T., Ginter, H., McCarthy, G., Nobre, A.C., Puce, A., Luby, M., & Spencer, D.D. (1994). Face recognition in human extrastriate cortex. *Journal of Neurophysiology*, *71*, 821–825.

Atkinson, R.C., & Juola, J.F. (1973). Factors influencing speed and accuracy of word recognition. In S. Kornblum (Ed.), *Attention and performance, IV* (pp. 583–611). New York: Academic Press.

Bartlett, J.C., & Fulton, A. (1991). Familiarity and recognition of faces in old age. *Memory and Cognition*, *19*, 229–238.

Bartlett, J.C., Hurry, S., & Thorley, W. (1984). Typicality and familiarity of faces. *Memory and Cognition*, *12*, 219–228.

Bartlett, J.C., Leslie, J.E., Tubbs, A., & Fulton, A. (1989). Aging and memory for pictures of faces. *Psychology of Aging*, *4*, 274–283.

Bartlett, J.C., Strater, L., & Fulton, A. (1991). False recency and false fame of faces in young adulthood and old age. *Memory and Cognition*, *19*, 177–188.

Bechara, A., Damasio, H., Tranel, D., & Anderson, S.W. (1998). Dissociation of working memory from decision making within the human prefrontal cortex. *Journal of Neuroscience*, *18*, 428–437.

Benson, D.F., & Stuss, D.T. (1990). Frontal lobe influences on delusions: A clinical perspective. *Schizophrenia Bulletin*, *16*, 403–411.

Benton, A. (1990). Facial recognition 1990. *Cortex*, *26*, 491–499.

Bradshaw, J.L., & Nettleton, N.C. (1981). The nature of hemispheric specialization in man. *Behavioral and Brain Sciences*, *4*, 51–91.

Brainerd, C.J., Reyna, V.F., & Kneer, R. (1995). False recognition reversal: When similarity is distinctive. *Journal of Memory and Language*, *34*, 157–185.

Bruce, V. (1988). *Recognising faces.* Hove, UK: Lawrence Erlbaum Associates Ltd.

Bruce, V., & Young, A. (1986). Understanding face recognition. *British Journal of Psychology*, *77*, 305–327.

Buckner, R.L. (1996). Beyond HERA: Contributions of specific prefrontal brain areas to long-term memory retrieval. *Psychonomic Bulletin and Review*, *3*, 149–158.

Cabeza, R., & Nyberg L. (1997). Imaging cognition: An empirical review of PET studies with normal subjects. *Journal of Cognitive Neuroscience*, *9*, 1–26.

Christodoulou, G.N. (1986). *The delusional misidentification syndromes.* Bibliotheca Psychiatrica No.164. Basel: Karger.

Courtney, S.M., Ungerleider, L.G., Keil, K., & Haxby, J.V. (1997). Transient and sustained activity in a distributed neural system for human working memory. *Nature*, *386*, 608–611.

Curran, T., Schacter, D.L., Norman, K.A., & Galluccio, L. (1997). False recognition after a right frontal lobe infarction: Memory for general and specific information. *Neuropsychologia*, *35*, 1035–1049.

Damasio, A.R., Tranel, D., & Damasio, H. (1990). Face agnosia and the neural substrates of memory. *Annual Review of Neuroscience*, *13*, 89–109.

Delbecq-Derouesné, J. Beauvois, M.F., & Shallice, T. (1990). Preserved recall versus impaired recognition: A case study. *Brain*, *113*, 1045–1074.

De Renzi, E., Perani, D., Carlesimo, G.A., Silveri, M.C., & Fazio, F. (1994). Prosopagnosia can be associated with damage confined to the right hemisphere—an MRI and PET study and a review of the literature. *Neuropsychologia*, *32*, 893–902.

Desimone, R. (1991). Face selective cells in the temporal cortex of monkeys. *Journal of Cognitive Neuroscience*, *3*, 1–18.

Dodson, C.S., & Johnson, M.K. (1993). Rate of false source attributions depends on how questions are asked. *American Journal of Psychology*, *106*, 541–557.

Ellis, A.W., Hillan, J.C., Cardno, A., & Kay, J. (1991). Processing of words and faces by patients with left and right temporal lobe epilepsy. *Behavioral Neurology*, *4*, 121–128.

Ellis, H.D., & Young, A.W. (1990). Accounting for delusional misidentifications. *British Journal of Psychology*, *157*, 239–248.

Eslinger, P.J., & Damasio, A.R. (1985). Severe disturbance of higher cognition after bilateral frontal lobe ablation: Patient EVR. *Neurology*, *35*, 1731–1741.

Fodor, J.A. (1983). *Modularity of mind.* Cambridge, MA: MIT Press.

Forstl, H., Burns, A., Jacoby, R., & Levy, R. (1991). Neuroanatomical correlates of misidentification and misperception in senile dementia of the Alzheimer type. *Journal of Clinical Psychiatry*, *52*, 268–271.

Glanzer, M., & Adams, J.K. (1985). The mirror effect in recognition memory. *Memory and Cognition*, *13*, 8–20.

Goldman-Rakic, P.S. (1996). The prefrontal landscape: Implications of functional architecture for understanding human mentation and the central executive. *Philosophical Transactions of the Royal Society of London (B)*, *351*, 1445–1454.

Grady, C.L., Macintosh, R.A., Horwitz, B., Maisog, J.M., Ungerleider, L.G., Mentis, M.J., Pietrini, P., Schapiro, M.B., & Haxby, J.V. (1995). Age-related reductions in human recognition memory due to impaired encoding. *Science*, *269*, 218–221.

Gross, C.G. (1992). Representation of visual stimuli in inferior temporal cortex. *Philosophical Transactions of the Royal Society of London (B)*, *335*, 23–30.

Haxby, J.V., Ungerleider, L.G., Horwitz, B., Maisog, J.M., Rapoport, S.I., & Grady, C.L. (1996). Face encoding and recognition in the human brain. *Proceedings of the National Academy of Science*, *93*, 922–927.

Hintzman, D.L., & Curran, T. (1994). Retrieval dynamics of recognition and frequency judgments: Evidence for separate processes of familiarity and recall. *Journal of Memory and Language*, *33*, 1–18.

Jacoby, L.L., & Dallas, M. (1981). On the relationship between autobiographical memory and perceptual learning. *Journal of Experimental Psychology: General*, *3*, 306–340.

Jacoby, L.L., & Kelley, C. (1992). Unconscious influences of memory: Dissociations and automaticity. In A.D. Milner & M.D. Rugg (Eds.), *The neuro-*

psychology of consciousness (pp. 201–233). London: Academic Press.
Jacoby, L.L., Kelley, C., Brown, J., & Jasechko, J. (1989). Becoming famous overnight: Limits on the ability to avoid unconscious influences of the past. *Journal of Personality and Social Psychology*, *56*, 326–338.
Janowski, J.S., Shimamura, A.P., & Squire, L.R. (1989). Memory and metamemory: Comparisons between frontal lobe lesions and amnesic patients. *Psychobiology*, *17*, 3–11.
Johnson, M.K. (1991). Reality monitoring: Evidence from confabulation in organic brain disease patients. In G.P. Prigitano & D.L. Schacter (Eds.), *Awareness of deficit after brain injury: Clinical and theoretical issues* (pp. 176–197). New York: Oxford University Press.
Johnson, M.K., Hashtroudi, S., & Lindsay, D.S. (1993). Source monitoring. *Psychological Bulletin*, *114*, 3–28.
Kanwisher, N., McDermott, J., & Chun, M.M. (1997). The fusiform face area: a module in human extrastriate cortex specialized for face perception. *Journal of Neuroscience*, *17*, 4302–4311.
Klatzky, R.L., Martin, G.L., & Kane, R.A. (1982). Semantic interpretation effects on memory for faces. *Memory and Cognition*, *10*, 195–206.
Koutstaal, W., & Schacter, D.L. (1997). Gist-based false recognition of pictures in older and younger adults. *Journal of Memory and Language*, *37*, 555–583.
Koutstaal, W., Schacter, D.L., Verfaellie, M., Brenner, C., & Jackson, E.M. (this issue). Perceptually based false recognition of novel objects in amnesia: Effects of category size and similarity to category prototypes. *Cognitive Neuropsychology*, *16*, 317–341.
Light, L.L., Kayra-Stuart, F., & Hollander, S. (1979). Recognition memory for typical and unusual faces. *Journal of Experimental Psychology: Human Learning and Memory*, *5*, 212–228.
Lindsay, D.S., & Johnson, M.K. (1989). The eyewitness suggestibility effect and memory for source. *Memory and Cognition*, *17*, 349–358.
Malloy, P.F., & Richardson, E.D. (1994). The frontal lobes and content-specific delusions. *Journal of Neuropsychiatry and Clinical Neurosciences*, *6*, 455–466.
Mandler, G. (1980). Recognizing: The judgment of previous occurrence. *Psychological Review*, *87*, 252–271.
McCarthy, G., Puce, A., Gore, J.C., & Allison, T. (1997). Face-specific processing in the human fusiform gyrus. *Journal of Cognitive Neuroscience*, *9*, 605–610.
McClelland, J.L., & Rumelhart, D.E. (1985). Distributed memory and the representation of general and specific information. *Journal of Experimental Psychology: General*, *114*, 159–188.
Metcalfe, J. (1993). Novelty monitoring, metacognition, and control in a holographic associative recall model: Implications for Korsakoff amnesia. *Psychological Review*, *100*, 3–22.
Metcalfe, J. (1994). A computational modeling approach to novelty monitoring, metacognition, and frontal lobe dysfunction. In J. Metcalfe & A.P. Shimamura (Eds.), *Metacognition: Knowing about knowing* (pp. 137–156). Cambridge, MA: MIT Press.
Milner, B., Corsi, P., & Leonard, G. (1991). Frontal lobe contribution to recency judgments. *Neuropsychologia*, *29*, 601–618.
Mishkin, M. (1982). A memory system in the monkey. *Philosophical Transactions of the Royal Society of London (B)*, *298*, 85–95.
Moscovitch, M. (1989). Confabulation and the frontal systems: Strategic versus associative retrieval in neuropsychological theories of memory. In H.L. Roediger III & F.I.M. Craik (Eds.), *Varieties of memory and consciousness: Essays in honour of Endel Tulving* (pp. 133–160). Hillsdale, NJ: Lawrence Erlbaum Associates Inc.
Moscovitch, M. (1994). Memory and working with memory: Evaluation of a component process model and comparisons with other models. In D.L. Schacter & E. Tulving (Eds.), *Memory systems 1994* (pp. 260–310). Cambridge, MA: MIT Press.
Multhaup, K.S. (1995). Aging, source, and decision criteria: When false fame errors do and do not occur. *Psychology and Aging*, *10*, 492–497.
Nyberg, L. Cabeza, R., & Tulving, E. (1996). PET studies of encoding and retrieval: The HERA model. *Psychonomic Bulletin and Review*, *3*, 135–148.
Ó Scalaidhe, S.P.O., Wilson, F.A.W., & Goldman-Rakic, P.S. (1997). Areal segregation of face-processing neurons in prefrontal cortex. *Science*, *278*, 1135–1138.
Parkin, A.J. (1998). The central executive does not exist. *Journal of the International Neuropsychological Society*, *4*, 518–522.
Parkin, A.J., Bindschaedler, C., Harsent, L., & Metzler, C. (1996). Pathological false alarm rates following

damage to the left frontal cortex. *Brain and Cognition*, *32*, 14–27.

Perrett, D.I., Hietanen, J.K., Oram, M.W., & Benson, P.J. (1992). Organization and function of cells responsive to faces in the temporal cortex. *Philosophical Transactions of the Royal Society of London (B)*, *335*, 23–30.

Perrett, D.I., Mistlin, A.J., Potter, D.D., Smith, P.A.J., Head, A.S., Chitty, A.J., Broennimann, R., Milner, A.D., & Jeeves, M.A.J. (1986). Functional organization of neurones processing face identity. In H.D. Ellis, M.A. Jeeves, F. Newcombe, & A. Young (Eds.), *Aspects of face processing* (pp. 187–198. Dordrecht, The Netherlands: Martinus Nijhoff.

Petrides, M. (1996). Specialized systems for the processing of mnemonic information within the primate frontal cortex. *Philosophical Transactions of the Royal Society of London (B)*, *351*, 1455–1462.

Puce, A., Allison, T., Asgari, M., Gore, J.C., & McCarthy, G. (1996). Differential sensitivity of human visual cortex to faces, letter strings, and textures: A functional magnetic resonance imaging study. *Journal of Neuroscience*, *16*, 5205–5215.

Rapcsak, S.Z., Kaszniak, A.W., Reminger, S.L., Glisky, M.L., Glisky, E.L., & Comer, J.F. (1998). Dissociation between verbal and autonomic measures of memory following frontal lobe damage. *Neurology*, *50*, 1258–1265.

Rapcsak, S.Z., Polster, M.R., Comer, J.F., & Rubens, A.B. (1994). False recognition and misidentification of faces following right hemisphere damage. *Cortex*, *30*, 565–583.

Rapcsak, S.Z., Polster, M.R., Glisky, M.L., & Comer, J.F. (1996). False recognition of unfamiliar faces following right hemisphere damage: Neuropsychological and anatomical observations. *Cortex*, *32*, 593–611.

Schacter, D.L. (1987). Memory, amnesia and frontal lobe dysfunction. *Psychobiology*, *15*, 21–36.

Schacter, D.L., Alpert, M.N., Savage, C.R., Rauch, S.L., & Albert, M.S. (1996a). Conscious recollection and the human hippocampal formation: Evidence from positron emission tomography. *Proceedings of the National Academy of Science*, *93*, 321–325.

Schacter, D.L., Curran, T., Galluccio, L., Milberg, W.P., & Bates, J.F. (1996b). False recognition and the right frontal lobe: A case study. *Neuropsychologia*, *34*, 793–808.

Schacter, D.L., Israel, L., & Racine, C. (1999). Suppressing false recognition in younger and older adults: The distinctiveness heuristic. *Journal of Memory and Language*, *40*, 1–24.

Schacter, D.L., Verfaellie, M., & Anes, M.D. (1997). Illusory memories in amnesic patients: Conceptual and perceptual false recognition. *Neuropsychology*, *11*, 331–342.

Schacter, D.L., Verfaellie, M., Anes, M.D., & Racine, C. (1998). When true recognition suppresses false recognition: Evidence from amnesic patients. *Journal of Cognitive Neuroscience*, *10*, 668–679.

Schacter, D.L., Verfaellie, M., & Pradere, D. (1996c). The neuropsychology of memory illusions: False recall and recognition in amnesic patients. *Journal of Memory and Language*, *35*, 319–334.

Searcy, J.H., Bartlett, J.C., & Memon, A. (in press). Age differences in accuracy and choosing in eyewitness identification and face recognition. *Memory and Cognition*.

Seeck, M., Mainwaring, N., Cosgrove, R., Blume, H., Dubuisson, D., Mesulam, M.-M., & Schomer, D.L. (1997a). Neurophysiologic correlates of implicit face memory in intracranial visual evoked potentials. *Neurology*, *49*, 1312–1316.

Seeck, M., Michel, C.M., Mainwaring, N., Cosgrove, R., Blume, H., Ives, J., Landis, T., & Schomer, D.L. (1997b). Evidence for rapid face recognition from human scalp and intracranial electrodes. *NeuroReport*, *8*, 2749–2754.

Sergent, J. (1984). An investigation into component and configural processes underlying face perception. *British Journal of Psychology*, *75*, 221–242.

Sergent, J., Ohta, S., & MacDonald, B. (1992). Functional neuroanatomy of face and object processing: A positron emission tomography study. *Brain*, *115*, 15–36.

Sergent, J., & Signoret, J.-L. (1992). Varieties of functional deficits in prosopagnosia. *Cerebral Cortex*, *2*, 375–388.

Shallice, T., & Burgess, P.W. (1991). Deficits in strategy application following frontal lobe damage in man. *Brain*, *114*, 727–741.

Shallice, T., & Burgess, P.W. (1996). The domain of supervisory processes and temporal organization of behavior. *Philosophical Transactions of the Royal Society of London (B)*, *351*, 1405–1411.

Snodgrass, J.G., & Corwin, J. (1988). Pragmatics of measuring recognition memory: Applications to

dementia and amnesia. *Journal of Experimental Psychology: General*, *117*, 34–50.
Stuss, D.T., & Benson, D.F. (1986). *The frontal lobes.* New York: Raven Press.
Tovée, M.J., & Cohen-Tovée, E.M. (1993). The neural substrates of face processing models: A review. *Cognitive Neuropsychology*, *10*, 505–528.
Ungerleider, L.G., Gaffan, D., & Pelak, V.S. (1989). Projections from inferior temporal cortex to prefrontal cortex via the uncinate fascicle in rhesus monkeys. *Experimental Brain Research*, *76*, 473–484.
Valentine, T., & Bruce, V. (1986). The effects of distinctiveness in recognising and classifying faces. *Perception*, *15*, 525–535.
Valentine, T., & Ferrara, A. (1991). Typicality in categorization, recognition and identification: Evidence from face recognition. *British Journal of Psychology*, *82*, 87–102.
Vokey, J.R., & Read, J.D. (1992). Familiarity, memorability, and the effect of typicality on the recognition of faces. *Memory and Cognition*, *20*, 291–302.
Wilson, F.A.W., Ó Scalaidhe, S.P., & Goldman-Rakic, P.S. (1993). Dissociation of object and spatial processing domains in primate prefrontal cortex. *Science*, *260*, 1955–1958.
Young, A.W., De Haan, E.H.F., & Newcombe, F. (1990). Unawareness of impaired face recognition. *Brain and Cognition*, *14*, 1–18.
Young, A.W., Ellis, H.D., Szulecka, T.K., & De Pauw, K.W. (1990). Face processing impairments and delusional misidentification. *Behavioral Neurology*, *3*, 153–168.
Young, A.W., Flude, B.M., Hay, D.C., & Ellis, A.W. (1993). Impaired discrimination of familiar from unfamiliar faces. *Cortex*, *29*, 65–75.
Young, A.W., Hay, D.C., & Ellis, A.W. (1985). The faces that launched a thousand slips: Everyday difficulties and errors in recognizing people. *British Journal of Psychology*, *76*, 495–523.

COGNITIVE NEUROPSYCHOLOGY, 1999, 16 (3/4/5), 293–315

FALSE RECOGNITION OF UNFAMILIAR PEOPLE: "SEEING FILM STARS EVERYWHERE"

Jamie Ward, Alan J. Parkin, Georgia Powell, Ella J. Squires, and Julia Townshend
University of Sussex, Brighton, UK
Veronica Bradley
Hurstwood Park Neurology Centre, Haywards Heath, UK

A patient (MR) is reported who is able to correctly recognise famous people as being familiar but has a strong tendency to falsely recognise unfamiliar people as being familiar. False recognition does not depend on the type of person involved (contemporary, historical, fictional) or the modality in which it is presented (face, spoken/written name). False recognition does not extend to vocabulary knowledge, to other proper name categories (e.g. places) or to news events. Several hypotheses are considered but discounted. False recognition does not reflect reliance on familiarity associated with parts of the stimuli as opposed to the whole. False recognition, instead, depends critically on the nature of the referent (i.e. whether it refers to a person or not) and not on the nature of the stimulus material. Thus, MR will not produce false recognition when asked to search for names that *refer* to song or book titles even when, in all other respects, the stimuli resemble the names of people (e.g. Eleanor Rigby, David Copperfield). It is suggested that this disorder stems from a top-down failure to regulate the person recognition system, such that inappropriate information is retrieved. The category specificity may reflect inappropriate use of meta-memory knowledge concerning the rate of potential new exemplars from the category of "people" relative to other categories.

INTRODUCTION

Memory researchers have recently become more interested in so-called false or illusory memory, in which subjects "remember" information that *was not* present at acquisition. Examples of this, in both the normal and neurological populations, include a tendency to falsely recognise nonpresented stimuli as being previously presented (normals: Roediger & McDermott, 1995; patients: Parkin, Bindschaedler, Harsent, & Metzler, 1996), misattributing the source of one's knowledge to another event (normals: Johnson, Hashtroudi, & Lindsay, 1993; patients: Janowsky, Shimamura, & Squire, 1989), or the recollection of an entire "fictitious" episode (normals: Hyman & Pentland, 1996; patients: Dalla Barba, 1993a—confabulation). Memory distortions such as these are of theoretical importance since they are assumed to derive from intrinsic properties of the normally functioning system and, as such, may shed light on the underlying mechanisms of veridical remembering (e.g. McClelland, 1995; Parkin, 1997; Roediger, 1996; Schacter, 1995; Schacter, Norman, & Koutstaal, 1998).

Several recent studies have documented pathological false recognition of distractor items in single

Requests for reprints should be addressed to Jamie Ward, Laboratory of Experimental Psychology, University of Sussex, Falmer, Brighton, BN1 9QG, UK [Tel: (01273) 678071; Fax: (01273) 678611; E-mail: jamiew@biols.susx. ac.uk].
This research was funded by a Human Frontiers grant (RG-126/97). We are grateful to Stephen Rapcsak and Chad Dodson for comments on an earlier draft, and to MR for his patience with many hours of testing.

probe recognition memory tasks in patients with frontal lobe lesions (Delbecq-Derouesné, Beauvois, & Shallice, 1990; Parkin et al., 1996; Parkin, Ward, Bindschaedler, Squires, & Powell, this issue; Schacter, Curran, Galluccio, Milberg, & Bates, 1996). For instance, patient JB was given a series of target unfamiliar faces to remember and was later given a single probe (yes/no) recognition memory test consisting of the previously seen targets and nonpresented distractors (Parkin et al., 1996). JB was able to correctly recognise the target faces as well as controls, but falsely recognised up to half of the distractors as being previously presented. He appeared to be as confident about his false recognitions as his true recognitions. This pattern was found for a variety of stimulus types (faces, abstract designs, words, nonwords). Parkin et al. (this issue) explained JB's pattern in terms of an episodic encoding deficit, such that he tends to encode more superficial features of stimuli, which tend to be shared by many items (including distractors), but fails to encode item-specific information. In support of this, JB was shown to benefit from encoding manipulations (orienting instructions) and does not show false recognition when asked to distinguish between famous and nonfamous people. That is, JB produces false recognition if given a series of faces to memorise and later asked to distinguish between seen and unseen faces (or names, words, etc.), but does not show false recognition when asked to distinguished between famous and nonfamous faces (or names). However, a number of patients have been reported in the literature who show the latter phenomenon. This study will also document such a patient.

First of all, it is important to distinguish between false recognition and misidentification. Following Rapcsak, Polster, Comer, and Rubens (1994), we define false recognition as an incorrect affirmative judgement of previous encounters with an unfamiliar person (or item), whereas misidentification is used when identity-specific semantic or name information is elicited by an unfamiliar person. There are clearly grey areas in between these definitions; for instance, if an unfamiliar person is falsely recognised as familiar but only very general semantic information is reported (e.g. appeared on TV). The term misidentification will be reserved for those instances in which it is clear with whom the unfamiliar person is being confused.

Young, Flude, Hay, and Ellis (1993) described a patient, JT, who was able to name and identify famous faces normally (given enough time) but showed a strong tendency to classify unfamiliar faces as familiar. He would often attribute semantic information to the unfamiliar faces (e.g. Russian politician) and would occasionally produce an outright misidentification of a specific named familiar person. However, when given the same items in the form of written names he was able to correctly reject all the nonfamous items. There was some evidence of perceptual problems in face processing, as shown by poor performance on the Benton test of matching unfamiliar faces across viewing conditions and poor recognition of familiar faces under speeded conditions. Young et al. (1993) concluded that JT had a malfunction of the face recognition units (FRUs). The FRUs are responsible for computing an index of similarity between an abstract face description at the structural encoding stage and stored representations of familiar faces (Bruce & Young, 1986). Although the precise nature of the FRU malfunction was not specified, subsequent studies of similar patients have suggested that such patients may adopt a feature-based processing style (Rapcsak et al., 1994).

Rapcsak et al. (1994) document two patients (WJ and BH) with right-hemisphere frontoparietal damage. Both patients had a tendency to falsely recognise unfamiliar faces as familiar, and would also produce outright misidentifications of both familiar and unfamiliar faces (BH also showed some tendency to falsely recognise voices). However, they performed normally with unfamiliar names. An important characteristic of their performance was a tendency to base familiarity judgements on parts of the face (e.g. nose, hairline) rather than the whole. This was found in other tasks involving faces (e.g. same–different matching tasks) and also in a nonfacial task, for instance, failing to identify a larger letter "E" when the letter is constructed out of smaller letter "O"s. Rapcsak et al. concluded that the patients were unable to process stimuli globally due to their right-hemisphere damage, and were relying on the left hemisphere, which processes the stimuli in component parts (see also Parkin & Williamson, 1987; Patterson & Bradshaw, 1975). In terms of Bruce and Young's (1986) functional architecture, Rapcsak et al. (1994) proposed that a failure of "global" structural encoding leads to individual facial features spuriously activating one or more FRUs, resulting in a false sense of familiarity. Rapcsak et al. also extended this explanation to JT (Young et al., 1993), whose performance was generally slow and severely affected by time constraints, suggestive of a serial, feature-by-feature strategy.

In addition to a difficulty in structural encoding, Rapcsak et al. (1994) postulated that their falsely recognising patients have a deficit to frontally associated decision mechanisms. This has been the focus of investigation in later studies by Rapcsak and colleagues (Rapcsak et al., 1998; Rapcsak, Polster, Glisky, & Comer, 1996; Rapcsak, Reminger, Glisky, Kaszniak, & Comer, this issue). Rapcsak et al. (1996) studied the relationship between false recognition of unfamiliar faces and prosopagnosia (i.e. impaired recognition of familiar faces) in 21 cases of right-hemisphere damage. Most patients demonstrated prosopagnosia without any false recognition tendency, and some patients showed both a tendency for false recognition and some evidence of prosopagnosia (as in the cases described earlier). However, one patient (Case 21; right prefrontal damage) was able to identify familiar faces at a normal level, was able to match faces across viewing conditions, had good recognition memory for faces (Warrington Recognition Memory Test; Warrington, 1984) but falsely recognised 40% of the unfamiliar faces as familiar. They concluded that this patient cannot be explained by degraded perceptual input to FRUs or damage to the FRUs themselves, but that there has been a breakdown of frontal/executive memory functions involved in strategic memory search, monitoring, and decision making. Specifically, Rapcsak et al. (1996; this issue) suggest that unfamiliar faces may evoke a false sense of familiarity because of physical resemblances to known people. In normal subjects, this uncertainty may be resolved by attempting to retrieve more detailed contextual information (e.g. their occupation, specific previous encounters) in order to support or discount the recognition judgement. Rapcsak et al. (this issue) assume that some frontal lobe patients, however, may not spontaneously initiate this memory search and therefore produce high levels of false recognition based on "gist" or familiarity information.

There are, however, a number of difficulties with this interpretation. First, if the face recognition system is intact, as they suggest, then we need to assume that the output of the system is under normal circumstances very noisy; such that many/most unfamiliar faces incorrectly trigger FRUs and require some frontal mediation[1]. Second, it is not clear to what extent their patients' false recognition deficits are face-specific, since performance on retrograde tests of memory with names or other material were not reported (although some patients show some material-specificity in anterograde recognition tests; BW—Rapcsak et al., this issue). The potential implications of such a result being that there is such a thing as "face-specific decision mechanism" within the frontal lobes.

This paper will address the issues raised by studying another patient (MR) with damage to the prefrontal cortex who also shows false recognition of people. This patient, like the ones described by Rapcsak et al. (1996, 1998, this issue), shows false

[1] Rapcsak et al. (this issue) suggest that face/person recognition is largely automatic and that frontal mechanisms are needed only in those circumstances in which there is a conflict/ambiguity to resolve. If this is the case, then the fact that these frontal patients produce false recognition levels of over 40% implies that normally over 40% of faces lead to some sort of conflict requiring frontal mediation. That is, the level of noise in the system is naturally very high. Obviously, there is *some* noise in the system. as shown by the fact that normals occasionally produce false recognition (Young, Hay, & Ellis, 1985). However, it seems unlikely to us that the face recognition system could naturally be over 40% error prone. It could be the case that the noise is *induced* by a top-down failure to regulate the system (for example, a failure to inhibit competing items or a failure to specify an appropriate termination of the search/recognition process), rather than a failure of a terminal "decision-making" or "problem-solving" device that is operating on an intrinsically noisy output. See later discussion.

recognition of unfamiliar people without prosopagnosia. However, MR's deficit is found for people's names as well as faces but does not extend to all other domains (e.g. place names). The implications to models of person recognition and the frontal lobes and memory will be discussed.

CASE BACKGROUND

MR is a 53-year-old, right-handed man previously employed as a professional photographer. His difficulties started in 1991, with a right homonymous quadrantinopia and spasms of the right arm and leg. A CT scan suggested a small lacunar infarct in the lentiform nucleus, and a diagnosis of stroke was originally offered. He began complaining of memory problems at this time, for both remote and recent memory. He was also concerned that he was remembering things that he had not done and recognising people that he did not know. For this reason he requested referral to a psychiatrist, in 1993, who concluded that these "memories" did not have a psychiatric origin. An MRI scan in 1995 showed an increased signal immediately above the body of the left lateral ventricle and adjacent to the left frontal horn. No evidence of basal ganglia infarct was seen. However, precise clinico-pathological correlations may not be possible in this case and, given that the MRI scan is somewhat old, we cannot unequivocally state that the lesion is restricted to the left frontal lobe. A diagnosis of multiple sclerosis (MS) was subsequently offered and confirmed by the presence of oligoclonal bands in the cerebriospinal fluid. MS is a disease of the nervous system resulting in demyelation followed by gliosis. There is no agreed cognitive profile for this disorder, although Richardson (1996) estimates that 10% of the MS population have memory impairments and deficits in executive function have also been reported (Canellopoulou & Richardson, 1998).

General Cognitive Abilities

MR is well oriented in space and time. On the Graded Naming Test (McKenna & Warrington, 1983) he scored 22/30 and 28.30 on two separate occasions, placing him in the "bright normal" and "superior" range. His performance on the Wechsler Adult Intelligence Scale-Revised (Wechsler, 1981) on two separate occasions is detailed in Table 1a. His most recent Full Scale IQ of 96 shows some general cognitive decline relative to his estimated pre-morbid IQ of 121 (NART; Nelson, 1985). He has a forwards digit span of 6 and backwards digit span of 4.

Memory

MR's performance on the Wechsler Memory Scale-Revised (WMS-R; Wechsler, 1984) on two separate occasions is detailed in Table 1b. MR shows a moderate impairment on every index of the scale and has shown signs of deterioration over the course of 2 years. On the Rey-Osterreith figure (Rey, 1964), his performance was normal on copying (40th percentile) but impaired on both immediate and delayed recall (<10th percentile).

MR's remote memory was assessed using the Autobiographical Memory Interview (Kopelman, Wilson, & Baddeley, 1990). His ability to recall personal semantic information (e.g. previous addresses) was borderline-to-poor (42.5/63; childhood = 15.5/21, early adult life = 8.5/21, recent life = 18.5/21). However, his ability to recall autobiographical incidents was in the acceptable-to-borderline range (18/27; childhood = 5/9, early adult life = 5/9, recent life = 8/9).

A somewhat different pattern of performance emerges on tests of recognition memory. In the Pictorial/Topographical Memory Test (Warrington, 1996) the subject is shown a series of scenes and is given a three-way forced-choice recognition test involving perceptually similar or perceptually distinct distractors. MR's scores of 56% (17/30) and 27% (8/30) on the perceptually distinct and perceptually similar conditions places him below the 1st percentile on both tests. On the Warrington Recognition Test (Warrington, 1984) he was at chance with both words (27/50) and faces (21/50). These scores are normally indicative of a dense amnesic syndrome. However, MR does not give the impression of being amnesic despite having significant

Table 1. *MR's Performance on the WAIS and WMS-R on Two Separate Occasions*

WAIS[a]			*WMS-R*[b]			
	1998	*1995*		*1998*	*1996*	*K*
Information	9	10	*Percentiles*			
Digit Span	9	6	Digits Forward	28	67	
Vocabulary	11	15	Digits Backward	51	29	
Arithmetic	10	5	Visual Span Forward	< 2	34	
Comprehension	9	16	Visual Span Backward	8	8	
Similarities	11	10	Logical Memory	18	29	
Picture Completion	11	9	Logical Memory Delay	12	26	
Picture Arrangement	8	7	Visual Reproduction	66	79	
Block Design	9	9	Visual Reproduction Delay	12	38	
Object Assembly	9	9	*Indices*			
Digit Symbol	7	6	Verbal Memory	82	91	(70)
Verbal IQ =	98	103	Visual Memory	86	103	(77)
Performance IQ =	93	96	General Memory	81	94	(68)
Full Scale =	96	100	Delayed Recall	79	87	(57)
			Attention/Concentrates	73	93	(91)

[a]Range = 1–19 for age-scaled scores; Mean score = 10.
[b]Mean scores for Indices = 100; K = mean score of 8 Korsakoff patients (Wechsler, 1984).

memory problems. For instance, he has no difficulty in identifying new members of the research team and is able to recall specific incidents from testing sessions.

He is also impaired on single probe recognition memory tests, and shows a pattern characterised by pathological false alarm rates. For instance, on the face recognition and abstract designs tests described by Parkin et al. (1996) he produced mean hit rates of 89% and 97% respectively (controls = 86% and 88%) and false alarm rates of 50% and 58% respectively (controls = 12 and 19%).

In short, MR has a memory deficit characterised by patchy retrieval of the past together with a severe deficit in recognition memory. These characteristics are often associated with frontal memory impairments (e.g. Parkin et al., this issue; Parkin, Yeomans, & Bindschaedler, 1994; Schacter et al., 1996).

Frontal Tests

Behaviourally, MR shows some signs of frontal damage. He sometimes has difficulty in organising complex action sequences (e.g. accidentally pouring milk into a teapot), indicative of frontal apraxia (e.g. Schwartz et al., 1995). On formal testing MR shows, at worst, only a mild impairment on tasks sensitive to frontal function.

On the Wisconsin Card Sorting Test (Nelson, 1976) he managed four categories and his difficulty was attributable to him forgetting what the current rule was (nine nonperseverative errors) rather than an inability to shift set (three perseverations). On the Stroop (Trenerry, Crosson, DeBoe, & Leber, 1989) he was at the 12th percentile. On the Hayling Sentence Completion Test (Burgess & Shallice, 1996b), which requires the subject to generate a non obvious answer to complete a sentence (e.g. "London is a very busy.."—car) he was in the moderate-average range. On the Brixton Spatial Anticipation Test (Burgess & Shallice, 1996a), which requires the subject to detect and use rules to predict locations, he was in the low-average range (21 errors). He scored seven (borderline impaired) and four (unimpaired) on the Cognitive Estimates Test (Shallice & Evans, 1978) when tested in 1995 and 1998 respectively. On the FAS test of verbal fluency (Benton & Hamsher, 1976) he scored 32 and 43 in 1995 and 1998 respectively. He was able to identify 11 and 16 alternate uses for 6 common objects on the Alternate Uses Test (Guildford, Christensen,

Merrifield, & Wilson, 1978) in 1995 and 1998 (unimpaired). He made no errors on trail-making (Reitan, 1971), his times being 60sec and 103sec in the no-switch and switch conditions respectively (unimpaired).

Recognition of Faces/People

This study was motivated by an observation that MR made during testing, stating that he often mistakes unfamiliar people for people who are famous or otherwise familiar to him. When coming across *unfamiliar* people in the street he would often remark to his wife "isn't that somebody?", thinking that it was either a personal acquaintance or somebody who is famous from TV. This would occur several times on a typical outing. He has previously approached people asking them which TV programme they are on, but has stopped doing this to avoid embarrassment. MR describes it as like "seeing film stars everywhere". When asked by the experimenter if he identifies these strangers as somebody in particular, recollecting a name or a specific film/programme, he states that this doesn't happen often (5–10% of occasions, according to self-report) and, instead, he just has a general idea of who the person is.

In contrast, when coming across *familiar* people in everyday settings he claims to be aware of who the person is (e.g. their name, occupation) and does not mistake them for somebody unfamiliar or another person known to him. However, he reports a consistent tendency for underestimating the time between the current encounter with this person and the last encounter (forward telescoping; e.g. Rubin & Baddeley, 1989); saying things like "isn't it funny that I should bump into you again, I only saw you yesterday", when in fact he hadn't seen them for a long while.

MR's perceptual processing of faces was assessed using the Mooney faces, a task involving visual closure in which the subject must point to the nose of an abstract/silhouette face (Parkin, 1998a). His score of 19/30 was normal for his age (12 controls, 44–59 years old; mean score = 24.30, SD = 5.15). MR was given the Sussex Test of Remote Memory for faces. (STORM-F; Parkin, 1998b) in which he was required to name faces from various decades. His score of 60% (37/60) was considered to be normal. Ten control subjects (mean age = 53.9) produced an average score of 66.5% (SD = 15.3). MR, like controls, showed no evidence of a temporal gradient (1950s = 6/12; 1950s = 9/12; 1970s = 7/12; 1980s = 8/12; 1990s = 7/12). His ability to generate imagery of faces was also good. He was given the "faces of celebrities" imagery test of Hanley, Young, & Pearson (1991) in which the subject must decide which of two named people (e.g. Robert Mitchum/Charles Bronson) looks most like a third named person (e.g. John Wayne). MR's score of 15/20 compares well with the controls reported by Hanley et al. (1991), (mean = 16.3, SD = 3.2). MR was given the Ekman and Friesen (1976) faces of facial expression, in which a single face should be matched to one of six written labels (happiness, surprise, fear, sadness, disgust, anger). MR was impaired on three out of six categories (impaired: fear = 1/10, sadness = 5/10, disgust = 4/10; unimpaired: anger = 6/10, happiness = 10/10, surprise = 9/10; controls from Calder et al., 1996).

MR's false recognition was initially investigated by giving him a series of 30 unfamiliar faces with no familiar faces present (as in Rapcsak et al., 1996) and asking him to decide who appears familiar and who does not. MR claimed that 73% (22/30) were familiar to him. He found the task frustrating, commenting "This can't be right. There must be somebody here who isn't famous. I get so desperate to try and find somebody who I feel that I haven't seen before".

In summary, preliminary assessments suggest that MR is not prosopagnosic (i.e. he can recognise familiar faces), although he does have some face-processing difficulties for expression. MR's false recognition of unfamiliar people forms the basis of this investigation.

This study was conducted from July–October 1998, during which time his physical and mental health was considered to be good and stable. He was fully mobile during this period and able to live an independent life, cooking and shopping for himself, and even organising visits abroad. MR has been lucid throughout testing and demonstrates a high level of awareness of his difficulties.

EXPERIMENTAL INVESTIGATION

We will first attempt to assess MR's false recognition deficit formally and then go on to assess in more detail whether his memory representations of known people have been compromised. We will then consider possible explanations of this phenomenon.

False Recognition of Unfamiliar People

Experiment 1: Famous Faces
In this experiment subjects are shown a sequence of faces one at a time and must decide whether a person is familiar or not (single probe frame decision).

Subjects. MR and 10 control subjects participated. Control subjects for this experiment, and all subsequent experiments (unless otherwise stated), were drawn from a larger pool of 20 subjects matched approximately to MR for age (45–60) and NART IQ (all had scores above 100). Each subject participated in at least one experiment, although no one subject participated in them all.

Materials and Procedure. This test consists of a modified single-probe version of Townshend's test of famous faces. The test contains 57 famous faces from the 1950s to the 1990s and 57 unfamiliar faces. The unfamiliar faces were matched on a one-to-one basis to the famous faces in terms of sex, approximate age, image size, and general appearance (e.g. wearing a hat, beard, posture). In this version of the test, the faces were printed on individual sheets and given to MR in a randomised order for a frame-decision.

Results and Discussion. He correctly recognised 98% (56/57) of the famous faces as familiar, but incorrectly recognised 77% (44/57) of unfamiliar faces as familiar. Control subjects produced true and false recognition rates of 85.3% (SD = 7.5) and 14.4% (SD = 11.2) respectively. We will adopt a 2 SD difference between MR and controls as a cut off measure of impairment throughout. As such, MR was impaired on unfamiliar face rejection ($z = -5.59$) but not familiar face recognition ($z = +1.69$).

The next experiments will assess whether this pattern is restricted to faces or extends to names.

Experiment 2: Contemporary Famous Names
Both of these tests have previously been described by Parkin et al. (1999) and had been given to JB, another frontal lobe patient, who does not show false recognition under these circumstances.

Method. The names of 40 famous people (e.g. Mary Quant) together with 40 nonfamous people (e.g. Alex Morrison) were scattered randomly onto a sheet of A4 paper and MR was asked to circle only the famous ones. This test was also administered in a separate session using spoken names instead of written names.

A harder version involved 40 real pop singers/groups (e.g. Leapy Lee) together with 40 unfamiliar singers/groups (e.g. Sharon Sugar) arranged randomly on to a single sheet of paper. The distractors were not truly fictitious, but were taken from record catalogues on the basis that they had never become famous. This was done to ensure that the names were as plausible as possible.

Results and Discussion. MR was unimpaired at identifying the written famous names and groups, with true recognition rates of 100% and 70% respectively (mean and SD of 10 controls: 96.0% [4.4] and 51.0% [10.0]). However, he showed a pathological tendency to classify the nonfamous names and groups as famous, with false recognition rates of 62.5% and 30.0% respectively (controls: 2.3% [3.4] and 2.0% [3.3]). The fact that MR's true recognition rate is significantly lower in the hard task [$\chi^2(1) = 11.09$, $P < .01$], as it was for controls [$t(9) = 14.5$, $P < .001$], suggests that this pattern of affirmative responding is not arbitrary but is related to the demands of the task. A similar pattern emerged with spoken famous and unfamiliar names: true recognition = 100% (40/40), false recognition = 45% (18.40).

Experiment 3: Historical Figures
Historical figures are likely to have different representational characteristics to contemporary people (e.g. Lucchelli, Muggia, & Spinnler, 1997). For

instance, they may be less likely to evoke a visual image and they are generally acquired earlier (in school years) than contemporary figures, who are acquired over the course of a lifetime. MR's performance with historical names was therefore assessed.

Method. Twenty British historical figures were selected (e.g. Duke of Wellington, Oliver Cromwell) and 20 distractor names were constructed to sound like plausible historical figures (e.g. Lady Jane Darnley, Horatio Felles). The names were randomly ordered and MR was required to circle those names who he considered to be famous historical figures.

Results and Discussion. MR claimed to have a good knowledge of history and indeed he was able to correctly recognise all (100%, 20/20) of the historical names. Controls ($N = 10$) correctly recognised 88.0% (SD = 5.9). However, he also produced an exceptionally high level of false recognition to the distractors (70%, 14/20) relative to controls (6.5%, SD = 4.1).

In short, Experiments 1–3 have demonstrated that MR falsely recognises unfamiliar people regardless of input modality (faces, spoken/written names), and without regard to the type of person involved (contemporary, historical). Although MR's levels of true recognition are normal, the next section will investigate whether this belies a more subtle difficulty in processing people in general.

Does False Recognition Stem from a Difficulty in True Recognition?

Although MR is able to recognise familiar people correctly it is possible that he has a difficulty in retrieving more detailed biographical information. This type of information may, under certain circumstances, be used as supporting evidence for fame judgements (e.g. Rapcsak et al., this issue). It is also conceivable that the opposite could be true, i.e. that MR might retrieve *too much* biographical detail to such an extent that the information is at best irrelevant and at worst confabulatory.

The experiments described next are designed to investigate in more detail the type of information on which MR might base his recognition judgements. Experiment 4 investigates whether false recognition can be attenuated by requiring him to make a semantic judgement (occupation decision) rather than a judgement based simply on familiarity.

Experiment 4: Familiarity vs. Occupation Judgement

If MR's false recognition arises primarily out of a general sense of familiarity without considering more differentiated knowledge (e.g. occupation), then it might be expected that false recognition could be reduced in an occupation judgement task.

Method. The names of 64 famous people were selected with equal numbers ($N = 16$) drawn from the categories of politics (P), music (M), films (F), and sport (S). An equal number of nonfamous names were created by recombining first names and surnames from a catalogue of bit-part or unknown actors/actresses. There were 34 men and 30 women in both the famous and nonfamous groups. The names were divided into two lists such that each list contained equal numbers of famous and nonfamous names and equal numbers of each occupation. Each list was randomised and printed (in three columns) on to a single piece of paper. For one of the lists, MR was instructed to circle those people who he thought was famous. For the other list, he was instructed to place a letter (either P, M, F, or S) next to those people who he thought was famous, according to their occupation. In a second session (1 week later) he was given the same lists again, but the instructions were reversed. Two groups of control subjects ($N = 10$ in each) participated, and performed either the occupation or familiarity judgement task.

Results and Discussion. Similar results were found across the two sessions and so the results were collapsed along this dimension. Table 2 shows that MR's false recognition is not suppressed by requiring him to make a judgement based on a semantic dimension (occupation) compared to overall famil-

Table 2. *Recognition Performance in Fame Decision (Familiarity Responding) versus Occupation Judgement (Semantic Responding)*

	Familiarity Responding			*Semantic Responding*		
	MR%	*Controls %*	*(SD)*	*MR%*	*Controls %*	*(SD)*
True recognition	98.4	93.4	(9.4)	96.9	96.4	(3.8)
Occupation errors[a]	N/A	N/A	N/A	1.6	5.9	(4.5)
False recognition	40.6	1.7	(1.6)	43.8	2.8	(3.4)

[a]Instances in which subjects correctly recognise a famous person as familiar but assigns the wrong occupation to them (N/A = not applicable).

iarity. He was just as willing to assign an occupation to nonfamous names (10 music, 7 film, 6 politics, 5 sport) as he was to simply identify the person as familiar. Thus, there is no evidence to suggest that taking into consideration factors other than general familiarity reduces false recognition. In contrast, MR's ability to correctly recognise famous people from names was unimpaired, as was his ability to recognise their occupation. The next experiment investigates whether MR can suppress false recognition when required to focus on uniquely specifying semantic information, as has been reported by Rapcsak et al. (in press) for their patients.

Experiment 5: Semantic Knowledge of Famous People

MR's ability to generate uniquely specifying semantic information from names and faces was investigated. Unfamiliar stimuli were also included in order to determine whether he would "retrieve" a false biography for these people.

Method. MR was given 35 spoken names of famous people, drawn from various decades and occupations, and 20 spoken names of unfamiliar people. In a separate session he was given 35 famous faces and 20 unfamiliar faces. He was instructed to provide as much biographical information about the person as he could, such that another person, given this biography, could unambiguously identify the person concerned. The recognised items were classified as (1) being uniquely identified, (2) as having a good idea who the person is but without unique identification, (3) as knowing only the occupation, or (4) as familiar without any further information being supplied. In the case of faces, a name was considered to provide unique specification. Examples of the scoring are given in Table 3.

Results and Discussion. The results are summarised in Table 3. MR often produces relatively detailed accounts of *unfamiliar* people and, in the case of faces, some misidentifications[2]. For instance, given the unfamiliar name *Michel Rapineaux* he came out with the description "A French singer who is half black and has braided hair. He had a hit a couple of years ago, but I can't remember what." MR is generally able to provide information to uniquely recognise *familiar* people. However, he occasionally produces information that is either irrelevant or incorrect. Thus he claimed that Richard Nixon liked to smoke cigars and that Mikhail Gorbachev had a wife who liked to spend a lot of money (perhaps retrieving information relating to Winston Churchill and President Marcos). He also occasionally produced information that had some grounding in reality but was nevertheless incorrect: For example, stating that Bob Geldof had something to do with Princess Diana's charity and that Saddam Hussein had been involved in the

[2] MR, in general, appears to make more false recognitions to faces than names. We suggest that this effect might arise out of the particular stimuli that were chosen rather than reflecting a greater impairment to faces. The faces that we used generally "looked famous" in that they were taken by professional photographers and were taken from a catalogue of bit-part or unknown actors/actresses. It is interesting to note that control subjects also produced higher false recognition to faces than names (e.g. Experiment 1 vs. 2), consistent with the idea that the face stimuli are intrinsically more potent at inducing false recognition.

Table 3. *Scoring Criteria and Response Distribution for Famous and Unfamiliar Person identification*

Scoring Criteria	*Description*
Uniquely specifying	E.g. "1950s singer with glasses who had a backing group called 'The Crickets' and had a hit with 'Peggy Sue'" [Buddy Holly]
Occcupation and some detail	Good idea of who the person is but not sufficient to identify uniquely. E.g. "An actor who was killed when he was young" [James Dean]
Occupation only	Supplying an occupation (e.g. politician, actress)
Familiarity only	Stating that a person (famous or unfamiliar) was familiar but supplying no further information.

Response Distribution

	Famous		*Unfamiliar*	
	Name	*Face*	*Name*	*Face*
	% (N)	*% (N)*	*% (N)*	*% (N)*
Percentage recognised	100 (35)	94 (33)	45 (9)	65 (13)
Uniquely specifying	80 (28)	86 (30	0 (0)	35 (7)
Occupation and some detail	20 (7)	9 (3)	30 (6)	20 (4)
Occupation only	0 (0)	0 (0)	0 (0)	5 (1)
Familiarity only	0 (0)	0 (0)	15 (3)	5 (1)

Falklands War. For the faces, two of the famous people were misidentified (George Best → George Harrison, Eric Cantona → "muscle man on original *Mission Impossible* series").

This experiment suggests that although MR is generally good at retrieving names and relevant semantic information, he also has a tendency to intrude extraneous information onto the definition. This may have little effect on familiar person recognition (since correct factual information will still predominate) but could have serious effects for rejecting unfamiliar people (since any retrieval of information is necessarily incorrect).

It is important to comment on the reason why MR still produced high false recognition in this task whereas the patients reported by Rapcsak et al. (this issue) apparently did not. Rapcsak et al. instructed their patients to respond "famous" only if they could remember the person's occupation *and name*. As we have already noted, MR very rarely produces a name for unfamiliar faces. If we were to apply the same criterion to MR, then his false face recognition would be a modest 7% (4/57, from a meta-analysis of three different tests) virtually identical to the 6% reported by Rapcsak et al. That is, the difference between MR and the Rapcsak patients may be more apparent than real. There is no convincing evidence that any of these patients fail to retrieve contextual detail spontaneously and rely, instead, on familiarity. It seems more probable to us that these patients do rely on semantic/contextual detail, but that this detail is retrieved in circumstances where it shouldn't (i.e. unfamiliar people) and that this can lead to false recognition judgements.

The experiment also shows that, in general, the amount of knowledge that MR retrieves about familiar people is greater than the amount of "knowledge" that he retrieves for unfamiliar people. If this is so, then recognition judgements that require a relative comparison between famous and unfamiliar items (i.e. forced choice) should prevent MR from accepting the unfamiliar ones.

Experiment 6: Famous Faces Forced Choice

This experiment consists of a forced-choice version of the test described in Experiment 1. Each famous face and its' matched (for age, sex and general appearance) unfamiliar face appeared side-by-side on a single sheet of paper and MR was required (1) to recognise which of the two faces is famous and (2) provide identifying (semantic/name) information. The famous face appeared equally often on the left and right.

MR's ability to recognise the famous faces was not strongly affected by decade of acquisition (1950s: 11/11; 1960s: 5/11; 1970s: 10/12; 1980s: 9/12; 1990s: 10/12) and so results were collapsed across this dimension. He chose the familiar face over the unfamiliar one in 77% (44/57) of instances, which is similar to controls (mean = 86.1%, SD = 12.9). Furthermore, he was able to provide uniquely identifying information on 47% (27/57) of occasions (22 names, 5 unique-semantic details), which again compares well with controls (mean = 59.0%, SD = 23.4).

Thus, MR is able to reject unfamiliar faces in favour of familiar ones in a forced-choice situation. This suggests that his memory for famous people is generally good and must differ, in some dimension, from his "false memory" for unfamiliar people.

Experiment 7: Famous Names Forced Choice

MR was given the famous names test, the pop singers test, and the historical figures test described earlier (Experiments 2–3) in a forced-choice format. That is, each target name was randomly paired with a distractor name and the subject was required to state which of the two names was famous. The pairs of names were printed side by side, with the target appearing equally often on the left and right. In this situation, MR was able to reject the distractors successfully in favour of the target. He scored 100% (40/40) with the famous names, 88% (35/40) with the pop stars, and 100% (20/20) with the historical names. Controls subjects ($N = 10$) produced scores of 99.5% (SD = 1.0), 79.8% (SD = 10.6), and 96.0% (SD = 4.6) respectively. Thus, when asked to make relative fame judgements (in forced-choice conditions) as opposed to absolute fame judgements (in single-probe conditions) MR does not falsely recognise unfamiliar people.

Does False Recognition Stem from Confabulation?

Confabulation may be defined as the retrieval of a fictitious information, without intent to deceive (e.g. Baddeley & Wilson, 1986; Berlyne, 1972; Kopelman, 1987; Moscovitch, 1995; Talland, 1965). This may consist of remembering entire fictitious episodes (e.g. Dalla Barba, 1993a; Dalla Barba, Cipolotti, & Denes, 1990) or fictitious semantic information (e.g. Dalla Barba, 1993b; Kopelman, Ng, & Van Den Brouke, 1997). It is, therefore, important to consider whether MR's false recognition stems from a wider confabulatory tendency. Observationally, MR does not give the appearance of confabulating either spontaneously or when provoked (e.g. the Autobiographical Memory Interview, described earlier). However, this was examined in more detail.

Experiment 8: Confabulation

MR was given a series of questions based on the confabulation battery of Dalla Barba (1993a, 1993b). He produced no confabulations on questions of personal semantic memory (e.g. "Are you married?," $N = 20$), general semantic memory (e.g. "Who is Bridget Bardot?," $N = 15$), episodic memory (e.g. "What did you do yesterday?," $N = 15$), orientation (e.g. "What is the month?," $N = 10$), or word definition (e.g. "Define *consume*," $N = 15$). If anything, MR's responses were vague rather than embellished (e.g. he could only remember one of his children's birth dates). The battery also includes questions that are designed to elicit an "I don't know" response, but may provoke a confabulation in some patients. For instance, "what country are the current world fencing champions?" (a "don't know" semantic question, $N = 10$) and "what did you have for dinner last February 3rd?" (a "don't know" episodic question, $N = 10$). MR produced only one affirmative response. He claimed to remember the last time that he heard the word "plug" (he had had an electrician in the day before).

Having said this, MR can recount incidences in which he has had what he terms a "false memory." For example, "My wife went out to work and while she was gone I promised that I would paint the door [points to it]. I got all the equipment out and started to paint. Halfway through, I dropped the brush on the carpet. I had to remove the carpet hairs from the brush and, because of the hairs on the brush, I cleaned it out properly with white spirit and then carried on painting until I finished." MR was unaware that the door had not been painted until his wife returned from work, and it was pointed out to him that there was no evidence that he had ever attempted to paint. In this instance it would appear that MR is making a source memory error (e.g. Johnson et al., 1993), confusing a memory of an intention for a memory of an event. The memory of the intention appears to contain an unusual amount of detail, which may give it an illusion of reality. MR even commented himself that "I felt so sure that I had done it because I can remember it in such detail." MR's acknowledgment of his error is unusual for many confabulating patients, who often continue to maintain belief in their memories in the face of implausibility (e.g. Moscovitch, 1995).

In short, the extent to which MR may be described as a confabulator is debatable and may be restricted to more acute phases of his illness, which we were unable to observe. The most important point is that MR's false recognition of unfamiliar people (often over 50%) is disproportionate to any confabulatory tendency that he may have, and an explanation of MR's deficit must be able to account for this fact.

Does False Recognition Extend to Other Categories?

This section will investigate whether MR's false recognition extends to other categories of stimuli. It has been suggested that proper names have different representational properties to common nouns, in that they represent unique items (see Valentine, Brennen, & Bredart, 1996, for a review). Proper names might also be learned in a different way (e.g. Hall, 1991). Indeed, a number of patients have been reported with either naming or semantic memory deficits that are exclusive to proper names (e.g. Hittmair-Delazer, Denes, Semenza, & Mantovan, 1994; Lucchelli & De Renzi, 1992; Semenza & Zettin, 1988, 1989). There is also some evidence for disproportionate sparing of proper names relative to common nouns in naming (e.g. Cipolotti, McNeil, & Warrington, 1993; Semenza & Sgaramella, 1993; but see Bredart, Brennen, & Valentine, 1997) and semantic memory tasks (e.g. Forde & Humphreys, 1995; McNeil, Cipolotti, & Warrington, 1994; Warrington & McCarthy, 1987). It is therefore of interest to know whether MR's difficulty with people is part of a wider proper name difficulty. Experiments 9 and 10 contrast MR's recognition of vocabulary with city names (a proper name category). Further investigations using other types of proper names are reported in Experiments 12–14.

Experiment 9: Vocabulary

Thirty real words of very low frequency (e.g. loquacity, osprey) were selected (Kuçera & Francis, 1967, count of 1 or unlisted words). Thirty nonwords were either created by the experimenter or taken from another test battery (Baddeley, Emslie, & Nimmo-Smith, 1992). The nonwords were all pronounceable and were designed to sound plausible (e.g. legify, florrical). All 60 items were printed on a single sheet and MR was instructed to circle only the real words.

His ability to identify real words (100%, 30/30) was at least as good as the controls (mean = 89.0%, SD = 11.9), and his false recognition level (7%, 2/30) was well within the control range (mean = 4.4%, SD = 8.0).

Experiment 10: Place Names

Thirty cities of the world were selected from an atlas (e.g. Jakarta, Bologna). Distractor items consisted of town and cities, listed in the atlas index, which had low populations and are outside of the UK, so they are unlikely to be known (e.g. Wabera, Raner). This was done to ensure that the distractors were as plausible as possible. It will be shown later that similar results are found with truly fictitious place names.

MR correctly recognised 93% (28/30) of the cities and did not falsely recognise any (0/30) of the distractors. Control subjects produced true and false recognition levels of 81.9% (SD = 16.6) and 4.0% (SD = 5.2) respectively. Thus, MR's false recognition of people is not part of a wider deficit affecting proper name categories. Finally, we will consider MR's recognition of news events.

Experiment 11: Shortened News Events Test (Kapur, 1989)

The test consisted of 20 brief descriptions of news events that had occurred from the 1960s to the 1990s (e.g. Kuwait invaded by Iraq) together with 20 descriptions of events that had never occurred but were nonetheless plausible (e.g. 10 Downing Street opens to the public). He was given the test twice: once in 1995 as part of a preliminary assessment, and again in 1998 during the same period in which this investigation was carried out. In 1995, he correctly identified all of the real events (20/20) but incorrectly claimed that 65% (13/20) of the fictitious events had occurred. Control subjects produced true and false recognition rates of 87.0% (11.8) and 12.0% (10.3) respectively. When tested again in 1998 he performed normally (true and false recognition rates of 95% and 10% respectively).

Experiments 9 and 10 showed that MR's false recognition deficit does not encompass all types of stimuli, nor does it encompass the category of proper names. The data from the news events is inconsistent and the reason for this is unclear. However, it is important to note that his performance with news events differs from his performance with people, in that the phenomena of false recognition of people has been highly consistent across different tests and sessions.

False Recognition: Familiarity of Parts or Nature of Referent?

People's names are generally composed out of parts that, in themselves, have an intrinsic familiarity value. For example, "Alex" and "Morrison" are both familiar names but "Alex Morrison" is not a familiar person. Similar arguments could be applied to faces: Thus a nose or hairline might appear familiar even though the face as a whole is not. Furthermore, it is conceivable that resolving these contradictions could be frontally mediated since attending to one dimension of a stimulus whilst suppressing task-irrelevant dimensions is considered to be a classic function of the frontal lobes (e.g. Stroop, WCST). Indeed, the patients reported by Rapcsak et al. (1994) who falsely recognised unfamiliar faces appeared to be relying on this type of part-based information. For instance, one patient (WJ) commented "That's a movie actor I know, I recognise the hair but I can't think of the name." If false recognition is based on incorrectly attributing familiarity to the parts rather than the whole, then it may well be expected that false recognition would not extend to other classes of stimuli that lack this internal structure. This could explain why MR did not falsely recognise the nonwords or city names in the earlier experiments. It could also explain why he did occasionally falsely recognise news events, since these are essentially combinations of familiar elements (countries, wars, bombs, etc.). This hypothesis can, however, be tested directly by constructing stimuli that do not refer to people but nevertheless are made up of meaningful parts: Certain place names, for instance, have this structure (e.g. Salt Lake City).

Experiment 12: Place Names Derived from Other Words

The names of 20 places in America that are name phrases (e.g. Salt Lake City, Fort Worth, Cape Cod) were selected and 20 fictitious place names with a similar structure were constructed (e.g. Blue Ridge City, Port Caroline, Cape Lincoln). The distractors were deemed to be fictitious on the basis that they were not listed in the index of a world atlas.

MR had little difficulty in correctly recognising the real place names (90%, 18/20) and he did *not* produce a high level of false recognition to the distractor places (15%, 3/20). Control subjects produced true and false recognition rates of 88.3% (SD = 15.6) and 12.8% (SD = 16.2) respectively. Thus, the hypothesis that MR is relying on part-based familiarity is not supported by this experiment.

An alternative explanation is that false recognition does not critically depend on the surface characteristics of the stimuli but depends, instead, on the status of the items that are being searched for (i.e. whether it refers to a person or not). If this is the case, then it might be expected that MR will *not* produce false recognition to unfamiliar peoples' names when the task instructions do not require him to recognise people (e.g. recognising names of songs or book titles), even when the surface properties of the targets resemble the names of people (e.g. Eleanor Rigby, David Copperfield).

Experiment 13: Pop Songs vs. Pop Singers/Groups
This experiment used the same set of distractors in two different conditions with either titles of pop songs as targets (condition "A"), or pop singers/groups as targets (condition "B"). If MR falsely recognises the distractors when asked to search for the singers/groups but not for songs then this suggests that false recognition is determined by the status of the time that is being sought (i.e. whether or not it refers to a person/persons) and not on the nature of the stimulus material itself (since this was equated for). If, however, MR falsely recognises under both conditions then this suggests that false recognition is determined by the general plausibility of the distractors and/or the similarity of distractors to targets.

Method. The names of 15 pop songs that sound like the names of people (e.g. Eleanor Rigby) were selected, together with the names of 15 real singers (e.g. Martha Reeves) and 15 fictitious names (e.g. Lindsay Leigh). In addition, the names of 15 pop songs that could plausibly be names of pop groups (e.g. Summertime Blues) were selected, together with the names of 15 real groups (e.g. Moody Blues) and 15 fictitious names (e.g. Downtown Blues). The test was presented over four sessions in an ABBA design. In the "A" sessions, MR was given the pop songs and distractor items and told to circle the items that corresponded to famous pop songs. In the "B" sessions, he was given the pop singers/groups and the same distractor items as before and told to circle the famous pop singers/groups. The lists in the two "A" sessions were identical, and similarly for "B" sessions. Ten control subjects were tested in the song condition.

Results and Discussion. Table 4 shows that MR's false recognition was significantly higher for the singers instruction than for the songs instructions [$\chi^2(1) = 5.29$, $P < .05$; collapsing across the name-like and not name-like stimuli], even though the distractor stimuli were identical in both instances. His level of true recognition was also higher for the pop singers than for the pop songs [$\chi^2(1) = 5.29$, $P < .05$; collapsing across the name-like and not name-like stimuli], but this result is harder to interpret given that different stimuli were used as targets. The results are consistent with false recognition being determined by the nature of the search strategy (impaired for people). However, given that overall levels of "yes" responding (both true and false recognition) were higher in one condition, a simple criterion shift could also be possible. The next experiment examines this further, using the same items as both targets and distractors, varying *only* the instructions.

Experiment 14: Book Titles
This experiment was similar to the latter, in that the critical factor varied was the instructions given. There were two types of target and distractor stimuli: book titles that are based on names (e.g. Oliver Twist) and book titles that are not (e.g. Pride and Prejudice). For the titles that resemble names, the instructions (but not the actual stimuli) were varied so that MR was instructed either to recognise fictional people or to recognise book titles. For the titles that do not resemble names, MR was given the same instructions (i.e. to recognise book titles) and stimuli throughout in order to establish a baseline level of variation across different testing sessions.

Method. Twenty well-known books in which the title bears an eponymous name (e.g. Oliver Twist, Anna Karenina) were selected and 20 fictitious names (e.g. Agnes Blythe, Nicholas Charles) acted as distractors. For comparison, 20 other well-known book titles that do not bear an eponymous name (e.g. Pride and Prejudice, Little Women) were selected and 20 fictitious titles (e.g. Love and Hope, Charity Fair) were devised. The 40 stimuli that resemble people's names were printed randomly on to a single sheet of paper and the 40 stimuli that do not resemble names were printed on a separate sheet. These same tests were presented to

Table 4. *True and False Recognition of Pop Songs versus Pop Singers (%), the Same Distractors Being Used in Both Conditions*

	MR				*Controls*
	Songs	*Singers*	*Singers*	*Songs*	*Mean (SD)*
Name-like					
False recognition (e.g. Lindsay Leigh)	0	27	20	0	0.0 (0.0)
True recognition (e.g. Eleanor Rigby/Carly Simon)	47	93	100	47	56.7 (14.1)
Not Name-like					
False recognition (e.g. Downton Blues)	13	30	27	13	2.7 (4.7)
True recognition (e.g. Yellow Submarine/Boomtown Rats)	40	60	73	67	63.3 (17.0)

MR in four sessions. For the name-like stimuli the instructions were varied in an ABBA design ("A" sessions required him to search for fictional people, "B" sessions required him to search for book titles). For the other stimuli, he was required to search for book titles in all four sessions. Ten control subjects were also run, and instructed to search for book titles for both types of stimuli.

Results. Table 5 shows that MR's false recognition depends critically on the instructions given to him. For the name-like stimuli, he was significantly more likely to show false recognition if asked to recognise literary characters than if asked to recognise book titles [$\chi^2(1) = 14.63$, $P < .001$]. In fact, his performance in the latter condition was no different to controls. These differences cannot be attributed to baseline shifts in false recognition tendency across sessions, since his performance did not vary for the titles which did not look like names. It is not clear why MR's level of false recognition is above that of controls for these stimuli. However, it should be noted that his false recognition tendency for these items (31%) is still less than for people (57% on average for Experiments 1–3).

The results from Experiments 13 and 14 support the conclusion that MR's false recognition is not driven purely by the stimulus material, but depends on the task configuration—i.e. whether he is instructed to search for people or not.

GENERAL DISCUSSION

This study has documented an unusual case of false recognition impairment in a patient (MR) with a demyelating illness centred on the frontal lobes. This patient falsely recognises unfamiliar people as being famous, regardless of input modality (Experiment 1: faces; Experiment 2–3: written words; Experiment 2: spoken words). The deficit extends to various kinds of people including contemporary (Experiments 1–3), historical (Experiment 4), and fictional (Experiment 14) people. False recognition is unlikely to reflect reliance on familiarity alone since it still occurs when MR is asked to retrieve general semantic knowledge (Experiment 4) or unique semantic knowledge (Experiment 5). Although MR often does retrieve incorrect semantic information for unfamiliar people, this is rarely uniquely specifying and is generally less rich than the information retrieved for famous people (Experiment 5). This may be used as a basis for rejecting distractors in forced-choice recognition experiments (Experiments 6–7) but may lead to false recognition under single-probe conditions. False recognition of people is disproportionate to any confabulatory tendency that he may have (Experiment 8). False recognition does not extend to vocabulary, place names, or news events (although there is some inconsistency for the latter; Experiments 9–12). False recognition, instead,

Table 5. *True and False Recognition of Name-like (e.g. Oliver Twist) and Non Name-like (e.g. Pride and Prejudice) Book Titles (%), as a Function of Task Instructions*

	MR				*Controls*
Instructions[a]:	*Books*	*People*	*People*	*Books*	*Mean (SD)*
Name-like					
False recognition (e.g. Agnes Blythe)	5	50	30	0	1.0 (3.2)
True recognition (e.g. Oliver Twist)	100	100	100	100	94.5 (6.9)
	MR				*Controls*
Instructions:	*Books*				*Mean (SD)*
Not Name-like					
False recognition (e.g. Pride and Prejudice)	30	30	30	35	0.5 (1.6)
True recognition (e.g. Love and Hope)	95	95	95	95	95.0 (4.1)

[a]The task instructions were varied for the name-like stimuli but were the same throughout for the non name-like stimuli.

appears to be determined more by the task requirements (i.e. whether the targets refer to people or not) than by the stimuli themselves (Experiments 13–14). This would appear to be more consistent with a top-down/frontal explanation of the disorder than a bottom-up explanation. Before considering in more detail possible explanations of this pattern, we will consider the similarities and differences to previous patients reported in the literature.

Comparisons with Other Patients

MR has no difficulty in recognising familiar people but has significant problems in rejecting unfamiliar people as unfamiliar. This provides a sharp contrast to patients with prosopagnosia and retrograde amnesia, who have difficulty in recognising familiar faces/people but are generally unimpaired at rejecting unfamiliar people (see A.W. Ellis & Young, 1988; McCarthy & Warrington, 1990; Parkin, 1996). That is, there is double dissociation between impairments of true and false recognition. In the case of retrograde amnesia it is possible that the storage of memory representations themselves have been compromised (e.g. Parkin, Montaldi, Leng, & Hunkin, 1990). Therefore the process of matching a stimulus, whether familiar or not, to a memory representation will tend to yield a null result. Similar arguments can be applied to prosopagnosics, in whom the information stored in face recognition units may be either lost or completely inaccessible (e.g. Bruyer et al., 1983; De Renzi, 1986). However, certain prosopagnosic patients may show false recognition of faces if perceptual processing is damaged in a particular way. For instance, if they are unable to attend to global characteristics of the perceptual input they may rely upon matching individual features to essentially intact memory representations of faces, resulting in spurious activation of FRUs and occasional misidentifications (Rapcsak et al., 1994; Young et al., 1993). Such an explanation cannot be applied to MR, who shows false recognition under a wide range of circumstances, including the auditory modality.

MR most strongly resembles Case 21 described by Rapcsak et al. (1996) and JS and BW described by Rapcsak et al. (1998, 1999). These patients showed false recognition without any evidence of prosopagnosia. JS and BW also showed evidence of impairments on single-probe episodic recognition tasks (Case 21 was not tested in this way). This led Rapcsak et al. (in press) to suggest that a similar deficit of reliance on gist/familiarity underlies both false recognition of unfamiliar people in fame decision and false recognition in episodic recognition tests. However, our data suggests that this may not be the case given that MR's difficulty in fame decision is, in some ways, qualitatively different from his performance in other recognition memory tasks (in that only the former is category-specific and can be eliminated by forced-choice requirements), and other patients show impaired single-probe episodic recognition but intact fame decision (Parkin et al., this issue). Thus it is possible that functionally different impairments underlie these disorders[3]. It is also hard to make direct comparisons with JS, BW, or Case 21 since data pertaining to name recognition and other classes of stimuli in retrograde test were not reported by Rapcsak et al. (1996, 1999).

MR also differs from patients with a delusional misidentification syndrome in that he does not mistake people, whether familiar of unfamiliar, for some other *specified* person (e.g. H.D. Ellis & Young, 1990). For instance, in the Capgras delusion (Capgras & Reboul-Lachaux, 1923) familiar people are mistaken for identical doubles and in the Fregoli delusion (Courbon & Fail, 1927) unfamiliar people are mistaken for familiar people in disguise. Ellis and Young (1990) account for the Fregoli delusion by assuming that modality-independent Person Identity Nodes (PINs) are inappropriately triggered and that defective decision mechanism fails to note the incongruity. However, the extent to which these syndromes are attributable to organic rather than psychiatric aetiology remains questionable (Fleminger & Burns, 1993).

Explanations and Implications

We have already discounted the possibility that MR relies solely on familiarity of parts, since he does not falsely recognise other types of stimuli that have a similar/identical structure to people's names. Several alternative explanations can be considered. (1) MR misattributes a percept or an affect for a memory. (2) MR has a category-specific deficit for people. (3) MR has a deficit to some control process that sets up the response criteria and/or retrieval description. We will consider each of these in turn.

1. The first explanation is that MR misattributes a percept/affect for a memory. These accounts draw on the assumption that deciding whether a given stimulus has been encountered before does not involve simply reading off an internal label, but involves a process of inference/attribution. Thus, stimuli that have been encountered before may be processed more quickly (e.g. Jacoby & Dallas, 1981), may evoke an affective tone (e.g. Kunst-Wilson & Zajonc, 1980), may be richer in detail (e.g. Johnson et al., 1993), and so forth. A false recognition may, therefore, arise if stimuli are processed too fluently, evoke an inappropriate affect, or result in the retrieval of inappropriate detail.

One explanation involving perceptual misattribution is in terms of interhemispheric asynchronism (Efron, 1963; Maudsley, 1889, cited in Sno & Linszen, 1990). A delay of information transmission between the two hemispheres may lead to the dominant hemisphere receiving the same information twice in succession, the second pass being attributed to a memory of the first. However, bottom-up explanations such as these seem incapable of accounting for the fact that false recognition is not found for all types of stimulus.

As for misattributing an affect for a memory, several researchers have proposed that familiar people are processed by both a conscious and unconscious route (Bauer, 1984; Tranel & Damasio, 1985). In the Bruce and Young (1986) model of person recognition, conscious and unconscious routes might correspond to retrieval of semantic/name information and retrieval of affective (including expression) information respectively. In order to explain MR's deficit, we might assume that an affective response is being inappropriately trig-

[3] This claim would be bolstered further if the opposite dissociation were reported (i.e. impaired fame decision, intact single-probe episodic recognition). However, this has yet to be documented.

gered by an unfamiliar person. There is indeed some evidence to suggest that MR is impaired in the emotional analysis of faces, and other patients with impaired emotion perception show false recognition of unfamiliar people (Broks et al., 1998). Broks et al. document four patients, two of whom (JC, RB) showed pathological false recognition of unfamiliar faces and names together with intact recognition of famous faces and names. However, give that these patients had a variety of other difficulties (e.g. naming, occupation judgement, views matching) it seems premature to conclude that there is a meaningful association between false recognition of people and impaired emotion perception. Furthermore, there are also documented cases of patients who are impaired in emotion perception who do not produce false recognition to unfamiliar people (SE—Broks et al., 1998; JB—Parkin, personal communication). Thus, impaired emotion perception, in itself, is not a sufficient explanation of MR's deficits.

2. The second explanation is that false recognition arises out of spurious retrieval/activation of PINs (Person Identity Nodes; Bruce & Young, 1986), which are essentially modality-independent pointers to a person's name and semantic details. Each known person may have their own PIN. If an unfamiliar person were to activate a number of different PINs spuriously then this would make false semantic information available. This is shown by MR's willingness to produce false recognition when asked to make occupation judgements (Experiment 4). The fact that several PINs may be active prevents an outright misidentification. Since PINs are not modality specific, this can account for false recognition from both names and faces. PINs are also specific to people, which could account for the fact that there is no false recognition of places, vocabulary, or news events.

There are, however, a number of difficulties with this explanation. First, it is not consistent with MR's left frontal pathology. One might expect, from lesion sites of other patients, that person-based semantic knowledge is located in right-temporal regions (A.W. Ellis, Young, & Critchley, 1989; Evans, Heggs, Antoun, & Hodges, 1995; Hanley, Young, & Pearson, 1989). Second, MR's false recognition seems to depend on the nature of the referent. To some extent, it is an empirical question whether the mental representation of *Oliver Twist* as a book is fundamentally different from *Oliver Twist* as a person (albeit fictional). However, such an account appears counter-intuitive and lacks parsimony. A more plausible explanation is that such effects arise out of the task configuration rather than the representations themselves. Thus, although false recognition of unfamiliar people may indeed arise from inappropriate retrieval/activity of PINs, this may reflect damage to modulatory control processes rather than damage to the person recognition system itself.

3. The final explanation involves the role of frontal control processes in recognition memory. Several theories have been proposed, including a role of the frontal lobes in setting up a focused retrieval description (Schacter et al., 1996), selection of suitable features at encoding (Parkin et al., this issue), utilising contextual information in recognition (Parkin et al., 1994), and decision making (Delbecq-Derouesné et al., 1990).

Rapcsak et al. (this issue) attribute false recognition of unfamiliar people in their patients, primarily, to a failure to spontaneously evoke a strategic memory search, which is used when the familiarity signal from the FRU system is uncertain. The strategic memory search might try to retrieve the person's occupation and other contextual information in those situations in which it does not become automatically available. However, this explanation does not appear to be entirely appropriate for MR, who will often retrieve semantic information either spontaneously or when provoked and does not appear to be relying on familiarity. It is not the case that MR fails to retrieve supporting information. On the contrary, he does attempt to retrieve such information, but he incorrectly retrieves information in those circumstances that should yield a null result (as did JT; Young et al., 1993). This information may then incorrectly lead him to accept the person as famous. He generally retrieves more detailed information for famous people than unfamiliar people, which explains why his level of true recognition is consistently higher than has level of false recognition. More convincing evidence that Rapcsak et al.'s (this issue) patients can utilise context but fail to do so spontaneously would come from a demonstration that these patients do not generate false semantic information from unfamiliar faces/names (since a null result should be the appropriate outcome of strategic memory search in this instance).

Rapcsak et al. (this issue) also consider a number of other frontal/executive processes which, when damaged, may result in false recognition. First, patients may have difficulty in monitoring and verifying the strength of the familiarity and context signals arising from the FRUs and PINs respectively. Second, patients may have a difficulty in criterion setting and decision making that may be based on meta-memory assumptions about the phenomenal characteristics of veridical remembering (e.g. the amount of detail to be retrieved in order for the memory trace to be accepted as genuine). The first explanation is hard to examine empirically since it not clear who or what is doing the monitoring and how this mechanism works. The second explanation is related to the one that we propose for MR. We suggest that MR has difficulties in setting up an appropriate response criterion, or that the retrieval description is too broadly specified. Thus, although he retrieves correct personal information (e.g. Richard Nixon was an American president sometime after Kennedy who was forced to resign because of a scandal), he also retrieves some irrelevant/erroneous information (e.g. Richard Nixon liked to smoke cigars), presumably because there is spurious activation of other memory representations of known people. In the case of an unfamiliar name/face, several different PINs of known people may be triggered which may be "blended" into a false identity. This could reflect a failure to inhibit irrelevant detail (e.g. Shimamura, 1995), or a failure to implement a "stop" command in retrieval (e.g. Papagno & Baddeley, 1997). Whilst this difficulty may not have detrimental consequences to recognition of famous people (since correct factual information predominates), it could have serious repercussions for unfamiliar people (since any spurious retrieval of information is necessarily incorrect).

Our hypothesis differs in emphasis from that of Rapcsak et al. (1996; this issue) in that they claim that the recognition process proceeds normally up to the point of some terminal decision-making or criterion-setting mechanism within the frontal lobes, whereas we suggest that the lower-level recognition procedure is proceeding abnormally (too many PINs being active) because of inappropriate *top-down* regulation by the frontal lobes. In this way, the frontal lobes are not "making decisions" (in a somewhat homuncular fashion), they are merely setting up appropriate conditions to enable a decision to be made. This account is in line with the SAS (supervisory attentional system) model of Norman and Shallice (1986; Shallice, 1988) in that it views the frontal lobes as controlling lower level activity, rather than being an end-point of processing. The frontal lobes may bias certain outcomes according to task demands and characteristics, meta-memory assumptions (generic properties of people relative to other kinds), the amount of information to be retrieved before recognition terminates (e.g. Papagno & Baddeley, 1997), and so forth.

Any explanation of MR's deficit must be able to take into account the specificity of his disorder—i.e. that it predominantly affects people. Brennen (1993) proposed one theory that accounts for representational differences between people (or specifically people's names) and other classes of items, which was termed the "plausible phonology hypothesis". He assumed that the potential number of new exemplars in the case of people was greater than for other classes, including places. Note that his hypothesis emphasises that it is the potential rate of new exemplars that is important (and new people are encountered more often than, say, new vocabulary) and not the current set size of exemplars (i.e. it is not simply a fan effect). Such a theory would appear to constitute a "meta-memory assumption" in that it is a generic characteristic of memory for people but it is not an intrinsic property of the memory representations themselves. Although Brennen explicitly rules out the suggestion that "set size of plausible phonology" is important for recognition memory, since the decision is assumed to be binary (unlike recall), it seems plausible to us that categories with a high potential rate of new exemplars (such as people) may be more biased towards false recognition than categories with a low potential rate of new exemplars.

In terms of existing models of person recognition (e.g. Bruce & Young, 1986), the results appear to suggest that recognition of people cannot be considered to be a completely bottom-up (or automatic) process. Top-down information may influence recognition at the level of the Person Identity Nodes (PINs) by setting up and/or regulating the retrieval specifications that form the basis of the recognition decision.

REFERENCES

Baddeley, A., Emslie, H., & Nimmo-Smith, I. (1992). *Speed and Capacity of Language Processing Test*. Bury St Edmunds, UK: Thames Valley Test Corporation.

Baddeley, A., & Wilson, B. (1986). Amnesia, autobiographical memory, and confabulation. In D.C. Rubin (Ed.), *Autobiographical memory*. New York: Cambridge University Press.

Bauer, R.M. (1984). Autonomic recognition of names and faces in prosopagnosia: A neuropsychological application of the guilty knowledge test. *Neuropsychologia*, *22*, 457–469.

Benton, A.L., & Hamsher, K.D. (1976). *Multilingual Aphasia Examination*. Iowa City: University of Iowa.

Berlyne, N. (1972). Confabulation. *British Journal of Psychiatry*, *120*, 31–39.

Bredart, S., Brennen, T., & Valentine, T. (1997). Dissociations between the processing of proper and common names. *Cognitive Neuropsychology*, *14*, 209–217.

Brennen. T. (1993). The difficulty with recalling people's names; The plausible phonology hypothesis. *Memory*, *1*, 409–431.

Broks, P., Young, A.W., Maratos, E.J., Coffey, P.J., Calder, A.J., Isaac, C.L., Mayes, A.R., Hodges, J.R., Montaldi, D., Cezayirli, E., Roberts, N., & Hadley, D. (1998). Face processing impairments after encephalitis: Amygdala damage and recognition of fear. *Neuropsychologia*, *36*, 59–70.

Bruce, V., Young, A.W. (1986). Understanding face recognition. *British Journal of Psychology*, *77*, 305–327.

Bruyer, R., Laterre, C., Seron, X., Feyereisen, P., Stryptstein, E., Pierrard, E., & Rectem, D. (1983). A case of prosopagnosia with some preserved covert remembrance of familiar faces. *Brain and Cognition*, *2*, 257–289.

Burgess, P.W., & Shallice, T. (1996a). Bizarre responses, rule detection and frontal lobe lesions. *Cortex*, *32*, 241–259.

Burgess, P.W., & Shallice, T. (1996b). Response suppression, initiation and strategy use following frontal lobe lesions. *Neuropsychologia*, *34*, 263–273.

Calder, A.J., Young, A.W., Rowland, D., Perrett, D.I., Hodges, J.R., & Etcoff, N.L. (1996). Facial emotion recognition after bilateral amygdala damage: Differentially severe impairment of fear. *Cognitive Neuropsychology*, *13*, 699–745.

Canellopoulou, M., & Richardson, J.T.E. (1998). The role of executive function in imagery mnemonics: Evidence from multiple sclerosis. *Neuropsychologia*, *36*, 1181–1188.

Capgras, J., & Reboul-Lachaux, J. (1923). L'illusion des sosies dans un delire sytematise chronique. *Bulletin de la Societe Clinique de Medecine Mentale*, *2*, 6–16.

Cipolotti, L., McNeil, J.E., & Warrington, E.K. (1993). Spared written naming of proper nouns: A case report. *Memory*, *1*, 289–311.

Courbon, P., & Fail, G. (1927). Illusion of Fregoli syndrome and schizophrenia. *Bulletin de la Societe Clinique de Medecine Mentale*, *15*, 121–125.

Dalla Barba, G. (1993a). Confabulation: Knowledge and recollective experience. *Cognitive Neuropsychology*, *10*, 1–20.

Dalla Barba, G. (1993b). Different patterns of confabulation. *Cortex*, *29*, 567–581.

Dalla Barba, G., Cipolotti, L., & Denes, G. (1990). Autobiographical memory loss and confabulation in Korsakoff's syndrome: A case report. *Cortex*, *26*, 525–534

De Renzi, E. (1986). Prosopagnosia in two patients with CT scan evidence of damage confined to the right hemisphere. *Neuropsychologia*, *24*, 385–389.

Delbecq-Derouesné, J., Beauvois, M.F., & Shallice. T. (1990). Preserved recall versus impaired recognition. *Brain*, *113*, 1045–1074.

Efron, R. (1963). Temporal perception, aphasia and déjà vu. *Brain*, *86*, 403–424.

Ekman, P., & Friesen, W.V. (1976). *Pictures of facial affect*. Palo Alto, CA: Consulting Psychologists Press.

Ellis, A.W., & Young, A.W. (1988). *Human cognitive neuropsychology*. Hove, UK: Lawrence Erlbuam Associates Ltd.

Ellis, A.W., Young, A.W., & Critchley, E.M.R. (1989). Loss of memory for people following temporal lobe damage. *Brain, 112*, 1469–1483.

Ellis, H.D., & Young A.W. (1990). Accounting for delusional misidentifications. *British Journal of Psychiatry, 157*, 239–248.

Evans, J.J., Heggs, A.J., Antoun, N., & Hodges, J.R. (1995). Progressive prosopagnosia associated with selective right temporal atrophy. *Brain, 118*, 1–13.

Fleminger, S., & Burns, A. (1993). The delusional misidentification syndromes in patients with and without evidence of organic cerebral disorder. A structured review of case reports. *Biological Psychiatry, 33*, 22–32.

Forde, E.M.E., & Humphreys, G.W. (1995). Refractory semantics in global aphasia: On semantic organisation and the access-storage distinction in neuropsychology. *Memory, 3*, 265–307.

Guildford, J.P., Christensen, P.R., Merrifield, P.R., & Wilson, R.C. (1978). *Alternate uses: Manual of instructions and interpretation*. Orange, CA: Sheridan Psychological Services.

Hall, D. (1991). Acquiring proper nouns for familiar and unfamiliar animate objects: Two-year-old's word-learning biases. *Child Development, 62*, 1142–1154.

Hanley, J.R., Young, A.W., & Pearson, N.A. (1989). Defective recognition of familiar people. *Cognitive Neuropsychology, 6*, 179–210.

Hanley, J.R., Young, A.W., & Pearson, N.A. (1991). Impairment of visuospatial sketchpad. *The Quarterly Journal of Experimental Psychology, 43A*, 101–125.

Hittmair-Delazer, M., Denes, G., Semenza, C., & Mantovan, M.C. (1994). Anomia for people's names. *Neuropsychologia, 32*, 465–476.

Hyman, I.E., & Pentland, J. (1996). The role of mental imagery in the creation of false childhood memories. *Journal of Memory and Language, 35*, 101–117.

Jacoby, L.L., & Dallas, M. (1981). On the relationship between autobiographical memory and perceptual learning. *Journal of Experimental Psychology: General, 3*, 306–340.

Janowsky, J.S., Shimamura, A.P., & Squire, L.R. (1989). Source memory impairment in patients with frontal lobe lesions. *Neuropsychologia, 27*, 1043–1056.

Johnson, M.K., Hashtroudi, S., & Lindsay, D.S. (1993). Source monitoring. *Psychological Bulletin, 114*, 3–28.

Kapur, N. (1989). *The Wessex Memory manual*. Southampton, UK: Wessex Neurological Centre.

Kopelman, M.D. (1987). Two types of confabulation. *Journal of Neurology, Neurosurgery and Psychiatry, 50*, 1482–1487.

Kopelman, M.D., Ng, N., & Van Den Brouke, O. (1997). Confabulation extending across episodic, personal and general semantic memory. *Cognitive Neuropsychology, 14*, 683–712.

Kopelman, M.D., Wilson, B.A., & Baddeley, A.D. (1990). *The Autobiographical Memory Interview*. Bury St Edmunds, UK: Thames Valley Test Company.

Kuçera, H., & Francis, W.N. (1967). *Computational analysis of present day American English*. Rhode Island: Brown University.

Kunst-Wilson, W.R., & Zajonc, R.B. (1980). Affective discrimination of stimuli that cannot be recognised. *Science, 207*, 557–558.

Lucchelli, F., & De Renzi, E. (1992). Proper name anomia. *Cortex, 28*, 221–230.

Lucchelli, F., Muggia, S., & Spinnler, H. (1997). Selective proper name anomia: A case involving only contemporary celebrities. *Cognitive Neuropsychology, 14*, 881–900.

Maudsley, H. (1889). The double brain. *Mind, 54*, 161–187.

McCarthy, R.A., & Warrington, E.K. (1990). *Cognitive neuropsychology: A clinical introduction*. London: Academic Press.

McClelland, J.L. (1995). Constructive memory and memory distortions: A parallel-distributed processing approach. In D.L. Schacter (Ed.), *Memory distortion*. Cambridge, MA: Harvard Press.

McKenna, P., & Warrington, E.K. (1983). *The Graded Naming Test*. Windsor, UK: Nelson.

McNeil, J.E., Cipolotti, L., & Warrington, E.K. (1994). The accessibility of proper names. *Neuropsychologia, 32*, 193–208.

Moscovitch, M. (1995). Confabulation. In D.L. Schacter (Ed.), *Memory distortion*. Cambridge, MA: Harvard Press.

Nelson, H.E. (1976). A modified card sorting test sensitive to frontal lobe deficits. *Cortex, 12*, 313–324.

Nelson, H.E. (1985). *National Adult Reading Test*. London: NFER-Nelson.

Norman, D.A., & Shallice, T. (1986). Attention to action. In R.J. Davidson, G.E. Schwartz, & D. Shapiro (Eds.), *Consciousness and self regulation*. New York: Plenum Press.

Papagno, C., & Baddeley, A. (1997). Confabulation in a dysexecutive patient: Implication for models of retrieval. *Cortex, 33*, 743–752.

Parkin, A.J. (1996). *Explorations in cognitive neuropsychology*. Oxford: Blackwell.
Parkin, A.J. (1997). The neuropsychology of false memory. *Learning and Individual Differences*, *9*, 341–357.
Parkin, A.J. (1998a). *The Mooney Faces*. Unpublished test, University of Sussex.
Parkin, A.J. (1998b). *The Sussex Test of Remote Memory (STORM)*. Unpublished test, University of Sussex.
Parkin, A.J., Bindschaedler, C., Harsent, L., & Metzler, C. (1996). Pathological false alarm rates following damage to the left frontal cortex. *Brain and Cognition*, *32*, 14–27.
Parkin, A.J., Montaldi, D., Leng, N.R.C., & Hunkin, N.M. (1990). Contextual cueing effects in the remote memory of alcoholic Korsakoff patients and normal subjects. *Quarterly Journal of Experimental Psychology*, *42A*, 585–596.
Parkin, A.J., Ward, J., Bindschaedler, C., Squires, E.J., & Powell, G. (this issue). False recognition following frontal lobe damage: The role of encoding factors. *Cognitive Neuropsychology*, *16*, 243–265.
Parkin, A.J., & Williamson, P. (1987). Cerebral lateralization at different stages of facial processing, *23*, 99–110.
Parkin, A.J., Yeomans, J., & Bindschaedler, C. (1994). Further characterization of the executive memory impairment following frontal lobe lesions. *Brain and Cognition*, *26*, 23–42.
Patterson, K., & Bradshaw, J.L. (1975). Differential hemispheric mediation of nonverbal visual stimuli. *Journal of Experimental Psychology: Human Perception and Performance*, *3*, 246–252.
Rapcsak, S.Z., Kaszniak, A.W., Reminger, S.L., Glisky, M.L., Glisky, E.L., & Comer, J.F. (1998). Dissociation between verbal and autonomic measures of memory following frontal lobe damage. *Neurology*, *50*, 1258–1265.
Rapcsak, S.Z., Polster, M.R., Comer, J.F., & Rubens, A.B. (1994). False recognition and misidentification of faces following right hemisphere damage. *Cortex*, *30*, 565–583.
Rapcsak, S.Z., Polster, M.R., Glisky, M.L., & Comer, J.F. (1996). False recognition of unfamiliar faces following right hemisphere damage: Neuropsychological and anatomical observations. *Cortex*, *32*, 593–611.
Rapcsak, S.Z., Reminger, S.L., Glisky, E.L., Kaszniak, A.W., & Comer, J.F. (this issue). Neuropsychological mechanisms of false facial recognition following frontal lobe damage. *Cognitive Neuropsychology*, *16*, 267–292.
Reitan, R.M. (1971). Trail Making Test results for normal and brain damaged children. *Perceptual and Motor Skills*, *33*, 575–581.
Rey, A. (1964). *L'examen clinique en psychologie*. Paris: Presses Universitaires de France.
Richardson, J.T.E. (1996). Memory impairment in multiple sclerosis: Reports of patients and relatives. *British Journal of Clinical Psychology*, *35*, 205–219.
Roediger, H.L. (1996). Memory illusions. *Journal of Memory and Language*, *35*, 76–100.
Roediger, H.L., & McDermott, K.B. (1995). Creating false memories: Remembering words not presented in lists. *Journal of Experimental Psychology: Learning, Memory and Cognition*, *21*, 803–814.
Rubin, D.C., & Baddeley, A.D. (1989). Telescoping is not time compression: A model of the dating of autobiographical events. *Memory and Cognition*, *17*, 653–661.
Schacter, D.L. (1995). Memory distortion: History and current status. In D.L. Schacter (Ed.), *Memory distortion*. Cambridge, MA: Harvard Press.
Schacter, D.L., Curran, T., Galluccio, L., Milberg, W.P., & Bates, J.F. (1996). False recognition and the right frontal lobe: A case study. *Neuropsychologia*, *34*, 793–808.
Schacter, D.L., Norman, K.A., & Koutstaal, W. (1998). The cognitive neuroscience of constructive memory. *Annual Review of Psychology*, *49*, 289–318.
Schwartz, M.F., Montgomery, M.W., Fitzpatrick-DeSalme, E.J., Ochipa, C., Coslett, H.B., & Mayer, N.H. (1995). Analysis of a disorder of everyday action. *Cognitive Neuropsychology*, *12*, 863–892.
Semenza, C., & Sgaramella, T.M. (1993). Production of proper names: A clinical case study of the effects of phonemic cueing. *Memory*, *1*, 265–280.
Semenza, C., & Zettin, M. (1988). Generating proper names: A case of selective inability. *Cognitive Neuropsychology*, *5*, 711–721.
Semenza, C., & Zerrin, M. (1989). Evidence from aphasia for the role of proper names as pure referring expressions. *Nature*, *342*, 678–679.
Shallice, T. (1988). *From neuropsychology to mental structure*. Cambridge, UK: Cambridge University Press.
Shallice, T., & Evans, M.E. (1978). The involvement of the frontal lobes in cognitive estimation. *Cortex*, *14*, 294–303.

Shimamura, A.P. (1995). Memory and frontal lobe function. In M.S. Gazzaniga (Ed.), *The cognitive neurosciences*. Cambridge, MA: MIT Press.

Sno, H.N., & Linszen, M.D. (1990). The déjà vu experience: Remembrance of things past? *The American Journal of Psychiatry*, *147*, 1587–1595.

Talland, G.A. (1965). *Deranged memory*. New York: Academic Press.

Tranel, D., & Damasio, A.R. (1985). Knowledge without awareness: An automatic index of facial recognition by prosopagnosics. *Science*, *228*, 1453–1454.

Trenerry, M.R., Crosson, B., DeBoe, J., & Leber, W.R. (1989). *Stroop Neuropsychological Screening Test*. Odessa, FL: Psychological Assessment Resources.

Valentine, T., Brennen, T., & Bredart, S. (1996). *The cognitive psychology of proper names*. London: Routledge.

Warrington, E.K. (1984). *Recognition Memory Test*. London: NFER-Nelson.

Warrington, E.K. (1996). *The Camden Memory Tests*. Hove, UK: Psychology Press.

Warrington, E.K., & McCarthy, R.A. (1987). Categories of knowledge. *Brain*, *110*, 1273–1296.

Wechsler, D. (1981). *Wechsler Adult Intelligence Scale-Revised*. New York: Psychological Corporation.

Wechsler, D. (1984). *Wechsler Memory Scale-Revised*. New York: Psychological Corporation.

Young, A.W., Flude, B.M., Hay, D.C., & Ellis, A.W. (1993). Impaired discrimination of familiar from unfamiliar faces. *Cortex*, *29*, 65–75.

Young, A.W., Hay, D.C., & Ellis, A.W. (1985). The faces that launched a thousand slips: Everyday difficulties and errors in recognising people. *British Journal of Psychology*, *76*, 495–523.

COGNITIVE NEUROPSYCHOLOGY, 1999, 16 (3/4/5), 317–341

PERCEPTUALLY BASED FALSE RECOGNITION OF NOVEL OBJECTS IN AMNESIA: EFFECTS OF CATEGORY SIZE AND SIMILARITY TO CATEGORY PROTOTYPES

Wilma Koutstaal and Daniel L. Schacter
Harvard University, Cambridge, USA

Mieke Verfaellie
Veterans Affairs Medical Center and Boston University School of Medicine, Boston, USA

Carolyn Brenner and Eric M. Jackson
Harvard University, Cambridge, USA

Previous research suggests that amnesics may show impaired semantically based false recognition under conditions where control participants show high levels of gist-based errors, but little or no impairment when controls show less robust false recognition. Using abstract novel objects, we examined perceptually based false recognition in amnesics under conditions designed to induce differing levels of false recognition in controls. Whereas amnesics showed significantly impaired false recognition for category prototypes, and numerically impaired false recognition when many perceptually similar exemplars were studied—conditions where controls showed high rates of illusory recognition—amnesics and controls showed lower, and comparable, levels of false recognition when few related exemplars were studied, or lures were at a far transformational distance from the prototype. Although amnesics may be able to extract some information regarding the perceptual "gist" of studied items, they appear to do so less efficiently than controls.

INTRODUCTION

The strategy of using illusory recollection as a means to probe the nature of memory encoding and retrieval processes has a long and diverse history in psychology (for general review and discussion see Estes, 1997; Johnson, Hashtroudi, & Lindsay, 1993; McClelland, 1995; Roediger, 1996; Schacter, 1995; Schacter, Norman, & Koutstaal, 1998a). Although many studies have focused on participants with intact memory, the uncovering of robust forms of false recollection, and the effort to understand the bases of illusory recollection have also prompted investigations of such errors in persons with impaired memory (for review, see Schacter, 1997; Schacter et al., 1998a).

Several studies have focused on amnesic patients: Individuals who, as a consequence of damage to medial temporal and diencephalic brain regions arising from a variety of possible causes (e.g.

Requests for reprints should be addressed to Wilma Koutstaal, Harvard University, Department of Psychology, 33 Kirkland Street, Cambridge, MA 02138, USA (Tel: (617) 495-3856; Fax: (617) 496-3122; E-mail: wk@wjh.harvard.edu).

This research was supported by National Institute on Aging grant AG08441, the Human Frontiers Science Program, and National Institutes of Mental Health grant R01 MH57681.

anoxia, encephalitis, Korsakoff's syndrome), show marked impairments in long-term memory for newly encountered facts and events, yet retain perceptual and linguistic functions within the normal range (Parkin & Leng, 1993; Squire, 1994). Importantly, these studies have revealed that, under some conditions, amnesics may prove to be *less* susceptible to illusory recollection than are individuals with intact memory, with their impairment in veridical memory in some way buffering them against the errors of illusory memory shown by control participants. In other instances, however, the reverse has been found: Under some conditions amnesics have shown *increased* rates of false recognition, proving to be more prone to such errors than are individuals with unimpaired memory.

One significant factor that may mediate which of these two patterns is observed—depressed versus elevated false recognition among amnesics relative to controls—is the extent to which the nonstudied lure items share semantic or conceptual features with previously encountered stimuli. Several recent studies have examined false recognition in amnesia under conditions where multiple items that are semantically or conceptually related to a particular theme word are presented (Schacter, Verfaellie, & Anes, 1997; Schacter, Verfaellie, Anes, & Racine, 1998b; Schacter, Verfaellie, & Pradere, 1996). A key observation from these studies is that under these conditions—where multiple items might serve to reinforce the conceptual or semantic gist of the list—amnesic patients show both impairment in correct recognition and *decreased* false recognition. For example, Schacter et al. (1996) compared the recognition performance of amnesics and controls in the converging verbal associates paradigm developed by Deese (1959) and Roediger and McDermott (1995). In this paradigm, participants are presented several lists of words, where each of the words in a given list is associatively related to a single (non presented) "critical lure" (e.g. participants might be asked to remember the words *bed*, *rest*, *awake*, *tired*, *dream*, etc., without being presented the word *sleep*, the critical lure to which each of these list words is associated). As expected, the average rate of veridical recognition of control participants (83%) substantially exceeded that of amnesics (46%); however, amnesics also showed impaired *false* recognition: Whereas controls falsely recognised 89% of the critical lures, amnesics' false recognition rate was 57%. Largely similar findings were reported by Schacter et al. (1998b), and by Schacter et al. (1997). In the latter study, using different word lists comprised of fewer semantic associates, amnesics showed impaired true recognition in two experiments and impaired false recognition in one experiment (Expt. 1) but not in another (Expt. 2); however, in the second experiment, control participants also showed particularly low levels of false recognition.

These observations of impaired false recognition in amnesics under conditions where multiple semantic associates are presented stand in marked contrast to an early report indicating that, compared to non-memory-impaired controls, amnesics might show *elevated* rates of false alarms under conditions where the lures are related to only one of the studied items (rather than multiple study items). In an early study, Cermak, Butters, and Gerrein (1973) found that, when only a single related item was presented in a continuous recognition paradigm, Korsakoff amnesics were more likely than alcoholic controls to show false recognition of new items that were similar to previously presented items. Compared to controls, Korsakoff amnesics showed significantly greater false recognition of associatively related words (e.g. study *table*, tested with *chair*), and also of homonyms (e.g. *bear–bare*); amnesics also showed a nonsignificant tendency to more often false alarm to synonyms (*robber–thief*) and to unrelated items than did controls. More recently, in the study by Schacter et al. (1996), amnesic patients demonstrated *both* a pattern of "impaired" false recognition of semantically related items for which many study items were presented, and increased baseline rates of false alarms for items that were unrelated to study items.

What might account for these differing patterns? Schacter et al. (1996) suggested that, when multiple related associates are presented, false recognition among the control participants depends on memory for the associative or semantic information that also supports veridical memory. They proposed that, because control participants were able to retain and integrate or "bind together" the studied items, they formed a strong and well-organised representation of the semantic gist of each set of associates—thereby rendering rejection of the semantically similar lures quite difficult, but also, and simultaneously, facilitating rejection of lures that were unrelated to any of the lists. In contrast, amnesic patients may have formed only a weak or degraded representation of the semantic gist of the list items. Such weak and less well-integrated representations would render amnesics less likely to show false recollection of the related lures, but also relatively less likely to reject unrelated new items successfully (which would not "fail to cohere" with their memory of the lists in the same manner that unrelated items for the control participants did). Based on these considerations, Schacter et al. predicted that, by systematically varying the number of related items that were presented, "it should be possible to specify a crossover point where amnesics shift from *enhanced* to *reduced* false recognitions" (Schacter et al. 1996, p. 329, emphasis added).

These outcomes each involved the false recognition of lures that were conceptually or semantically related to the studied items. Importantly, however, in contrast to these converging findings from studies involving similarity of meaning, the findings relating to the effects of *perceptual* similarity on false recognition of amnesics are notably less clear. Whereas some studies have suggested that amnesics may also show impaired false recollection when items share perceptual similarity (Schacter et al., 1997), other studies have not found a deficit (Kolodny, 1994) or—in instances where perceptual features of studied stimuli are recombined to form new items (Kroll, Knight, Metcalfe, Wolf, & Tulving, 1996, Expt. 2; also cf. Reinitz, Verfaellie, & Milberg, 1996)—have even reported significantly higher false recognition among amnesic individuals[1].

Evidence that perceptually based false recognition in amnesics also might be depressed compared to that found for control participants was reported by Schacter et al. (1997). In addition to conditions manipulating the conceptual similarity of studied items, these researchers included a condition in which they manipulated the perceptual similarity of words, exposing amnesic and control participants to some study lists where the words shared a high level of orthographic and phonemic similarity (e.g. for the related lure *fate*, the study list words were *fade*, *fame*, *face*, *fake*, *mate*, *hate*, *late*, *date*, and *rate*, Experiment 1) or were all rhyming words (Experiment 2). In both experiments, amnesics showed impaired true recognition for such perceptually similar items, and also impaired false recognition (after correcting for baseline levels of false alarms). In one experiment, the level of corrected false recognition of amnesics did not exceed chance; in the second, both amnesics and controls showed above-chance levels of corrected false recognition, but perceptual false recognition of amnesics fell significantly behind that of controls.

[1] The studies of Kroll et al. (1996) and Reinitz et al. (1996) are of particular interest in that, in agreement with many researchers, they underscore the notion that the hippocampal system may play a key role in allowing the "cohesion" or "binding" of different elements into a single trace (e.g. Moscovitch, 1994; Rudy & Sutherland, 1994; Schacter, Church, & Bolton, 1995; Shapiro & Olton, 1994; Sutherland & Rudy, 1989). For example, Reinitz et al. (1996) found that both amnesics and controls often falsely recognised compound words that were comprised of a conjunction of words embedded in previously studied items (e.g. study "*tooth*paste" and "heart*ache*;" test with the lure "*toothache*"); however, whereas controls showed substantially greater veridical recognition for actually studied items (that is, items that preserved both the elements and their relation with one another), amnesics showed largely similar levels of false recognition of recombined conjunction lures and veridical recognition of the target words. These researchers proposed that amnesics may have especial difficulty retaining information concerning *global stimulus structure*, so that although they can remember individual features or parts of items, they have marked deficits in tasks that require access to information about how the parts or features are interrelated to one another. Similar findings of especially heightened susceptibility to conjunction errors among amnesics were reported by Kroll et al. (1996), both for words comprised of recombined syllables (e.g. study "val*ley*" and "*bar*ter," test with "*barley*") and for schematic pictures of faces. Nonetheless, it is also important to note that, unlike the experiments of both Kroll et al. (1996) and Reinitz et al. (1996), in the present study, the lures were not created by recombining previously presented features but were comprised of new elements that were perceptually similar—but not identical—to presented items. Because of this difference, we focus on studies where perceptual similarity was manipulated without the recombination of previously studied elements.

Although suggestive, these findings are somewhat difficult to interpret because the manipulation of perceptual similarity involved familiar words, and thus may have invoked both semantic and perceptual processing. This is especially important as these findings conflict with the outcome of a study in which perceptual similarity was manipulated for abstract novel materials that did not possess prior semantic associations. Kolodny (1994) examined recognition performance of amnesics and controls for "random dot patterns"—patterns that were each comprised of nine simple black dots, arrayed in different statistically determined configurations (cf. Posner, Goldsmith, & Welton, 1967; Posner & Keele, 1968). Participants saw multiple exemplars derived from three different "prototype" patterns and then were given a yes/no recognition test for items that had been presented previously, as well as for new items derived from the prototypes and the prototypes themselves. False recognition of amnesics numerically exceeded that of controls, with false recognition of amnesics (69%) actually somewhat greater than true recognition (59%); in contrast, controls showed the reverse pattern (52% false recognition, 67% true recognition). A similar pattern—with amnesics showing numerically greater false recognition (73%) than controls (63%)—was observed for a subset of the new items that were prototypes or low-level distortions of the prototype, that is, items for which, all else being equal, perceptually based similarity- or gist-based responding might be expected to be most pronounced. Moreover, a second experiment reported by Kolodny (1994), involving pictures with representational content (e.g. paintings with religious or biblical themes), but where lures probably shared both conceptual and perceptual similarity with target items, again showed elevated false recognition among amnesics compared to controls.

Does false recognition derived from the perceptual similarity of lures with previously encountered target items differ in some way from that derived from shared semantic similarity? Direct comparisons of these studies are hampered by the many methodological differences across the paradigms. Also, because the Kolodny (1994) dot pattern study did not include an estimation of baseline levels of false recognition, comparisons with the results of Schacter et al. (1997) using perceptually similar words are difficult. Nonetheless, the differing patterns for these studies clearly suggest the need for further evidence regarding the influence of perceptual similarity on illusory recognition in amnesics relative to controls. Evidence is particularly needed under conditions where: (1) the stimuli are novel objects or patterns for which contributions from pre-existing semantic knowledge are minimised, and (2) factors that manipulate the degree to which general similarity might contribute to performance are used. The possibility that there might be a cross-over pattern in the level of false recognition shown by amnesics versus controls as a function of the degree of false recognition induced among controls is especially of interest because documenting such a pattern for novel perceptually related stimuli would provide evidence for the similarity of gist extraction mechanisms across perceptual and conceptual domains.

The experiment reported here was designed to address these issues. We examined false recognition errors arising from perceptual similarity in a paradigm where the stimuli were abstract novel objects: complex, multi-featured shapes constructed from a prototype. We employed two forms of manipulation that—based on findings from other experiments—are known to affect "general similarity" (Curran, Schacter, Norman, & Galluccio, 1997) or "gist based" (Brainerd, Reyna, & Kneer, 1995; Reyna & Brainerd, 1995) false recognition responding in controls. One manipulation was *category size*. Robust effects of category size have been found in several previous studies of false recognition in individuals with intact memory functioning, with higher rates of false recognition found following the presentation of increasing numbers of semantically related words (e.g. Arndt & Hirshman, 1998; Robinson & Roediger, 1997; Shiffrin, Huber, & Marinelli, 1995), categorised pictures of everyday objects (e.g. Koutstaal & Schacter, 1997; Koutstaal, Schacter, Galluccio, & Stofer, in press), and abstract patterns (e.g. Homa, Cross, Cornell, Goldman, & Schwartz, 1973; Omohundro, 1981). The second manipulation involved the degree of perceptual similarity of the lures: *transformational distance* from a category prototype. High rates of false recognition of prototype items have been reported among individuals with unimpaired memory (e.g. Franks & Bransford, 1971; Solso & Raynis, 1979), with false recognition rates decreasing with decreasing similarity to the prototype.

Based on the findings from Kolodny (1994), one might expect no impairment among amnesics compared to controls in false recognition of perceptually related items (at least for the uncorrected data), and equivalent or even enhanced false recognition of the prototypes. However, based on the findings of Schacter et al. (1997) using perceptually similar words, and also on the findings from studies that used multiple semantically related items (Schacter et al., 1996, 1997, 1998b)—all of which pointed to impaired gist-memory among amnesics—it might be expected that amnesics would show a deficit in false recognition relative to controls, particularly under conditions where there was an opportunity for a *strong* build-up of gist (for example, for categories where many related items were presented during the study phase, and for category prototypes). In contrast, under conditions promoting a less strong build-up of gist in control participants (for example, where only one or a few related exemplars had been presented, or for exemplars at a far distance from the category prototypes), one would not necessarily expect false recognition of amnesic individuals to fall behind that of control participants. When only a few categorically related exemplars had been presented, control participants would not have formed a robust gist-like representation of the category, and so should not be strongly inclined to show false recognition of lure items from the category because of their general similarity to studied items (cf. Homa et al., 1973; Koutstaal & Schacter, 1997; Koutstaal et al., in press; Omohundro, 1981; Robinson & Roediger, 1997). Further, when only a few categorically related items had been presented, controls may be more able to retain, and draw upon, more "item-specific" representations of the actually presented items so as to differentiate studied from nonstudied items and thus successfully "oppose" or "suppress" false recognition responses (cf. Schacter et al., 1998a, b). For these items, the combination of a less robust gist representation, and possibly greater retention of item specific information, among the control participants might result in similar levels of false recognition for amnesics and controls; indeed, as in the case of Cermak et al. (1973), for the smaller category sizes, false recognition among amnesics might even exceed that of controls.

METHOD

Participants

Twelve amnesic patients (9 male, 3 female) and 12 individuals with intact memory functioning (8 male, 4 female) took part in the experiment. Both amnesics and their controls were screened at the Memory Disorders Research Center of the Boston Veterans Affairs Medical Center. A subgroup of six amnesic patients were of mixed aetiology (anoxia, encephalitis, and thalamic infarct) and six had a diagnosis of alcoholic Korsakoff's syndrome. All patients were matched to a corresponding control participant on the basis of age, education, and verbal IQ (Wechsler Adult Intelligence Scale-Revised); the Korsakoff patients were matched to individuals with a history of alcoholism (alcoholic controls) whereas mixed aetiology patients were matched to controls with no history of alcoholism (non-alcoholic controls). Table 1 presents the characteristics of the individual amnesic patients, including their performance on the Wechsler Memory Scale-Revised and, where available, anatomical lesion information. Individual lesion data for the Korsakoff patients is not available; however, several of these patients took part in a larger magnetic resonance imaging study (Jernigan, Schafer, Butters, & Cermak, 1991) that used quantitative image-analytic methods to compare Korsakoff patients to age-matched alcoholic controls and age-matched normal controls. In this study, on a group level, and relative to a larger normative sample of 55 normal volunteers, both alcoholic controls and Korsakoff patients showed considerably reduced diencephalic grey matter volumes; however, the volume loss of Korsakoff patients was

Table 1. *Characteristics of Amnesic Patients*

Patient: Aetiology	*Age*	*Ed*[c]	*Verbal IQ*[d]	*WMS-R*[e] *GM*	*Delay*	*Atn*
CW: Thalamic infarct: bilateral anterior nuclei[a]	56	12	87	79	80	89
AB: Encephalitis: mild diffuse cortical atrophy[b]	58	16	105	76	51	92
PD: Anoxia: enlarged ventricles, diffuse cortical atrophy[b]	60	20	109	65	61	89
JM: Anoxia: bilateral hippocampal complex[b]	48	12	89	70	52	92
PS: Anoxia: bilateral hippocampal complex[b]	39	14	95	90	50	115
RL: Anoxia	68	18	103	68	66	93
Mean	54.8	15.3	98.0	74.7	60.0	95.5
AA: Korsakoff	70	9	93	76	62	109
LB: Korsakoff	63	11	90	99	61	99
PB: Korsakoff	71	14	87	82	60	93
RD: Korsakoff	67	12	83	66	50	99
WR: Korsakoff	69	7	88	76	53	96
RM: Korsakoff	77	14	112	91	68	95
Mean	69.5	11.2	92.2	81.7	59.0	98.5

Anatomical lesion information is provided where available.
[a] Lesions assessed by CT.
[b] Lesions assessed by MRI.
[c] Ed = years of formal education.
[d] Verbal IQ from the Wechsler Adult Intelligence Scale (Revised).
[e] WMS-R = Wechsler Memory Scale-Revised; scores are presented separately for the indices of general memory (GM), delay, and attention (Atn). The WMS-R does not provide scores below 50, and 50 was the lowest score used to compute means.

significantly greater than that of alcoholic controls in anterior regions of the diencephalon; in addition, relative to alcoholic controls, Korsakoff patients showed significant reductions in grey matter in mesial temporal structures and orbitofrontal cortex.

The controls for the mixed amnesic subgroup had a mean age of 50.7 years, with an average of 14.2 years of education and a verbal IQ of 104.2. Alcoholic controls had a mean age of 67.5, an average of 12.8 years of education, and an average verbal IQ of 99.2.

Design

The experimental design included a between-subjects factor of group (amnesic vs. control) and two within-subjects factors: transformational distance and category size. Transformational distance had three levels for studied items (near, middle, far) and four levels for nonstudied items (prototype, near, middle, far). Category size had four levels for studied items: one, three, six, or nine related items presented at study (termed single, small, medium, and large categories respectively) and five levels for nonstudied items: the four levels above, plus "novel" category items for which no related items were presented at study; these latter items provided an estimate of baseline levels of false alarms. In addition, non-categorised items (termed "unrelated," see following) were included both as studied items and as new items.

Stimuli

The stimuli were colour depictions of complex, multi-featured, abstract objects, created using a computer graphics program (Aldus Freehand). Most of the stimuli were "categorised" items, generated by first creating a novel prototype according to a specific set of construction rules (described later), and then generating additional exemplars that belonged to the same category through manipulations that distorted the initial prototype in greater or lesser degree. Also, non-categorised or "unrelated" items were created that did not follow the rules of construction for the categorised items.

Prototypes for 18 different categories were first created according to a set of construction rules. Each prototype consisted of a large central form (the "main" component) together with three smaller features. All of the prototypes were two-dimensional and were created so as to form a single, unified object with multiple parts. The prototypes were created so as to be as dissimilar from one another as possible. Each category had a set of four unique features associated with it; these features were assigned in all possible groupings of three to create four "prototypes" per category, with the only difference between the prototypes for a given category being the features they contained. Specifically, using the letters *a*, *b*, *c*, and *d* to designate the four possible features of a category, the prototypes for a given category consisted of one—invariant—main component, with superimposed features of either *abc*, *abd*, *acd*, or *bcd*. The features associated with a given category were selected to possess some "pairwise" similarity (i.e. the features within a category comprised two pairs of two features, with the features in each pair being relatively similar to one another). The placement of features on the main unit was constant for a given feature, such that if the different prototypes of a category shared a given feature, it appeared in a similar place.

The initial prototypes were then manipulated in various prescribed ways, including alterations of shape, colour, outline, and size, to create additional exemplars that possessed varying degrees of similarity to the prototypes. These manipulations specified particular types and ranges of manipulations and were applied in an algorithmic fashion to items within each category. The placement of features on these exemplars was also altered, but within a specified range (e.g. a given feature would generally appear more towards the top or side of an object, but its precise placement varied somewhat).

Pilot research that examined yes/no recognition of the exemplars derived from these algorithmically applied alterations suggested that the items were too similar to one another: Participants were largely unable to discriminate studied from nonstudied exemplars. Accordingly, the stimuli were further altered to increase the within-category distinctiveness of the stimuli. This involved several further steps: first, each item in a category was further manipulated in a specified manner (e.g. one exemplar's shape was "bent" a certain amount, another exemplar's outline was increased in thickness, etc.); then, following these manipulations, three items within each category that were still relatively similar to one another were selected for additional alterations that rendered the three items less similar to one another and to other exemplars within the category. These latter alterations employed overall manipulations (e.g. rendering the entire shape into a somewhat "swirled" or "warped" shape) and, if necessary, were followed by yet a further manipulation in which particular portions of the shape were altered. Finally, because these further alteration procedures resulted in non systematic variations in the initial "distance metric" for the exemplars, the similarity of the new items to the prototypes was assessed by asking six raters to place the exemplars in each category on a distance metric corresponding to how similar they were to the prototype. The transformational distance of a given item was then determined by the average of the six raters' judgements, in conjunction with the further ratings of two of the experimenters (EJ and WK) in cases where the judges' ratings did not point to a clear outcome. In addition, the two exemplars that comprised the clearest representatives of the three distances (near, middle, and far) were chosen to comprise the critical stimulus items (to be counterbalanced across study and test status; see following).

Examples of the categorised items are provided in Fig 1. Shown in the upper two panels are

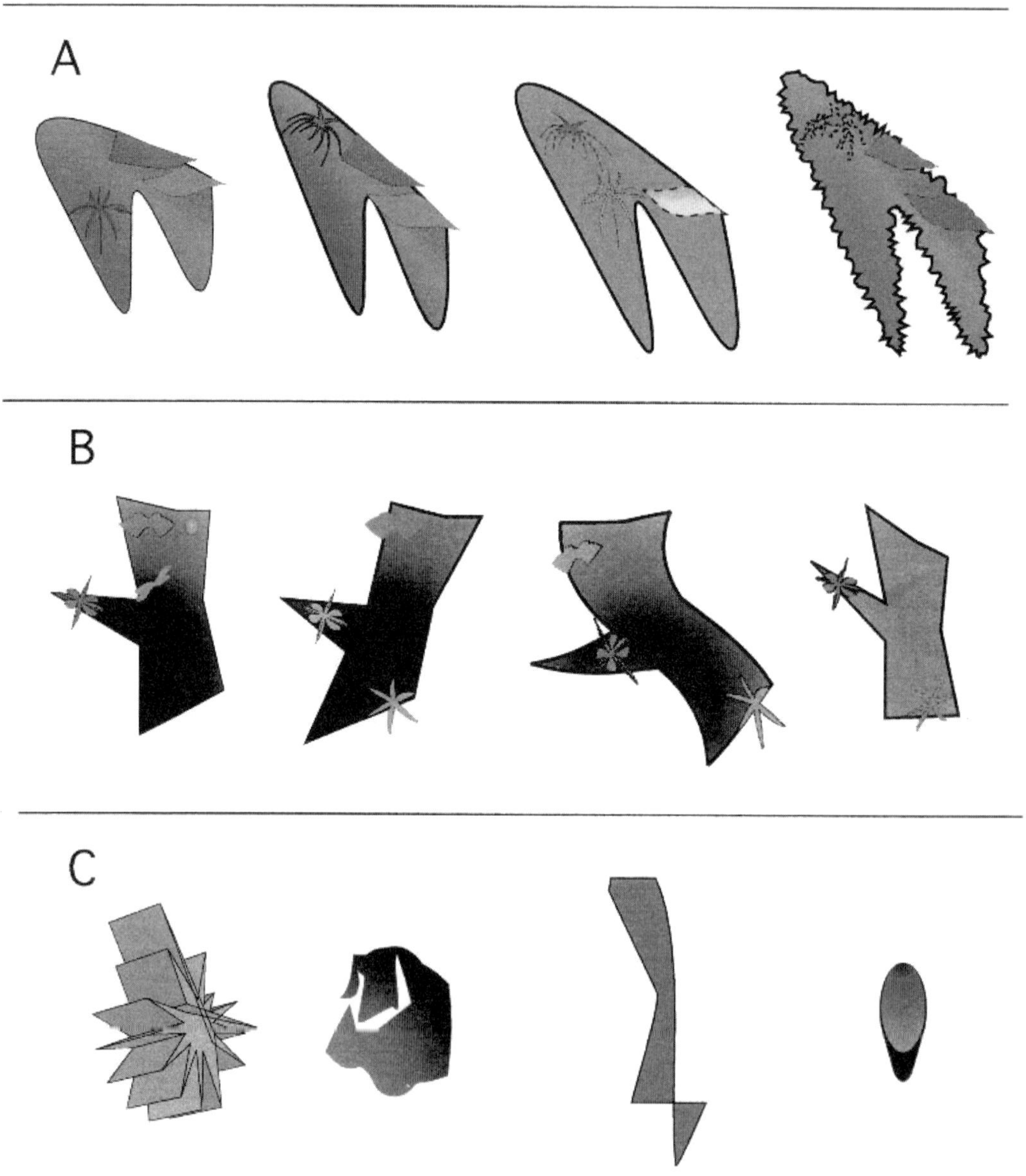

Fig. 1. *Examples of categorised stimuli (A, B) and unrelated items (C). The upper two panels show examples from two different categories including, from left to right, a category prototype, and items from the near, middle, and far transformational distances respectively. Note that, although, for illustrative purposes here, the stimuli are shown in black and white, the stimuli as shown to participants were presented in colour, with colour comprising an important attribute that was varied both within and across categories.*

exemplars from two categories including (from left to right) a prototype, and items from the near, middle, and far distances. In addition, examples of unrelated items are shown in the bottom panel; unrelated items were never comprised of four components and could be either two- or three-dimensional figures.

For each category, the critical exemplars of each distance were randomly assigned to one of two sets (A or B). These sets were subsequently used for counterbalancing the critical exemplars across studied and nonstudied status. In order to avoid confounding the number of related exemplars that were presented at *study* with the number of items that were *tested*, only a subset of all the items in each category was tested: for the three-, six-, and nine-item categories, three old items (one from each distance) and four new items (one from each distance, plus the prototype) were tested; for categories where only one item was presented, only this single target item (always a middle distance item), and two new items (one from the middle distance, plus the prototype) were tested. Category size at study was manipulated by systematically excluding some of the noncritical items depending on the category size to be used: no noncritical items were excluded for nine-item categories, but a given set of three noncritical items (one at each distance) was excluded for six-item categories, and six noncritical items (two at each distance) were excluded for three-item categories. For categories where only one item was presented at study, only one middle distance item from the critical items was presented (from Set A or Set B, depending on the counterbalancing condition).

Templates for the study and test lists were created such that, within each third of the list, the number of items from each category type, category size (including singles, and unrelated items), and transformational distance (near, middle, far) were balanced; in addition, for the test lists, the number of novel items and prototypes was also balanced across the test thirds. Finally, additional templates were created employing different orderings of the items within each of the test thirds.

For counterbalancing purposes, the 18 categories were assigned to 6 stimulus subsets comprised of 3 categories each; these subsets were used to determine, across subjects, whether a given category was shown as studied items or as novel items, with 1 stimulus subset assigned to each of the large, medium, small, and novel category-size conditions (each of which were thus represented by 3 categories), and 2 stimulus subsets assigned to the single condition (thus represented by 6 categories). Counterbalancing across subjects ensured that each category occurred in each of the 6 conditions once, with each category represented once with the "A" and "B" exemplars as the studied, and nonstudied, exemplars. Thus a counterbalancing required 12 subjects. Amnesics and their matched controls were assigned the same counterbalancing lists.

Procedure

The overall procedure involved three phases, including a study phase, in which participants were exposed to the stimuli under an incidental encoding task, a brief retention interval, and the test phase. All participants were tested individually, in a single session of approximately 40 to 50 minutes. The stimuli at both study and test were presented via a powerbook computer with a colour monitor, using the PsyScope experimental presentation program. The stimuli appeared in the centre of the screen, with prompts for responding to the encoding task or the recognition test displayed beneath.

In the study phase, participants were shown a total of 78 items (72 critical items, preceded and followed by 3 buffer items; critical items = 27 large, 18 medium, 9 small, 6 single, and 12 unrelated items). Each item was presented for 6 seconds, and participants were asked to rate the "overall complexity" of the stimulus on a 9-point scale, where "1" indicated the stimulus was not at all complex and "9" indicated it was extremely complex. In making their complexity ratings, participants were instructed to consider all aspects of the stimulus, including both different dimensions of the stimulus (e.g. shape, colour, size, and outline) and all of the components of the stimulus. Participants entered their complexity ratings on the computer keyboard, using the number keys 1–9. The study items were preceded by a brief practice session that included items from two further categories not employed in the experiment and additional unrelated items.

The study phase was followed by a 5-minute retention interval, during which participants performed an unrelated number search task. In the test phase, participants were shown a subset of the items shown in the study phase, together with new items, and were asked to designate each item as "old" (previously presented) or "new" (never previously presented). The test list included 117 items, of which 45 were "old" and 72 were "new." The old items consisted of 3 items from each of the studied categories, with the exception of the single categories, where only the single studied item was presented, plus the 12 unrelated items (i.e. old items = 3 × 3 large category items, 3 × 3 medium category items, 3 × 3 small category items, 6 × 1 single category items, and 12 unrelated items). The new items were comprised of 3 related lure items from each of the studied categories (or, for the single categories, 1 new item), together with one prototype from each category; in addition there were 3 items plus the prototype from each of 3 novel categories, and 12 new unrelated items.

RESULTS

All analyses are first presented combining across the two amnesic subgroups (i.e. combining across the mixed aetiology and Korsakoff subgroups), with results first considered as a function of transformational distance, and then as a function of category size. Thereafter, the two subgroups are briefly considered separately. The Appendix presents the central true and false recognition outcomes for individual patients in both the mixed aetiology and Korsakoff groups. The results for the unrelated items are presented first. To increase the normality of the distributions, and to make "equal differences equally detectable" (Rosenthal & Rosnow, 1991; Snedecor & Cochran, 1989), all analyses of proportions were performed after arcsine transformation.

Combined Groups

Unrelated Items

We first considered performance for the unrelated items, that is, items that were markedly different from the categorised items and that did not follow the basic rules of construction for category items (see Table 2). For these items, amnesics showed substantially impaired veridical recognition: means of 65% vs. 43% for controls and amnesics respectively, $F(1,22) = 5.02$, $MSe = 0.09$, $P = .04$. False alarms to unrelated items were numerically, but not significantly, more frequent for amnesics (.24) than controls (.18), $F < 1$. After correcting for these (nonsignificant) baseline differences in false alarms to unrelated lures, veridical recognition of control participants also significantly exceeded that of amnesics, $F(1,22) = 10.52$, $MSe = 0.05$, $P = .004$.

Analyses by Distance

Table 3 presents the proportion of "old" responses given to studied items (true recognition) and nonstudied items (false recognition) for amnesics and controls, with responses shown separately as a function of distance from the prototype (near, middle, far). Also shown are the proportion of "old" responses to the prototypes (averaged for study categories comprised of three, six, and nine items), and the baseline rate of false alarms to novel items. (Note that the results for "single" items, for which only one categorised item was presented at study and which was always from the "middle" distance, are not considered here but are considered in the subsequent section considering the effects of category size.)

Table 2. *Recognition Responses for Unrelated (Noncategorised) Items*

	Hits	*False Alarms*	*Hits – False Alarms*
Amnesic	.43	.24	.20
Korsakoff	.40	.14	.26
Mixed	.46	.33	.13
Control	.65	.18	.47
Alcoholic	.56	.18	.38
Non-alcoholic	.74	.18	.56

Table 3. *True and False Recognition Responses by Transformational Distance*

	True Recognition				*False Recognition*					
	Near	*Middle*	*Far*	*Mean*	*Near*	*Middle*	*Far*	*Mean*	*Prototype*	*Novel*
Amnesic	.60	.59	.56	.58	.58	.50	.39	.49	.52	.35
Korsakoff	.65	.69	.56	.63	.56	.54	.50	.53	.61	.35
Mixed	.56	.50	.56	.54	.61	.46	.28	.45	.43	.35
Control	.80	.80	.62	.74	.69	.62	.41	.57	.72	.38
Alcoholic	.85	.82	.69	.78	.72	.65	.46	.61	.72	.47
Non-alcoholic	.74	.78	.56	.69	.65	.59	.35	.53	.72	.28

Items for categories where only one item was shown at study are omitted because for these categories all exemplars were from the middle distance. The prototype means shown are also based only on categories where three, six, or nine exemplars were shown. Novel indicates the baseline level of false alarms to "novel" category exemplars (0 exemplars shown at study).

From Table 3 it can be seen that, whereas true recognition of amnesics was largely unaffected by the distance of studied exemplars from the prototype (means of .60, .59, and .56 for near, middle, and far respectively), true recognition of the controls was more strongly affected by distance. Control participants showed a high level of correct recognition for near and middle distance items (.80) but considerably reduced recognition for items that were far from the prototype (.62). Table 3 also shows that false recognition for both amnesics and controls declines with increasing distance, but with controls showing higher false recognition for near and middle distance items (means for near, middle, and far respectively, for amnesics of .58, .50, and .39, compared to .69, .62, and .41 for controls). Importantly, from Table 3 it can also be seen that the group differences in false recognition are most pronounced for the prototypes. Relative to the controls, amnesics show a false recognition impairment of 20% for the prototype items compared to an impairment of 11%, 12%, and 2% for lures from the near, middle, and far distances respectively. Amnesics and controls showed moderately high and very similar baseline rates of false alarms: "old" responses to novel category items of .35 and .38 respectively. False alarms to these novel category items—that is, items that followed the same general rules as all of the categorised items but were not from the categories that were presented—provide a measure of participants' general willingness to respond "old" under conditions of uncertainty, but where the stimuli share broad similarity with the types of items that were studied.

The true and false recognition scores following correction for differences in baseline levels of false alarms (Hits − Novel Category False Alarms, and Related False Alarms − Novel Category False Alarms, or "novel-corrected" scores) are shown in Table 4. Focusing first on the true recognition results, an initial 2 (Group: amnesic or control) × 3 (Distance: near, middle, far) analysis of variance (ANOVA) on the novel-corrected true recognition scores showed a significant effect of Distance, $F(2,44) = 4.36$, $MSe = 0.03$, $P = .02$, but no effect of Group, $F = 2.1$, and no Group × Distance interaction, $F < 1.6$. Pairwise comparisons showed that, averaging across groups, novel-corrected true recognition for near and middle distance items exceeded that of far distance items (smallest $F = 6.66$), but near and middle distance items did not differ from one another ($F < 1$). Combining the near and middle distance items and comparing novel-corrected true recognition for these items with that for the far distance items, and also including Group as a factor, again showed a main effect of Distance, $F(1,22) = 10.49$, $MSe = 0.02$, $P = .004$; however, in this more focused analysis, the differentially enhanced performance of the controls for the near and middle distance items was more strongly apparent: $F(1,22) = 4.08$, $MSe = 0.02$, $P = .06$ for the Group × Distance interaction.

Next considering false recognition, a 2 (Group) × 4 (Distance: prototype, near, middle,

Table 4. *Novel-corrected True and False Recognition Responses by Transformational Distance*

	True Recognition				*False Recognition*				
	Near	*Middle*	*Far*	*Mean*	*Near*	*Middle*	*Far*	*Mean*	*Prototype*
Amnesic	.26*	.25*	.21*	.24*	.24*	.15*	.04	.14*	.17*
Korsakoff	.30*	.34*	.21*	.28*	.21*	.19*	.15	.18*	.26*
Mixed	.21*	.15	.21[a]	.19[a]	.26*	.12	− .07	.10	.08
Control	.42*	.42*	.25*	.36*	.31*	.25*	.03	.20*	.35*
Alcoholic	.38*	.34*	.21[a]	.31*	.25*	.18[a]	− .01	.14[a]	.25*
Non-alcoholic	.46*	.50*	.28*	.41*	.37*	.32*	.07	.25*	.45*

Items for categories where only one item was shown at study are omitted because for these categories all exemplars were from the middle distance. The prototype means shown are also based only on categories where three, six, or nine exemplars were shown.

* $P < .05$ for comparisons against zero.

[a] Marginal effects: $.05 < P < .10$ for comparisons against zero.

far) ANOVA performed on the novel-corrected false recognition scores revealed a main effect of Distance, $F(3,66) = 15.34$, $MSe = 0.02$, $P < .0001$, no effect of group, $F < 1.5$, and a slight trend toward a Group × Distance interaction, $F(3,66) = 2.04$, $MSe = 0.02$, $P = .12$. Pairwise comparisons showed that, except for the prototype and near items, novel-corrected false recognition decreased regularly with increasing distance from the prototype (prototype = near > middle > far; for the near, middle, and far comparisons, smallest $F = 5.77$). Critically, however, although there was no overall effect of group, an analysis restricted to the novel-corrected false recognition scores for the *prototypes* alone revealed significantly impaired false recognition among amnesics relative to controls, $F(1,22) = 4.36$, $MSe = 0.05$, $P = .05$.

Analyses by Category Size

Table 5 presents the proportion of "old" responses for the amnesic and control groups separately as a function of category size (one, three, six, or nine related exemplars shown at study) for both studied items ("true recognition") and nonstudied items ("false recognition"). Also shown are the proportion of old responses to novel items (i.e. the baseline measure of false alarms). In order to reduce the number of comparisons, and to increase the power of individual comparisons, we combined the two relatively smaller category sizes (one and three related items presented) and the two relatively larger categories (six and nine related items presented), contrasting the two larger and two smaller categories.

We first considered veridical recognition as a function of category size after correcting for novel false alarms (see Table 6). For novel-corrected true recognition, a 2 (Group) × 2 (Category Size: larger vs. smaller) ANOVA revealed no overall effect of Group, $F = 1.9$, an effect of Category Size, $F(1,22) = 12.52$, $MSe = 0.01$, $P = .002$, and a Group × Category Size interaction, $F(1,22) = 4.71$, $MSe = 0.01$, $P = .04$. Overall, novel-corrected veridical recognition was greater for larger (.32) than smaller (.23) categories, but this difference was largely carried by control participants (.24 vs. .20 for amnesics compared to .41 vs. .25 for controls).

We next conducted a similar 2 (Group) × 2 (Category Size: larger vs. smaller) analysis on the novel-corrected false recognition scores. This analysis showed a main effect of Category Size, $F(1,22) = 14.51$, $MSe = 0.02$, $P = .001$, with no effect of Group, $F < 1$, and no Category Size × Group interaction, $F = 2.0$. False recognition was greater for lures from many-exemplar categories (.21) than for lures from few-exemplar categories (.07), with both amnesics and controls showing this pattern (for amnesics, .17 vs. .08, difference of 9%; for controls, .26 vs. .06, difference of 20%).

Table 5. *True and False Recognition Responses by Category Size*

	True Recognition					*False Recognition*									
	Category Items					*Category Items*					*Prototype*				
	9	*6*	*3*	*1*	*Mean*	*9*	*6*	*3*	*1*	*Mean*	*9*	*6*	*3*	*1*	*Novel*
Amnesic	.62	.56	.57	.53	.57	.55	.48	.44	.40	.47	.56	.44	.56	.29	.35
Korsakoff	.76	.57	.56	.56	.61	.67	.50	.43	.42	.50	.72	.61	.50	.25	.35
Mixed	.48	.54	.59	.50	.53	.43	.46	.46	.39	.44	.39	.28	.61	.33	.35
Control	.81	.76	.65	.60	.70	.68	.58	.45	.42	.53	.86	.70	.61	.32	.38
Alcoholic	.83	.82	.70	.64	.75	.65	.63	.56	.50	.58	.89	.61	.67	.36	.47
Non-alcoholic	.78	.70	.59	.56	.66	.70	.54	.35	.33	.48	.83	.78	.56	.28	.28

False recognition responses to the prototype are also shown separately as a function of category size (nine, six, three, or one item shown at study). Also shown are false alarms to "novel" items.

We also considered novel-corrected false recognition of the prototypes separately as a function of the number of exemplars that were studied. A 2 (Group) × 2 (Category Size: larger vs. smaller) ANOVA revealed a marginal effect of Group, with controls tending to show greater overall false recognition of the prototypes on this measure than amnesics, $F(1,22) = 3.34$, $MSe = 0.08$, $P = .08$. (Note that, because this analysis includes single categories, it differs somewhat from the analyses reported earlier for transformational distance, which excluded the single item categories, and where amnesics were significantly impaired on this measure.) There was also a main effect of Category Size, $F(1,22) = 10.51$, $MSe = 0.05$, $P = .004$, and a trend toward a Group × Category Size interaction, $F(1,22) = 4.10$, $MSe = 0.05$, $P = .06$. Comparing the level of novel-corrected false recognition of the prototypes for the amnesics versus controls within each category size separately showed that amnesics were significantly impaired in false recognition of prototypes from large categories, $F(1,22) = 4.92$, $MSe = 0.12$, $P = .04$, marginally impaired in false recognition of prototypes from medium categories, $F(1,22) = 2.75$, $MSe = 0.15$, $P = .11$, and not impaired for prototypes from small or single-item categories, *F*s < 1.

Table 6. *Novel-corrected True and False Recognition Responses by Category Size*

	True Recognition					*False Recognition*									
	Category Items					*Category Items*					*Prototype*				
	9	*6*	*3*	*1*	*Mean*	*9*	*6*	*3*	*1*	*Mean*	*9*	*6*	*3*	*1*	*Mean*
Amnesic	.27*	.21*	.23*	.18*	.22*	.20*	.13*	.10	.06	.12*	.21[a]	.10	.21*	– .06	.12*
Korsakoff	.41*	.23[a]	.21[a]	.21[a]	.26*	.32*	.15	.08	.07	.16*	.38*	.26[a]	.15	– .10	.17*
Mixed	.13	.19	.25*	.15	.18[a]	.08	.12	.12	.04	.09	.04	– .07	.26*	– .01	.06
Control	.43*	.38*	.27*	.22*	.33*	.30*	.21*	.08	.04	.16*	.49*	.32*	.24*	– .06	.25*
Alcoholic	.36*	.34*	.23	.17	.28*	.18*	.16	.08	.03	.11	.42*	.14	.20*	– .11	.16[a]
Non-alcoholic	.50*	.43*	.32*	.28*	.38*	.43*	.26[a]	.07	.06	.20*	.56*	.50*	.28*	1.3E-4	.33*

Results are shown for true and false recognition following correction for baseline levels of false alarms to novel category items.

* $P < .05$ for comparisons against zero.

[a] Marginal effects: $.05 < P < 10$ for comparisons against zero.

Subgroup Analyses

From the means shown in Table 3 and Table 5 it can be seen that, in absolute terms, the Korsakoff patients generally showed higher levels of both true and false recognition than did mixed amnesics (average true recognition for all four category sizes for Korsakoff vs. mixed amnesics respectively of .61 vs. .53, average false recognition of .50 vs. .44). Korsakoff patients also showed greater false recognition of the prototypes than did mixed amnesics, with this effect especially pronounced for items for which nine or six related exemplars had been studied (Korsakoff patients, means of .72 and .61; mixed amnesics, means of .39 and .28 respectively). However, a largely similar pattern was found for the two subgroups' respective *control groups*, with the alcoholic controls on average showing numerically higher true recognition than did the mixed aetiology controls (means for all four category sizes of .75 vs. .66 respectively) and also higher false recognition (means of .58 vs. .48). An exception, however, concerned unrelated items (see Table 2), where alcoholic controls showed relatively less true recognition than did mixed controls (.56 and.74 respectively).

Because the alcoholic controls also showed an especially high rate of false alarms to novel items (.47 compared to .35 for the Korsakoff amnesics), after correction for baseline levels of false alarms, there were relatively small and unsystematic differences in corrected true and false recognition for the Korsakoff group compared to their controls (e.g. for all four category sizes, overall novel-corrected true recognition of .26 vs. .28 for Korsakoff patients and alcoholic controls respectively; overall novel-corrected false recognition of .16 vs. .11; likewise, for false recognition of the prototypes, novel-corrected false recognition averages of .26 vs. .25 respectively). In contrast, mixed amnesics and their controls showed a less pronounced difference in baseline rates of false alarms to novel categorised items (.35 and .28 respectively).

Focusing on the performance of the mixed amnesia subgroup, Table 3 and Table 5 show that the recognition performance of the mixed amnesic patients was quite consistent with the expectation that, under conditions of relatively little or weak gist, amnesics might show levels of false recognition similar to, or exceeding, that shown by controls. False recognition of the mixed amnesics numerically exceeded that shown by controls for *novel items* (.35 vs. .28), for *single-item category lures* (.39 vs. .33) and for *three-item category lures* (.46 vs. .35). However, also as expected, under conditions of relatively greater build-up of gist, this pattern reversed, with the control participants showing higher levels of false recognition than the mixed amnesics for larger category sizes, where either six or nine items had been presented (for six-item categories, false recognition of .46 vs. .54 for mixed amnesics versus their controls respectively; for nine-item categories, .43 vs. .70). This difference was also observed for the prototypes, where the false recognition rate of mixed amnesics fell nearly 30% behind their controls (combining across categories of three, six, and nine items, means of .43 vs. .72). Indeed, within the prototypes themselves, a similar "crossover" in performance as a function of category size (and presumably "gist") was observed, with mixed amnesics falling well behind their controls in false recognition of the prototypes for the six- and nine-item categories (.39 vs. .83, and .28 vs. .78 respectively) but with the pattern reversed for the three-item and single-item categories (.61 vs. .56, and .33 vs. .28, respectively).

For the novel-corrected data, subgroup analyses revealed no significant differences for the Korsakoff amnesics compared to their controls. For the mixed amnesics, significant or nearly significant differences in novel-corrected true recognition were found for near-distance items [means of .21 vs. .46, $F(1,10) = 4.98$, $MSe = 0.05$, $P = .05$]; for middle-distance items [means of .15 vs. .50, $F(1,10) = 4.64$, $MSe = 0.09$, $P = .06$]; items from large categories [means of .13 vs. .50, $F(1,10) = 9.64$, $MSe = 0.05$, $P = .01$]; and for unrelated items [means of .13 vs. .56, $F(1,10) = 13.01$, $MSe = 0.05$, $P = .005$]. For novel-corrected false recognition, significant or nearly significant differences were found for middle-distance items [means of .12 vs. .32, $F(1, 10) = 3.66$, $MSe = 0.04$, $P = .08$]; for items from large categories [means of .08 vs. .43, $F(1,10) = 5.27$, $MSe = 0.08$, $P = .04$]; prototypes for large categories [means of .04 vs. .56, $F(1,10) = 6.55$, $MSe = 0.16$, $P = .03$]; prototypes for medium categories [means of − .07 vs. .50, $F(1,10) = 10.09$, $MSe = 0.12$, $P = .01$]; and for the prototypes from large, medium, and small categories combined [means of .08 vs. .45, $F(1,10) = 7.31$, $MSe = 0.06$, $P = .02$]. The pattern of depressed false recognition for the larger categories and for prototypes was quite consistent across patients (see individual patient data in the Appendix): for the larger category sizes, and for the near/middle transformational distances, five of the six mixed aetiology patients showed false recognition scores that fell below the mean of the controls; for the prototypes, all of the mixed aetiology patients showed lower false recognition rates than the mean for their controls.

GENERAL DISCUSSION

A central finding of this experiment is that amnesics may show *either* substantial impairment of perceptually based false recognition, or virtually no impairment, depending on the nature of the experimental conditions and the extent to which they allow the extraction of gist information among control participants. Under some conditions—particularly those that allow maximal strengthening of gist-based representations in controls—amnesics showed a substantial impairment of perceptually based false recognition for pictures of novel abstract objects for which they had no pre-existing semantic or conceptual knowledge. However, under conditions where control participants showed relatively less robust false recognition, false recognition of amnesics was also less impaired. The deficit in amnesics' false recognition was especially apparent for the prototypes. For the control participants, the prototypes elicited the highest levels of false recognition that were observed for any of the experimental conditions, with rates of false recognition that matched, or for some conditions exceeded, those seen for true recognition. Yet for these items, amnesic patients showed a substantial and reliable deficit in false recognition.

Although this pattern was observed both in the overall group analysis (associated with a false recognition deficit of 18% after taking baseline false alarms into account), and in the analysis for the mixed aetiology subgroup alone (associated with a novel-corrected false recognition deficit of 37%), the unusually high baseline level of false alarms among the alcoholic control group largely eliminated the pattern observed for the uncorrected or absolute scores in the subgroup of Korsakoff patients. Thus the conclusions for this subgroup are less clear. Ignoring the baseline differences, Korsakoff and mixed aetiology patients generally showed not dissimilar patterns for transformational distance. Korsakoff patients showed comparatively greater false recognition "deficits" for the prototype and near and middle distance items (deficits of .11, .16, and .11) than for far distance items (deficit of − .04); mixed aetiology patients did not show a very marked deficit for near items (.04) but showed strong deficits for middle distance items (.13) and an extremely marked deficit for the prototypes (.29) with little deficit for far distance items (.07). For the factor of category size, however, mixed aetiology amnesics showed more systematic "gist-related" deficits than did Korsakoff patients.

The nature of this "gist-related" pattern of deficits in mixed amnesics is perhaps most clearly seen by comparing the differences in false recognition of mixed amnesics versus their controls for the various categories. These differences were positive, showing numerically higher false recognition for amnesics than for controls, for each of five categories involving few items: novel items, single items, single item prototypes, small category items, and small category prototypes (differences of + 7%, + 6%, + 5%, + 11% and + 5% respectively); in marked contrast, for medium and large category items, and medium and large category prototypes, the differences were all negative and, in several instances, of substantial magnitude (− 8%, − 27%, − 50%, and − 44%), now in each case showing higher false recognition for controls than for amnesics or "impaired false recognition" for amnesics. A focused comparison, contrasting the performance of mixed amnesics versus their controls for the former set of items, drawn from "low-gist" conditions, against those for the latter set of items drawn from "high-gist" conditions, yielded no effect of Group, $F < 1$, a main effect of Gist (high gist = .55, low gist = .39), $F(1,10) = 9.15$, $MSe = 0.02$, $P = .01$, and a highly significant Group × Gist interaction, $F(1,10) = 14.40$, $MSe = 0.02$, $P = .004$.

This interaction provides clear evidence for a "crossover" in the false recognition performance of amnesics versus control participants as a function of the number of categorically related items that had been encountered previously. Moreover, consistent with the proposal made earlier by Schacter et al. (1997), the across-group difference tracks with the *magnitude of the false recognition effect in the control group*, with mixed aetiology amnesics showing the greatest deficits under conditions where gist-based responding among their normal controls is most robust, namely for the large categories (.70) and medium categories (.54) and especially for the prototypes from these categories (.83 and .78 respectively). Mixed amnesics showed no such deficit, however, for the small or single item categories, where gist-based responding among controls was also much lower (.35 and .33 respectively).

What might account for these differential patterns, with amnesics showing little or no impairment under some conditions (few or far transformational distance exemplars) and substantial impairment under others (many or near transformational distance exemplars)? A pattern of this form might emerge if amnesics showed uniformly little effect of the manipulations of category size or transformational distance but controls were sensitive to these manipulations—acquiring an increasingly strong sense of familiarity with the categories as more exemplars were encountered, and more often incorrectly succumbing to this sense of familiarity if a lure item was similar to many previously encountered items, or if it was similar to (or actually was) the most representative or "prototypical" instance of the category. On this account, a differential pattern of impairment across the different conditions would emerge because, in the control participants, general familiarity with the categories was relatively weak in some conditions (and thus matched that of amnesics) but continued to accumulate in other conditions (and thus exceeded that of amnesics).

This simple account, however, does not appear to provide a sufficiently modulated portrayal of the data. Although, overall, the performance of amnesic patients was less affected by the factors of transformational distance and category size than was found for control participants, amnesics were not entirely immune to the influence of perceptual gist or general similarity information. Combining across the two amnesic subgroups, amnesics' overall level of false recognition for the category lures (.47) significantly exceeded their baseline level of false alarms to novel category items (.35), $F(1,11) = 7.37$, $MSe = 0.01$, $P = .02$. Further, at least in numerical terms, amnesics showed some "gist-like systematicity" in their false recognition responses to categorised lures, showing numerically greater false recognition of categorised lure items that were closer in similarity to the prototypes (means of .58, .50, and .39 for near, middle, and far distance items respectively) and also for lures for which a larger number of related items had been presented at study (.55, .48, .44, and .40 for study categories comprised of nine, six, three, and one items respectively). This result suggests that amnesics were able to retain at least some "category-specific" information regarding the stimulus items, and that this information—like that for controls—was influenced by the factors of transformational distance and category size, albeit to a lesser degree.

The obtained pattern of results, therefore, can be better understood in terms of a differential build-up of gist information in the amnesics compared to the controls. If category specific information was extracted and/or retained less efficiently by amnesics than by control participants, this difference might be least evident in cases where controls also were able to construct only relatively weak gist representations (as when few category exemplars were presented), but might emerge more strongly as the gist representations of controls became increasingly robust. Given the relatively low levels of within-category discriminability shown by both amnesics (on average, approximately 10%) and controls (less than 20% for the categorised items, excluding the prototypes), it is likely that this category-specific information was of a relatively global and "coarse" form, most often involving general familiarity with the nature of "category-like" items rather than specific or richly detailed recollection.

This account of the differences in false recognition between amnesics and controls is based on the notion that an impairment in gist extraction might selectively affect performance for large category sizes and near transformational distance exemplars. The same pattern of results, however, might emerge if control participants had stronger gist representations for the smaller category sizes or far transformational distance exemplars, but if controls—unlike amnesics—were able to *counteract* false recognition responses successfully for these items (cf. Schacter et al., 1998b). That is, it is possible that individuals in the control group actually had a stronger gist-like representation than did amnesics for the smaller categories (as they apparently did for the larger categories), but they were able to oppose or suppress gist-based responding for these items by relying on more detailed, item-specific memory (which might, for example, suffer from less interference when few rather than many overlapping exemplars had been studied, cf. Schacter et al., 1998a).

The overall pattern of performance by the control participants argues against a strong contribution from this factor. For a "selective suppression" account of this form to be viable, it would be expected that control participants would demonstrate a high level of item-specific memory in those conditions in which suppression was occurring. Such "item-specific" memory might be shown in various ways, but one measure—readily obtained from the present data—is participants' ability to discriminate studied items from similar but not studied lures (i.e. hits minus related false alarms). Overall, controls showed somewhat greater ability than did amnesics to discriminate studied targets from related category lures. Yet, contrary to what would be expected on the basis of a selective suppression account, amnesics and controls showed numerically *less* pronounced differences in such within-category discriminability for the far distance items (True Target − Related False Target means of .17 for amnesics compared to .21 for controls) than for middle distance items (means of .09 vs. .18) or near distance items (means of .02 vs. .11). Similarly, for the factor of category size, the differences in within category discriminability for amnesics versus controls were not noticeably more pronounced for the smaller categories (means of .13 and .19 for amnesics and controls) than for the larger categories (means of .07 vs. .15 for amnesics and controls).

One qualification concerning the differential patterns of false recognition for amnesics versus controls that we observed concerns the levels of false recognition that emerged for lures at a far transformational distance from the prototype, and for lures from smaller categories, where participants were exposed to only one or three target items per category. For these conditions, neither amnesics nor controls showed rates of false recognition significantly above those found for novel category lures (on average, for both combined groups, false recognition of far distance items was approximately 4% greater than for novel category lures and between 6% and 8% for the smaller categories; also see Table 4 and Table 6, where asterisks indicate the conditions where novel-corrected true recognition and novel-corrected false recognition exceeded chance levels). On the one hand, this pattern is of concern because, where false recognition rates are at floor or at near-floor levels, it would be difficult to detect a difference between the amnesic and control groups. On the other hand, and while acknowledging this as a legitimate concern, it might also be noted that the absolute levels of false recognition for the far distance lures and smaller category lures were not inconsiderable, ranging between .28 and .50 for the four subgroups for far distance items, and between .33 and .56 for the smaller category sizes. Further, the near-equivalence of false recognition rates in these cases to the false alarm rate observed for lures from novel categories—that is, items that followed the same general rules of construction as the studied categorised items, false recognition rates of .28 to .47—may reflect a real functional equivalence: The overall levels of general familiarity of novel category lures would not be expected to differ radically from that for lures from categories where only one or three related exemplars had been presented. Still, it is possible that, especially under conditions involving lower baseline levels of false recognition, some differences in the false recognition rates of amnesics versus controls might be observed for these conditions.

These considerations—which have thus far been confined to categorised items—have emphasised the parallels in the memory processes shown by amnesics and controls, with amnesics showing similar but less efficient gist extraction than that shown by individuals with intact memory. However, the emergence of clear group differences for the *non-categorised* or unrelated items, where the memory performance of controls far exceeded that of amnesics, suggests that, in addition to building up coarse or global forms of category information, control participants were also able to encode and retain more detailed, item-specific information. Evidence for this latter form of more detailed or specific recollective information—and the need to differentiate it from other forms of information—especially derives from a comparison of participants' corrected true recognition for the *unrelated* items versus their recognition of items for which a *single* categorised item was presented. These two conditions were similar in that, for both conditions, only one item of a given sort was presented at study; however, whereas the single items followed the rules of construction for the categorised items (and were themselves category items), the unrelated items did not follow those rules and were noticeably different from the categorised items. Whereas amnesic and control participants showed essentially identical novel-corrected veridical recognition for the single categorised items (.18 and .22 respectively), corrected veridical recognition of the two groups diverged markedly for the unrelated items. For the unrelated items, amnesics achieved a very similar score to that seen for single items ("unrelated-corrected" mean of .20) but control participants—now presumably responding on the basis of detailed item-specific information—showed significantly higher levels of recognition (.47). An analysis contrasting corrected veridical recognition of the single versus unrelated items for the two groups yielded a significant interaction of group with item type, $F(1,22) = 5.62$, $MSe = 0.03$, $P = .03$, indicating reliably differential patterns of responding for these item types for amnesics versus controls.

The above pattern of findings, with controls showing greater item-specific memory for non categorised items, and also—in the case of the prototypes—greater gist-based false recognition, raises a question regarding the extent to which item-specific memory and gist memory might covary. Is decreased gist-based false recognition an inevitable consequence of decreased item-specific memory? Although generalisations across different paradigms and different populations need to be made very cautiously, it might be noted that, contrary to this suggestion, across a number of studies we have observed several different relations between indices that probably primarily reflect item-specific memory (veridical recognition of single or unrelated "one-of-a-kind" items) and gist-based false memory (false recognition of lures that are perceptually and/or conceptually similar to target items). For example, in other experiments using the same abstract novel objects as in the present experiment but comparing older and younger adults, we observed largely *equivalent* levels of gist-based false recognition in older and younger adults even though, like the control participants in the present study, younger adults demonstrated greater item-specific memory (as indexed by performance for unrelated items) than did older adults. In a paradigm involving categorised pictures of everyday objects, we found that older adults show reliably *greater* gist-based false recognition than younger adults together with *decreased* item-specific memory, as measured by their recognition of unrelated items, or items from categories where only a single related item was presented (Koutstaal & Schacter, 1997; Koutstaal et al., in press). Further, matching older and younger adults on their level of item-specific memory, by requiring younger participants to perform a secondary task during the initial encoding of the pictures (Koutstaal, Schacter, & Brenner, 1998), did not eliminate the age-difference in gist-based responding: Under these conditions, the two age groups showed similar levels of item-specific memory but older adults continued to show greater gist-based false recognition. These varied patterns of gist-based false recognition in relation to item-specific memory for older versus younger adults suggest that the two forms of responding may be determined by multiple factors and, though they may sometimes covary (as they did here), at other times they may not. (For more general discussion and findings concerning the bases underlying true and false recognition, and the conditions under which they may or may not covary, see Arndt & Hirshman, 1998). These multiple patterns also make it hazardous to predict whether, if the amnesic patients and control participants were led to have similar levels of item-specific memory (by, for example, testing control participants after a longer study-to-test interval), they would show false recognition similar to that of the amnesics. Although an increased study-to-test interval might decrease item-specific memory in the control participants, it is possible that false recognition of categorised items, particularly category prototypes, would remain relatively preserved (cf. McDermott, 1996; Payne, Elie, Blackwell, & Neuschatz, 1996; Reyna & Brainerd, 1995), with controls still more often falsely recognising these items than amnesics.

Theoretical Implications

Overall, the outcomes of the present experiment are consistent with the predictions based on prior studies using multiple conceptually or perceptually related words where, under conditions where controls showed high levels of illusory recognition, amnesics also showed substantial deficits in false recognition. The present demonstration of a significant impairment in perceptually based false recognition of prototypes among amnesics using novel abstract visual stimuli extends these earlier findings, showing that impairments in amnesic patients may be observed in cases where the stimuli have no pre-existing semantic associations and where the extraction of similarities depends on representational and associational processes that occur entirely within the experimental session itself.

The parallel patterns found for both perceptually similar items (this study; Schacter et al., 1997) and for semantically or conceptually similar items (Schacter et al., 1996, 1997, 1998b), with amnesics showing "impaired" false recognition under conditions where individuals with intact memory show high levels of false recognition but not under conditions where cognitively intact individuals show less pronounced levels of false recognition, suggest that some of the processes underlying false recognition may be similar across these broad types of similarity. In particular, both forms of false recognition appear, at least in part, to derive from—and also to reflect—limits on the "exact" or "verbatim" encoding, retention, and/or retrieval of information. In both domains, increasing convergence or overlap of the stimulus items, whether in terms of semantic or associative attributes (e.g. Robinson & Roediger, 1997; Vogt & Kimble, 1973) or perceptual features (e.g. Franks & Bransford, 1971; Solso & Raynis, 1979), may act to increase the likelihood of false recognition of nonstudied items that possess similar characteristics.

Nonetheless, these findings do not imply that the processes are entirely parallel across the perceptual and conceptual domains. Although we have underscored the congruencies in the processes relating to these broad types of similarity in regard to certain aspects, particularly in relation to the number of related items that are presented, and their "distance" from a central prototype, other aspects of the processing of perceptually and conceptually similar materials are quite likely to differ. Thus, depending on the particular paradigm used, specific factors may contribute differently to false recognition (or other forms of memory errors, such as false recall) in the conceptual versus perceptual domains. For example, with semantically or associatively related items, such as the converging associates used in the Deese/Roediger-McDermott paradigm where all of the items converge upon a single critical lure, errors may arise from a form of inferential and elaborative processing at the time of encoding and/or retrieval in a way that differs from that for novel perceptually similar items, where pre-existing associative and thematic information is less likely to be strongly evoked. Further, whereas the convergence of items in semantic paradigms (during either study or test) may lead to explicit phenomenological awareness of the nonstudied lure because this item is generated or automatically activated in response to the multiple semantically related items (cf. Gallo, Roberts, & Seamon, 1997; McDermott & Roediger, 1998; Read, 1996; Roediger & McDermott, 1995), the convergence of visually similar items, particularly novel patterns or shapes, is unlikely to result in the "generation" of a "lure" in quite the same way: Although a given exemplar might remind an individual of earlier presented similar target items, participants would appear to be unlikely to generate "novel" variants or exemplars of the targets spontaneously (in part because pre-existing associational support for such generation is lacking). This suggests that direct "source confusions" between items that are presented and items that are implicitly or consciously generated during study (did I hear or read this word versus only think it?) may be more likely to arise for semantically or associatively related words than for perceptually similar items.

Although a number of studies have focused on the effects of *either* perceptual similarity or conceptual similarity on false recognition, the relations between perceptual and conceptual similarity, including the possibility that they may have additive effects, have been much less explored. In the paradigm using categorised pictures of everyday objects that we have used to explore false recognition in older and younger adults (Koutstaal & Schacter, 1997; Koutstaal et al., in press), the objects within a particular category (e.g. cats, chairs, or teddy bears) may share both considerable perceptual similarity (general shape, colour, etc.) and also conceptual (semantic and lexical) information; however, in this paradigm, perceptual and conceptual similarity are confounded and the relative roles of each in false recognition can be assessed only indirectly, by considering the consequences of shifting attention to the different components, or similar manipulations. More direct evidence for the possible additive effects of perceptual and conceptual similarity has been provided by Henkel and Franklin (1998). These researchers found higher rates of source monitoring errors in a judgement task requiring participants to differentiate between visually presented versus imagined items if the items both physically resembled one another and belonged to the same functional category (e.g *bagel–doughnut*) than if items shared primarily only conceptual similarity (e.g. *pants–shirt*) or primarily only physical similarity (e.g. *magnifying glass–lollipop*). The possible effects of combining both perceptual and conceptual similarity on false recognition performance, including false recognition of amnesic patients versus controls, have not been explored.

Although our finding that amnesics showed significantly depressed false recognition for prototypes based on perceptual similarity is consistent with the results from previous studies of false recognition in amnesia using conceptually related words (Schacter et al., 1996, 1997, 1998b), or orthographically and phonologically similar words (Schacter et al., 1997), this outcome clearly appears to be inconsistent with the findings reported by Kolodny (1994), particularly those of the random-dot pattern study, where amnesics showed false recognition rates that exceeded those of controls, even for items that were prototypes or low distortion exemplars of the categories. As noted previously, the absence of baseline rates in that study makes comparisons difficult, and it is possible that—after correction—the results from the two studies would be less discrepant. In addition, the studies differed in many respects. One factor, in particular, that recent research has suggested may have been important is the number of times that the target items were presented: Whereas target items were presented only once in the present study, targets were presented repeatedly in the Kolodny study. This latter factor is important because repeated presentation of the targets may have allowed control participants—at least to some extent—to *suppress* false recognition of the lures. Although, within the current experiment, we found little evidence of "suppression-like" processes, other experiments using the semantic converging associates paradigm have demonstrated suppression among younger persons with intact memory when the target items have been presented repeatedly (Kensinger & Schacter, this issue; McDermott, 1996)—possibly because such repetition facilitates the encoding and retention of greater amounts of item-specific information, or otherwise encourages more careful monitoring of recognition responding. Importantly, in a study comparing the effects of repeated study presentation on the false recognition of amnesics versus controls, Schacter et al. (1998b) found that whereas repeated presentations of semantic associates lead to decreasing false recognition in controls, amnesics showed either increasing rates of false recognition across trials (Korsakoff patients) or fluctuating levels of false recognition (amnesic patients of mixed aetiology). These findings raise the possibility that the repeated target presentations in the study by Kolodny may have acted both to decrease false recognition among controls (albeit not too successfully given that, in absolute terms, the rates of false recognition were not inconsiderable) and either to exacerbate, or at least to maintain, false recognition in amnesic individuals.

From a broader theoretical perspective, our results showing impaired gist-based false recognition of prototypes in amnesics bear upon two more general questions about the nature of preserved versus impaired memory functions in amnesics. One issue concerns the relation between *categorisation or classification tasks*—that is, tasks involving the acquisition and transfer of knowledge concerning the classification of novel stimuli, including the ability to correctly assign novel items to classes based on experience with other category members—and *recognition memory*, involving the explicit recollection of stimuli or events. Previously reported evidence showing a dissociation in the performance of amnesics relative to control participants on these two types of task, with amnesics showing impaired recognition memory but intact or near-normal levels of categorisation learning (Knowlton & Squire, 1993; Kolodny, 1994; Squire & Knowlton, 1995; also cf. Knowlton, Mangels, & Squire, 1996; Knowlton, Ramus, & Squire, 1992; Knowlton, Squire, & Gluck, 1994), has provoked considerable discussion and research concerning the factors underlying this dissociation, especially whether it is necessary to invoke separate memory systems to account for the difference, or if other accounts (e.g. Nosofsky, 1988; Nosofsky & Zaki, 1998) are possible. Our finding of impaired gist-based false recognition of prototypes in amnesics appears to provide additional evidence for the distinction between the processes or structures that support categorisation performance, and those that underlie recognition (in this case, illusory, rather than veridical recognition). Indeed, a growing set of evidence suggests that, in contrast to intact classification performance, including intact classification of perceptually based prototypes (Knowlton & Squire, 1993; Kolodny, 1994; Squire & Knowlton, 1995), amnesic patients show impaired false recognition of "prototypical" but not-presented target items, with such deficits found for semantically similar words (Schacter et al., 1996, 1997, 1998b), perceptually similar words (Schacter et al., 1997), and—in the present study—perceptually similar novel abstract patterns. On the one hand, it is not known if amnesics would show normal or near-normal classification performance for complex abstract stimulus patterns of the form used here, as has been found for the random dot patterns (Knowlton & Squire, 1993; Kolodny, 1994; Squire & Knowlton, 1995) and artificial grammar strings (Knowlton et al., 1992; Knowlton & Squire, 1994) used by previous investigators. On the other hand, the findings of the current study, taken together with those of the several earlier studies employing semantically and perceptually similar words, suggest that different processes, and possibly different representations, may support "gist-based false recognition"—manifested during a task requiring the making of explicit recognition decisions upon the basis of an episodic query of the past—and categorisation performance, requiring the designation of items as belonging or not belonging to a specific category, without any direct or necessary involvement of recollection. Although the factors underlying the dissociation between amnesics' recognition versus classification performance are likely to be a subject of continuing investigation, a clear implication of the present findings is that differences in the performance of amnesics and control participants as manifested in illusory or *false* recognition also comprise one part of the overall data set for which a satisfactory account must be offered.

Finally, and also in a broader perspective, it might be noted that our results provide evidence against early proposals suggesting that, whereas conceptual or semantic processing is impaired in amnesia, perceptual processing—not only for implicit tests, but also for explicit tests—might be *unimpaired* in amnesia (Blaxton, 1989, 1995). We found that, under certain conditions, perceptually based false recognition was clearly and significantly impaired in amnesics, thereby demonstrating that the processes involved in the explicit false recollection of abstract perceptual patterns—like that of conceptual information—may also be impaired in amnesics. These findings are thus consistent with our earlier findings, using perceptually related words (Schacter et al., 1997), and with other recent reports indicating that explicit memory of amnesics is impaired, not only for tests that emphasise conceptual processing, such as free or cued recall, but also on tests that draw more extensively upon perceptual processes, such as graphemic cued recall (Cermak, Verfaellie, & Chase, 1995) and word fragment cued recall (Vaidya, Gabrieli, Keane, & Monti, 1995). That, in the present study, this perceptual memory impairment should assume the apparently paradoxical guise of *fewer* false recognition errors in amnesic individuals than in control participants shows, yet again, the versatility and generality of the strategy of using false recollection to uncover the nature of the retrieval and encoding processes operating in veridical memory.

REFERENCES

Arndt, J., & Hirshman, E. (1998). True and false recognition in MINERVA2: Explanations from a global matching perspective. *Journal of Memory and Language, 39*, 371–391.

Blaxton, T.A. (1989). Investigating dissociations among memory measures: Support for a transfer-appropriate processing framework. *Journal of Experimental Psychology: Learning, Memory, and Cognition, 15*, 657–668.

Blaxton, T.A. (1995). A process-based view of memory. *Journal of the International Neuropsychological Society, 1*, 112–114.

Brainerd, C.J., Reyna, V.F., & Kneer, R. (1995). False recognition reversal: When similarity is distinctive. *Journal of Memory and Language, 34*, 157–185.

Cermak, L.S., Butters, N., & Gerrein, J. (1973). The extent of the verbal encoding ability of Korsakoff patients. *Neuropsychologia, 11*, 85–94.

Cermak, L.S., Verfaellie, M., & Chase, K.A. (1995). Implicit and explicit memory in amnesia: An analysis of data-driven and conceptually driven processes. *Neuropsychology, 9*, 281–290.

Curran, T., Schacter, D.L., Norman, K.A., & Galluccio, L. (1997). False recognition after a right frontal lobe infarction: Memory for general and specific information. *Neuropsychologia, 35*, 1035–1049.

Deese, J. (1959). On the prediction of occurrence of particular verbal intrusions in immediate recall. *Journal of Experimental Psychology, 58*, 17–22.

Estes, W.K. (1997). Processes of memory loss, recovery, and distortion. *Psychological Review, 104*, 148–169.

Franks, J.J., & Bransford, J.D. (1971). Abstraction of visual patterns. *Journal of Experimental Psychology, 90*, 65–74.

Gallo, D.A., Roberts, M.J., & Seamon, J.G. (1997). Remembering words not presented in lists: Can we avoid creating false memories? *Psychonomic Bulletin and Review, 4*, 271–276.

Henkel, L.A., & Franklin, N. (1998). Reality monitoring of physically similar and conceptually related objects. *Memory and Cognition, 26*, 659–673.

Homa, D., Cross, J., Cornell, D., Goldman, D., & Schwartz, S. (1973). Prototype abstraction and classification of new instances as a function of number of instances defining the prototype. *Journal of Experimental Psychology, 101*, 116–122.

Jernigan, T.L., Schafer, K., Butters, N., & Cermak, L.S. (1991). Magnetic resonance imaging of alcoholic Korsakoff patients. *Neuropsychopharmacology, 4*, 175–186.

Johnson, M.K., Hashtroudi, S., & Lindsay, D.S. (1993). Source monitoring. *Psychological Bulletin, 114*, 3–28.

Kensinger, E.A., & Schacter, D.L. (this issue). When true memories suppress false memories: Effects of ageing. *Cognitive Neuropsychology, 16*, 399–415.

Knowlton, B.J., Mangels, J.A., & Squire, L.R. (1996). A neostriatal habit learning system in humans. *Science, 273*, 1399–1402.

Knowlton, B.J., Ramus, S.J., & Squire, L.R. (1992). Intact artificial grammar learning in amnesia: Dissocia-

tion of classification learning and explicit memory for specific instances. *Psychological Science, 3*, 172–179.
Knowlton, B.J., & Squire, L.R. (1993). The learning of categories: Parallel brain systems for item memory and category knowledge. *Science, 262*, 1747–1749.
Knowlton, B.J., & Squire, L.R. (1994). The information acquired during artificial grammar learning. *Journal of Experimental Psychology: Learning, Memory, and Cognition, 20*, 79–91.
Knowlton, B.J., Squire, L.R., & Gluck, M.A. (1994). Probabilistic classification learning in amnesia. *Learning and Memory, 1*, 106–120.
Kolodny, J.A. (1994). Memory processes in classification learning: An investigation of amnesic performance in categorization of dot patterns and artistic styles. *Psychological Science, 5*, 164–169.
Koutstaal, W., & Schacter, D.L. (1997). Gist-based false recognition of pictures in older and younger adults. *Journal of Memory and Language, 37*, 555–583.
Koutstaal, W., Schacter, D.L., Galluccio, L., & Stofer, K.A. (in press). Reducing gist-based false recognition in older adults: Encoding and retrieval manipulations. *Psychology and Aging.*
Koutstaal, W., Schacter, D.L., & Brenner, C. (1998). *Dual task demands and gist based false recognition of pictures in younger and older adults.* Manuscript submitted for publication.
Kroll, N.E.A., Knight, R.T., Metcalfe, J., Wolf, E.S., & Tulving, E. (1996). Cohesion failure as a source of memory illusions. *Journal of Memory and Language, 35*, 176–196.
McClelland, J.L. (1995). Constructive memory and memory distortions: A parallel distributed processing approach. In D.L. Schacter, J.T. Coyle, G.D. Fischbach, M.M. Mesulam, & L.E. Sullivan, (Eds.), *Memory distortion: How minds. brains. and societies reconstruct the past* (pp. 66–90). Cambridge, MA: Harvard University Press.
McDermott, K.B. (1996). The persistence of false memories in list recall. *Journal of Memory and Language, 35*, 212–230.
McDermott, K.B., & Roediger, H.L. III (1998). Attempting to avoid illusory memories: Robust false recognition of associates persists under conditions of explicit warnings and immediate testing. *Journal of Memory and Language, 39*, 508–520.
Moscovitch, M. (1994). Memory and working with memory: Evaluation of a component process model and comparisons with other models. In D.L. Schacter & E. Tulving (Eds.), *Memory systems 1994* (pp. 269–310). Cambridge, MA: MIT Press.
Nosofsky, R.M. (1988). Exemplar-based accounts of relations between classification, recognition, and typicality. *Journal of Experimental Psychology: Learning, Memory, and Cognition, 14*, 700–708.
Nosofsky, R.M., & Zaki, S.R. (1998). Dissociations between categorisation and recognition in amnesic and normal individuals: An exemplar-based interpretation. *Psychological Science, 9*, 247–255.
Omohundro, J. (1981). Recognition vs. classification of ill-defined category exemplars. *Memory and Cognition, 9*, 324–331.
Parkin, A.J., & Leng, N.R.C. (1993). *Neuropsychology of the amnesic syndrome.* Hillsdale, NJ: Lawrence Erlbaum Associates Inc.
Payne, D.G., Elie, C.J., Blackwell, J.M., & Neuschatz, J.S. (1996). Memory illusions: Recalling, recognising and recollecting events that never occurred. *Journal of Memory and Language, 35*, 261–285.
Posner, M.I., Goldsmith, R., & Welton, K.E. (1967). Perceived distance and the classification of distorted patterns. *Journal of Experimental Psychology, 73*, 28–38.
Posner, M.I., & Keele, S.W. (1968). On the genesis of abstract ideas. *Journal of Experimental Psychology, 77*, 353–363.
Read, J.D. (1996). From a passing thought to a false memory in 2 minutes: Confusing real and illusory events. *Psychonomic Bulletin and Review, 3*, 105–111.
Reinitz, M.T., Verfaellie, M., & Milberg, W. (1996). Memory conjunction errors in normal and amnesic subjects. *Journal of Memory and Language, 35*, 286–299.
Reyna, V.F., & Brainerd, C.J. (1995). Fuzzy-trace theory: An interim synthesis. *Learning and Individual Differences, 71*, 1–75.
Robinson, K.J., & Roediger, H.L. III (1997). Associative processes in false recall and recognition. *Psychological Science, 8*, 231–237.
Roediger, H.L. III. (1996). Memory illusions. *Journal of Memory and Language, 35*, 76–100.
Roediger, H.L. III, & McDermott, K.B. (1995). Creating false memories: Remembering words not presented in lists. *Journal of Experimental Psychology: Learning, Memory, and Cognition, 21*, 803–814.
Rosenthal, R., & Rosnow, R.L. (1991). *Essentials of behavioral research: Methods and data analysis.* New York: McGraw-Hill.
Rudy, J.W., & Sutherland, R.J. (1994). The memory-coherence problem, configural associations, and the hippocampal system. In D.L. Schacter & E.

Tulving (Eds.), *Memory systems 1994* (pp. 119–146). Cambridge, MA: MIT Press.

Schacter, D.L. (1995). Memory distortion: History and current status. In D.L. Schacter, J.T. Coyle, G.D. Fischbach, M.M. Mesulam, & L.E. Sullivan (Eds.), *Memory distortion: How minds, brains. and societies reconstruct the past* (pp. 1–43). Cambridge, MA: Harvard University Press.

Schacter, D.L. (1997). False recognition and the brain. *Current Directions in Psychological Science, 6*, 65–70.

Schacter, D.L., Church, B., & Bolton, E. (1995). Implicit memory in amnesic patients: Impairment of voice-specific priming. *Psychological Science, 6*, 20–25.

Schacter, D.L., Norman, K.A., & Koutstaal, W. (1998a). The cognitive neuroscience of constructive memory. *Annual Review of Psychology, 49*, 289–318.

Schacter, D.L., Verfaellie, M., & Anes, M.D. (1997). Illusory memories in amnesic patients: Conceptual and perceptual false recognition. *Neuropsychology, 11*, 331–342.

Schacter, D.L., Verfaellie, M., Anes, M.D., & Racine, C. (1998b). When true recognition suppresses false recognition: Evidence from amnesic patients. *Journal of Cognitive Neuroscience, 10*, 668–679.

Schacter, D.L., Verfaellie, M., & Pradere, D. (1996). The neuropsychology of memory illusions: False recall and recognition in amnesic patients. *Journal of Memory and Language, 35*, 319–334.

Shapiro, M.L., & Olton, D.S. (1994). Hippocampal function and interference. In D.L. Schacter & E. Tulving (Eds.), *Memory systems 1994* (pp. 87–117). Cambridge, MA: MIT Press.

Shiffrin, R.M., Huber, D.E., & Marinelli, K. (1995). Effects of category length and strength on familiarity in recognition. *Journal of Experimental Psychology: Learning, Memory, and Cognition, 21*, 261–287.

Snedecor, G.W., & Cochran, W.G. (1989). *Statistical methods* (8th ed.). Ames, IA: Iowa State University Press.

Solso, R.L., & Raynis, S.A. (1979). Prototype formation from imaged, kinesthetically, and visually presented geometric figures. *Journal of Experimental Psychology: Human Perception and Performance, 5*, 701–712.

Squire, L.R. (1994). Declarative and nondeclarative memory: Multiple brain systems supporting learning and memory. In D.L. Schacter & E. Tulving (Eds.), *Memory systems 1994* (pp. 203–231). Cambridge, MA: MIT Press.

Squire, L.R., & Knowlton, B.J. (1995). Learning about categories in the absence of memory. *Proceedings of the National Academy of Sciences. USA, 92*, 12470–12474.

Sutherland, R.J., & Rudy, J.W. (1989). Configural association theory: The role of the hippocampal formation in learning, memory, and amnesia. *Psychobiology, 17*, 129–144.

Vaidya, C.J., Gabrieli, J.D.E., Keane, M.M., & Monti, L.A. (1995). Perceptual and conceptual memory processes in global amnesia. *Neuropsychology, 9*, 580–591.

Vogt, J., & Kimble, G.A. (1973). False recognition as a function of associative proximity. *Journal of Experimental Psychology, 99*, 143–145.

APPENDIX

Novel-Corrected True and False Recognition Data for Individual Patients

	True Recognition				*False Recognition*					
	Category Size		*Distance*		*Category Size*		*Distance*			
Patient: Aetiology	*Larger*	*Smaller*	*Near/ Middle*	*Far*	*Larger*	*Smaller*	*Proto-type*	*Near/ Middle*	*Far*	*Novel*
CW: Thalamic infarct: bilateral anterior nuclei[a]	.42	.39	.47	.25	.14	.11	.25	.25	−.08	.42
AB: Encephalitis: mild diffuse cortical atrophy[b]	.00	.14	.06	.17	−.11	−.08	−.17	−.06	−.28	.50
PD: Anoxia: enlarged ventricles, cortical atrophy[b]	.50	.53	.45	.67	.39	.47	.33	.56	.44	.00
JM: Anoxia: bilateral hippocampal complex[b]	.03	.08	.08	.14	.25	.00	.14	.25	−.08	.42
PS: Anoxia: bilateral hippocampal complex[b]	.03	.00	−.03	.03	−.14	−.03	−.08	.08	−.42	.75
RL: Anoxia	.00	.06	.06	.00	.06	.00	.00	.06	.00	.00
Patient Mean	.16	.20	.18	.21	.10	.08	.08	.19	−.07	.35
Control Mean	.46	.30	.48	.28	.34	.07	.45	.34	.07	.28
AA: Korsakoff	.33	.19	.28	.00	.28	.20	.22	.22	.33	.33
LB: Korsakoff	.39	.45	.39	.39	.22	.33	.39	.17	.28	.50
PB: Korsakoff	.11	.14	.11	.28	.06	−.11	.28	.11	−.17	.17
RD: Korsakoff	.03	.03	.03	−.03	.25	.00	.20	.14	.31	.58
WR: Korsakoff	.61	.28	.72	.33	.33	.11	.22	.39	.11	.00
RM: Korsakoff	.45	.17	.39	.28	.28	−.08	.28	.17	.06	.50
Patient Mean	.32	.21	.32	.21	.24	.07	.26	.20	.15	.35
Control Mean	.35	.20	.36	.21	.17	.06	.25	.21	−.01	.47

Means for prototypes are based on items from category sizes of three, six, and nine items; larger = average of six- and nine-item categories; smaller = average of one- and three-item categories. False alarms for novel category items are shown at the far right; all scores shown here have been corrected for these baseline differences in false alarms. Anatomical lesion information is provided where available.

[a] Lesions assessed by CT.

[b] Lesions assessed by MRI.

COGNITIVE NEUROPSYCHOLOGY, 1999, 16 (3/4/5), 343–359

FALSE RECALL AND FALSE RECOGNITION: AN EXAMINATION OF THE EFFECTS OF SELECTIVE AND COMBINED LESIONS TO THE MEDIAL TEMPORAL LOBE/DIENCEPHALON AND FRONTAL LOBE STRUCTURES

Brenda Melo

University of Toronto and Rotman Research Institute, Baycrest Centre for Geriatric Care, North York, Canada

Gordon Winocur

University of Toronto, Rotman Research Institute, Baycrest Centre for Geriatric Care, North York, and Trent University, Peterborough, Canada

Morris Moscovitch

University of Toronto and Rotman Research Institute, Baycrest Centre for Geriatric Care, North York, Canada

The present experiment examined the false recall and false recognition of nonstudied words that are preceded by a list of strong associates in patients with amnesia due to damage restricted to medial temporal lobe or diencephalic regions (MTL/D amnesics), in nonamnesic patients with damage restricted to the frontal lobes (FL nonamnesics), and in amnesic patients with damage to the frontal lobes in addition to medial temporal lobe damage (FL amnesics). We used the Deese/Roediger and McDermott paradigm (Deese, 1959; Roediger & McDermott, 1995) in which people frequently claim that nonstudied words appeared on a presented list. At immediate free recall, the results taken together showed that MTL/D amnesic patients and FL nonamnesic patients produced higher levels of false memory than did controls. At recognition both types of amnesic patients produced less false recognition than either frontal-lobe patients or controls. The results are consistent with the hypothesis that abnormally high levels of false memories are related to the following three conditions: (1) partial memory for the word lists, (2) the ability to extract the semantic gist of the list, and (3) a deficit in strategic monitoring processes.

INTRODUCTION

Since the pioneering studies of Sir Frederic Bartlett (1932), psychologists have conceptualized memory as a constructive process that can be prone to errors, distortions, and illusions (for a review, see Roediger & McDermott, 1995; Schacter, 1996). Clearly, understanding memory distortion has many important implications for everyday life. For example, how accurate is memory and under what conditions is it subject to distortion? In recent years, there have been a growing number of investigations of

Requests for reprints should be addressed to Brenda Melo, Rotman Research Institute, Baycrest Centre for Geriatric Care, 3560 Bathurst St, North York, Canada M6A 2E1 (Tel: (416) 785-2500, ext. 2708; E-mail: melo@psych.utoronto.ca).

This research was supported by a Medical Research Council Grant (MRC- 6694). We also thank Marilyne Ziegler for her technical assistance.

phenomena that illuminate reconstructive aspects of remembering, such as source amnesia, false recognition, false recall, and confabulation (Anisfeld & Knapp, 1968; Belli, Lindsay, Gales, & McCarthy, 1994; Cermak, Butters, & Gerrein, 1973; Craik, Morris, Morris, & Loewen, 1990; Johnson, 1991; Johnson, Hashtroudi, & Lindsay, 1993; Johnson, O'Connor, & Canton, 1997; Knowlton & Squire, 1995; Kopelman, Ng, & Van Den Brouke, 1997; Kroll, Knight, Metcalfe, Wolf, & Tulving, 1996; Loftus & Palmer, 1974; Moscovitch, 1989, 1995; Moscovitch & Melo, 1997; Norman & Schacter, 1997; Reinitz & Milberg, 1996; Roediger & McDermott, 1995; Schacter, 1996; Schacter, Buckner, Koutstaal, Dale, & Rosen, 1997a; Schacter, Koutstaal, Johnson, Gross, & Angell, 1997b; Schacter, Verfaellie, & Anes, 1997c, Schacter, Verfaellie, Anes, & Racine, 1998; Schacter, Verfaellie, & Pradere, 1996c; Schnider, von Daniken, & Gutbrod, 1996; Shimamura & Squire, 1987; Stuss, Alexander, Lieberman, & Levine, 1978).

A version of a list-learning paradigm, originally designed by Deese (1959) and recently revived and modified by Roediger and McDermott (1995), has been used to investigate false recall and false recognition in normal subjects and amnesic patients (Roediger & McDermott, 1996, 1995; Schacter et al. (1996c). In this paradigm, participants study a list of words (e.g. bed, rest, dream, slumber) that are strong associates of a nonstudied critical item (e.g. sleep), and are then asked to recall the list words. Deese reported that subjects often produced the nonstudied critical items on the recall test. That is, they exhibited false memories for the nonstudied but strongly associated items. Roediger and McDermott (1995) replicated the false recall effect initially reported by Deese, and extended it to recognition memory. After studying associates of nonpresented target words such as *sweet*, participants frequently claimed with high confidence that *sweet* had appeared previously on the study list. Moreover, when asked to make remember/know judgements (Tulving, 1985), indicating whether they specifically recalled having studied a word during list presentation ("remember"), or thought that a word was on the list because it seemed familiar ("know"), people claimed to "remember" nonpresented associates nearly as often as they claimed to "remember" words that had actually appeared on the list (Roediger & McDermott, 1995).

Using this paradigm, Schacter et al. (1996c) reported that amnesic patients with Korsakoff's syndrome or other aetiologies (anoxia, encephalitis, thalamic infarct) recalled fewer targets from previously presented words than did controls. More importantly, they found that both types of amnesic subjects were less likely to show false recognition of nonpresented critical lures than were controls, although they made more false alarms to unrelated lures than controls did. To Schacter et al. (1996c) the latter finding suggested that false recognition of nonpresented associates derives from retention of associative or semantic information that also supports veridical recognition of presented words—information that is not available to amnesic patients. They contend that control subjects bind together studied items and generated associates, thereby forming and retaining a well-organised, focused representation of the semantic gist of the study list. Related test distractors that match this semantic gist representation (e.g. sweet) are likely to be falsely recognised; unrelated distractors that do not match it are likely to be correctly rejected. They suggest further that amnesic patients do not form and/or retain a focused semantic representation of gist.

Schacter et al.'s (1996c) explanation accounts for the finding that amnesic patients showed reduced false recognition of related distractors. When few, if any, of the associates (true targets) are remembered, as in the case of amnesia, there is effectively no medial temporal lobe output that can be prone to distortion (i.e. there is little opportunity for a related test item to match a semantic gist representation). Their explanation also accounts for amnesics' inflated false recognition of unrelated distractors. Whereas control subjects can use their semantic gist representation to reject unrelated distractors that do not match it, amnesic patients are less able to do so. Schacter et al. combined Korsakoff and other amnesic patients into a single group and they concluded that retention and/or retrieval of semantic gist information depends on memory-related structures in the medial temporal lobes and diencephalon that are damaged in amnesia. It is important to bear in mind that Korsakoff's amnesics typically have significant frontal lobe involvement. Thus, interpretation of these data must take into account the strong possibility that frontal lobe impairment contributed to the false memory effects. Moreover, given the aetiologies of the other patients, frontal lobe deficits cannot be ruled out.

Further evidence that medial temporal lobe and frontal lobe structures are implicated in false memory comes from a PET study of normal subjects (Schacter et al., 1996b). This study showed that the medial temporal lobe was activated as much during recognition of false targets as of true targets, suggesting that output from the medial temporal lobe is a contributing factor to false memory. Frontal lobe activation, although apparent on all trials, was greater during false than true recognition. This indicates that distortions are a feature of normal memory because output from the medial temporal lobe is not always accurate even in normal people and frontal lobe monitoring may not always be adequate to distinguish accurate from inaccurate output.

Other studies implicate the frontal lobes in false memory phenomena. Damage to the ventromedial aspect of the frontal lobes and basal forebrain are often associated with the most flagrant form of memory distortion, namely confabulation. Patients who confabulate misremember the time and other contextual aspects of actual events and sometimes concoct improbable and bizarre scenarios that could not have occurred (Berlyne, 1972; Dalla Barba, 1993; De Luca & Cicerone, 1991; De Luca & Diamond, 1995; Johnson, 1991; Johnson et al., 1997; Kopelman et al., 1997; Moscovitch, 1989, 1995; Moscovitch & Melo, 1997). Moscovitch and his colleagues have proposed that the prefrontal cortex is necessary for strategic search, monitoring, verification, and organisation of the automatic output from medial temporal lobe structures. According to this view, confabulation may arise as a result of impairment to strategic search and monitoring processes that depend on prefrontal regions. This defective search process may produce misleading cues that elicit inappropriate memories (Burgess & Shallice, 1996; Moscovitch, 1995; Moscovitch & Melo, 1997). Furthermore, when monitoring is defective, the faulty output from the medial temporal lobe system emerges unedited as a confabulatory response (Burgess & Shallice, 1996; Moscovitch & Melo, 1997).

Recently, the frontal lobes have also been implicated in false recognition (Curran, et al., 1997; Schacter, Curran, Galluccio, Milberg, & Bates, 1996a; Schacter, et al., 1998). Schacter et al. (1996a) studied a 65-year-old man, BG, who suffered an infarction restricted to the right frontal lobe. From their description of this case study, it was clear that BG does not spontaneously generate extensive confabulations, shows no signs of amnesia, and is generally alert, attentive, and cooperative. He does, however, exhibit a striking pattern of false recognition that provides useful clues concerning the role of frontal lobe regions in illusory memories. Parkin and colleagues (Parkin, Bindschaedler, Harsent, & Metzler, 1996) have reported a patient with *left* frontal lobe damage who makes excessive numbers of false alarms and resembles patient BG in many respects. In two recent studies (Norman & Schacter, 1997; Schacter et al., 1997b), normal old people, whose medial temporal lobe and prefrontal structures tend to be compromised, were found to be more susceptible than younger adults to false memory effects.

Taken together, these findings support the idea that memory distortion is exaggerated when output from the medial temporal lobes is inaccurate and monitoring by the prefrontal cortex is impaired. Under normal conditions, production of false recall and false recognition in the Deese/Roediger and McDermott paradigm (Deese, 1959; Roediger & McDermott, 1995) has been linked to three cognitive processes: (1) partial memory for the study lists, (2) the ability to extract the semantic gist of the lists, and (3) poor monitoring that makes decisions about specific items in a given list prone to error. The first two processes are believed to be subserved, at least in part, by medial and lateral temporal lobe structures respectively, and the second and third may both be dependent on the prefrontal cortex.

Exaggerated production of false memories will be linked to an overdependence on semantic gist in the absence of memory for specific items and/or an impaired ability to monitor information. A deficiency in the ability to extract semantic gist will lead to an abnormally low level of false memory.

While our review suggests that medial temporal lobe/diencephalic structures and frontal lobe structures are implicated separately in memory distortion, no study has examined the effects of damage to each of these regions alone or in combination. Accordingly, we administered the false memory paradigm, as described by Schacter et al., (1996c), to three groups of patients: (1) amnesics with damage to medial temporal lobe or diencephalic structures (MTL/D amnesics); (2) nonamnesic patients with damage restricted to the frontal lobes (FL nonamnesics); and (3) amnesics with damage to the frontal lobes in addition to medial temporal lobe damage (FL amnesics). Three predictions follow if the three previously mentioned criteria are necessary for increased production of false recall and false recognition: (1) MTL/D amnesics are expected to exhibit poor veridical memories but increased false memories on immediate testing because impoverished output from memory structures forces excessive reliance on semantic gist without access to critical specific details. At longer delays even the gist may be degraded, resulting in a decline in all memories. (2) FL nonamnesic patients are also expected to exhibit exaggerated memory distortion because of a failure to monitor the output from MTL/D structures. However, their memory for target items should be at or near normal levels. (3) Assuming that the FL amnesics, who in our study have frontal lobe damage or impairment, are functionally comparable to those of Schacter et al. (1996c), we predict the same pattern that they observed, namely poor memory for targets and fewer false memories. This pattern probably results from the combination of severe memory loss and poor strategic processing that may add another factor, namely preventing these patients from deriving the semantic gist or, from using it effectively. It is also possible that the primary locus of damage differs in FL nonamnesic and the FL amnesic groups, with the former being more dorsolateral and the latter being more ventromedial, involving the basal forebrain regions.

METHOD

Participants

Table 1 shows, for each subject, the aetiology, probable or confirmed site of brain damage as determined by MRI, CAT, or SPECT scans, and demographic data. The participants in this study included 14 people with brain damage (6 females, 8 males). Eight were amnesic patients with various aetiologies and considerable variability in the nature and extent of their damage. Four of the amnesic patients had damage restricted to medial temporal lobe or diencephalic regions (MTL/D amnesics). The other four amnesic patients had confirmed lesions in frontal lobe regions in addition to damage in MTL regions (FL amnesics). Of these four amnesic patients, three were classified as confabulators, depending on their behaviour in real life and on their performance on a modified version of the Crovitz cue-word test (Crovitz & Schiffman, 1974) that elicited confabulations (see Moscovitch & Melo, 1997, for a detailed description of this test). These patients had probable or confirmed lesions in the ventromedial aspect of the prefrontal cortex. The average age of the MTL/D amnesics was 53 years and their mean education level was 16.7 years. The FL amnesics had a mean age of 56 and an average of 12.5 years of education.

Table 2 shows the results of psychometric tests for the amnesic patients. The intellectual functioning of the entire group of amnesics was in the average range, as indicated by a mean Full Scale IQ of 92.3 on the Wechsler Adult Intelligence Scale-Revised. In contrast, they consistently exhibited severe deficits on a variety of explicit memory tasks from the Wechsler Memory Scale-Revised. They obtained a mean General Memory Index of 69 and a mean Delayed Memory Index of 53.

The other six patients had focal lesions restricted to the frontal lobes (FL nonamnesics). Although complete psychometric test scores were not

Table 1. *Patient Demographics*

Patient	*Sex*	*Age*	*Edu*[a]	*Hand*	*Aetiology*	*Lesion Location*
MTL/D Amnesics						
DA	M	45	17	RH	Herpes encephalitis	Bilateral medial temporal lobe
CC	M	60	20+	RH	Astrocytoma/hydrocephalus	3rd ventricle; diencephalon
PT	F	52	14	RH	Right temporal lobe artery malformation	Right temporal lobe
JF	F	53	16	RH	Seizures, specific aetiology unknown	Bilateral medial temporal lobe
Mean		53	16.7			
FL Amnesics						
KC	M	45	15	RH	Traumatic brain injury	Bilateral medial temporal lobe, right frontoparietal, right occipital
FE	F	60	15	LH	ACommA aneurysm clipped	Left orbitofrontal and dorsolateral frontal
RC	M	61	10	RH	Cerebral vascular accident	Bilateral orbitofrontal including ventromedial frontal
GE	M	59	10	RH	Occlusion of intracerebral artery	Bilateral frontal including ventromedial and anterior regions
Mean		56	12.5			
FL Nonamnesics						
CB	F	29	12	RH	Epilepsy/resection frontal corticectomy	Right dorsolateral frontal
DW	M	59	13	RH	Cystic meningioma—dural base	Right frontal convexity at level of lateral sphenoid ridge
PK	F	35	16	LH	Traumatic brain injury	Right frontal
ED	F	65	7	RH	ACommA aneurysm clipped	Right frontal from A1 to A2, large left-frontobasal lesions
DS	M	60	16	RH	ACommA aneurysm clipped	Right inferior medial frontal
SP	M	35	16	RH	Brain tumour	Right frontal
Mean		47	13.3			

[a] Years of education.

available for these patients, they were screened on the basis of previous clinical testing and only patients who were not classified as confabulators, who did not exhibit severe memory impairment, and who were reported to have average intellectual functioning were included in this study. In Table 2 we report limited neuropsychological data relating to the frontal executive functioning of the patients in the three groups. These data suggest that the FL amnesic and the FL nonamnesic patient groups are impaired on a test of Verbal Fluency and on the Wisconsin Card Sorting Task. In contrast, the performance of the MTL/D amnesics on these tests suggest that they have preserved frontal executive functioning. The average age of the FL nonamnesic patients was 47, and their mean education level was 13.3 years.

The control group consisted of 14 individuals (6 females, 8 females) matched to patients on the basis of age, education, handedness, and sex.

Materials

The materials consisted of 24 lists of 16 words identical to those used by Roediger and McDermott (1995). Each list contained 15 words to be presented for study and a target word (critical lure) that was not presented for study. The study words were all highly associated to the critical lure and ordered such that the strongest associates occurred first in the list. In order to counterbalance the list order, the 24 lists were subdivided into 3 sets of 8 lists. The lists were presented auditorily via a desktop computer equipped with Soundblaster software.

Table 2. *Psychometric Test Scores*

	WAIS-R				*WMS-R*		*RMT*						*WCST*	
Patient	*VIQ*	*PIQ*	*FSIQ*	*NART*	*Gen*	*Del*	*Words*	*%ile*	*Faces*	*%ile*	*Sem Flu*	*Verbal Flu*	*Err*	*#*
MTL/D Amnesics														
DA	121	106	117	115	74	< 50	21	<5th	25	<5th	25th–75th	25th–75th	16	6
CC	115	95	106	118	95	< 57	35	5th	34	<5th	25th–75th	25th–75th	15	6
PT	96	77	87	115	50	62	20	<5th	12	<5th	25th–75th	25th–75th	12	4
JF			111	109	82	61	42	25th	36	<5th	25th–75th	96th	13	6
Means	111	93	105	114	75	60	30		27					
FL Amnesics														
KC	96	79	88	109	61	< 50	27	<5th	29	<5th	25th–75th	1st–3rd	34	3
FE	90	78	85	107	66	51	27	<5th	23	<5th	25th–75th	11th–22nd	33	4
RC	86	81	83	94	70	51	40	10th	39	10th	5th–8th	5th–8th	42	0
GE	88	85	86	93	60	< 50	39	<25th	28	<5th	25th–75th	11th–22nd		
Means	90	81	86	101	64	51	33		30					
FL Nonamnesics														
CB				98							25th–75th	25th–75th		
DW				110							25th–75th	11th–22nd		
PK											25th–75th	25th–75th		
ED				90							5th–8th	1st–3rd	71	2
DS				115							25th–75th	96th	39	3
SP				107							5th–8th	5th–8th		

WAIS-R: Wechsler Adult Intelligence Scale-Revised; NART: National Adult Reading Test; WMS-R: Wechsler Memory Scale-Revised; RMT: Recognition Memory Test; WCST: Wisconsin Card Sorting Test; VIQ: Verbal IQ; PIQ: Performance IQ; FSIQ: Full Scale IQ: Gen: General; Del: Delayed; Sem Flu: Semantic Fluency; Verb Flu: Verbal Fluency; Err: Perseverative Errors; #: No. of Categories.

Design and Procedure

Because one purpose of this study was to replicate Schacter et al.'s (1996c) findings with amnesic patients, all participants were tested in the two conditions used in that experiment (i.e. Study + Recall condition and Study + Arithmetic condition, administered in two sessions separated by at least 1 week). Half of the subjects received the Study + Recall condition during the first session and the Study + Arithmetic condition during the second session. For the other half, this order was reversed.

In each condition a set of 8 lists was used. The remaining eight lists were not studied. Four of the latter appeared on the recognition test that accompanied the Study + Recall condition, whereas the other four appeared on the recognition test that accompanied the Study + Arithmetic condition. Lists were counterbalanced so that they were used equally often in the Study + Recall condition, in the Study + Arithmetic condition, and as nonstudied lists. Nonstudied lists were counterbalanced across the two recognition tests. Before presentation of each study list, the subjects were told that they would hear several lists of words via speakers attached to a desktop computer and that they should try and remember the words. The words were recorded in a female voice and were presented at a rate of one word every 1.5 seconds. Immediately following presentation of a study list, participants were asked to say out loud as many of the words as they could remember (Study + Recall condition) or to perform simple addition and multiplication problems (Study + Arithmetic condition). Approximately 1 minute was given for the completion of either of these tasks, after which the next study list was presented. Eight study lists were presented during a single session. Presentation of all 8 study lists took approximately 20 minutes.

The recognition test was administered approximately 2 minutes after completion of the recall or arithmetic task that followed the final study list. The recognition test contained 48 words, 24 studied words and 24 nonstudied words. The studied words were obtained by selecting for each of the eight study lists the items in serial positions 1, 8, and 10. The nonstudied words consisted of the critical lures corresponding to each of the eight studied lists, the critical lures corresponding to four nonstudied lists, and the items in serial positions 1, 8, and 10 of these nonstudied lists. The words were presented all at once in columns on a computer screen.

Subjects were asked to indicate for each word whether they had heard it earlier in any of the lists. They were instructed to move down the columns using the cursor key and to select (by pressing a different key—the space bar) only those words they had heard previously. For each of the words they selected, they were then asked to indicate whether they remembered or knew the word by typing an "R" (remember) or a "K" (know) beside the word. Instructions for the remember/know judgement were similar to those used by Roediger and McDermott (1995) and Schacter et al. (1996c). Participants were told to make a remember judgement if they could specifically recollect hearing a word—that is, they could actually travel back in their minds to the precise moment of hearing and studying the word and remember something about that event. It was explained that such recollection might include remembering something about the speaker's voice or about the thoughts they had when they heard the word. They were told that a know judgement should be made if they believed or knew that a word was presented earlier but they could not recollect anything specific about the word or its occurrence. An analysis of remember responses in this experiment tells us little more than the analysis of old responses. This, in addition to the fact that we have small numbers of subjects in each group, did not allow us to interpret the remember/know data and so they will not be discussed further in this paper.

RESULTS

Free Recall

Due to the limited number of subjects in each group, nonparametric analyses were conducted using primarily the Mann-Whitney *U* test and the

Wilcoxin Signed Rank test. The mean proportion of study list words and critical lures produced by the three patient groups and control subjects on the free recall test averaged across the eight target lists is presented in Figs. 1 and 2. As expected, both groups of amnesic patients recalled on average a smaller proportion of study list words than did their matched controls. The difference between the proportion of targets recalled by MTL/D amnesics (.32) and their controls (.49) was not significant ($Z = 1.742$, $P < .5$). However, FL amnesics recalled a significantly smaller proportion of targets (.24) than did their controls (.52) ($Z = 2.309$, $P < .05$). MTL/D amnesics and FL amnesics did not differ significantly from each other ($Z = 1.307$, $P < .5$) with respect to the proportion of target words recalled. Although the proportion of study list words recalled by control subjects (.47) was slightly higher than the proportion of study list words recalled by frontal lobe patients (.41) this difference was not significant ($Z = 1.123$, $P < .5$). There was also no significant difference between the proportion of study list words recalled by FL nonamnesics and that recalled by MTL/D amnesics ($Z = 1.307$, $P < .5$). The difference between the proportion of study list words recalled by FL nonamnesic patients and that recalled by FL amnesics was significant ($Z = 2.032$, $P < .05$).

Contrary to Schacter et al. (1996c) who found that MTL/D amnesic patients produced a much smaller proportion of critical lures than did controls, we found that these patients intruded a larger proportion of critical lures (.63) than did controls (.34) although this difference was not significant ($Z = 1.637$, $P < .5$). FL amnesics intruded a smaller proportion of critical lures (.19) than did controls

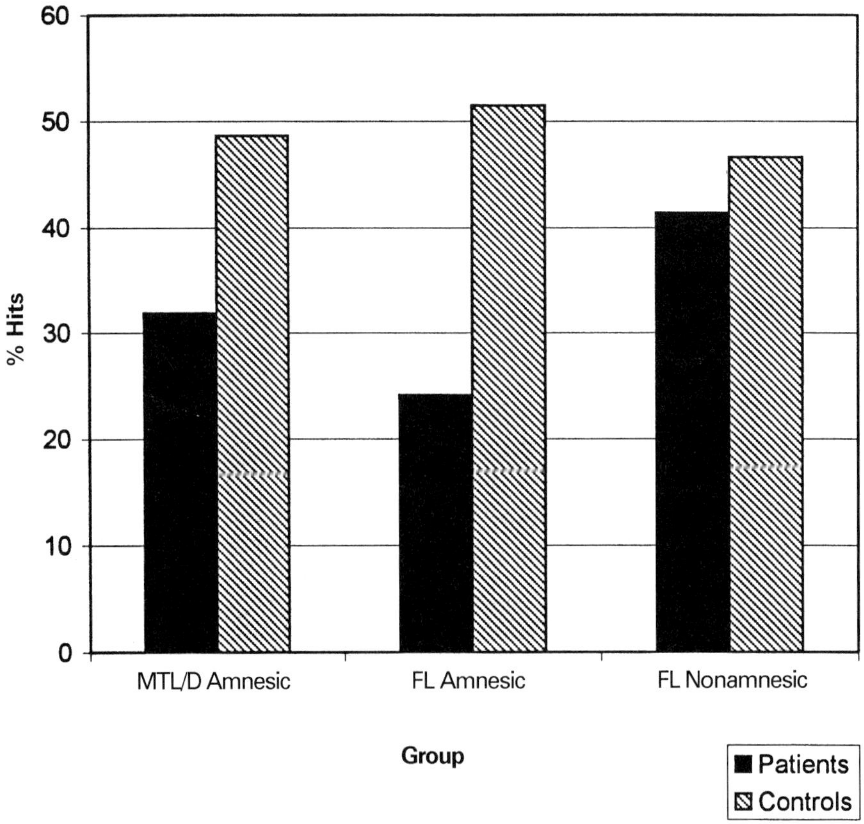

Fig. 1. *Percentage of study list words produced by patients and controls.*

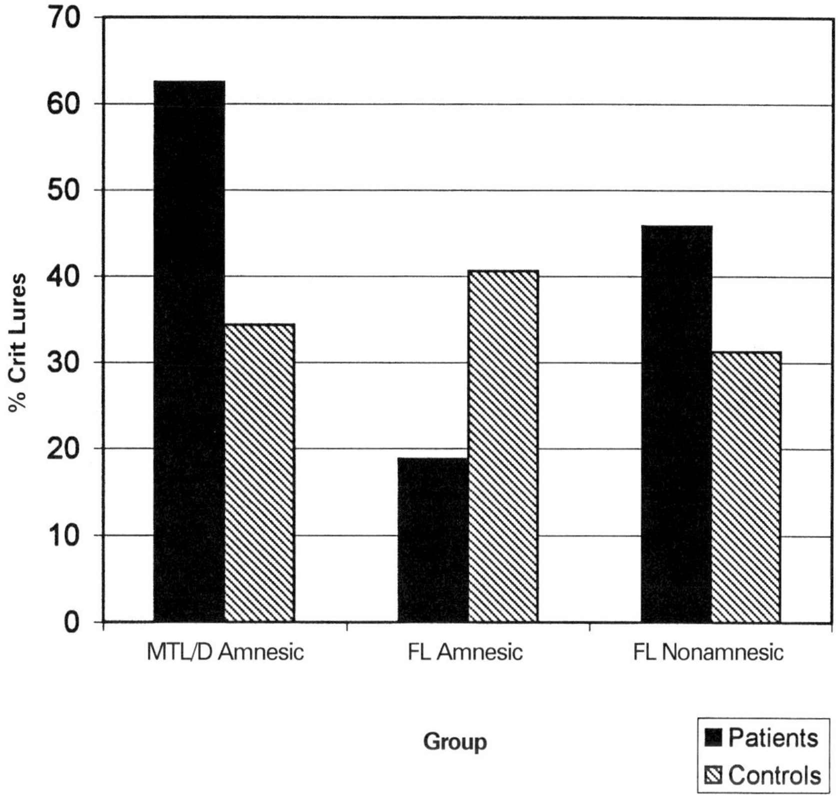

Fig. 2. *Percentage of critical lures intruded by patients and controls.*

(.41). This difference approached significance ($Z = 2.097$, $P = .057$). They also intruded a significantly smaller proportion of critical lures than did MTL/D amnesics ($Z = 2.352$, $P < .05$) (see Fig. 2). The FL nonamnesic patients intruded a larger proportion of critical lures (.46) than did controls (.31), although this difference was nonsignificant ($Z = 0.900$, $P < .5$). The proportion of critical lures intruded by FL nonamnesic patients was not significantly different from MTL/D amnesics ($Z = 1.328$, $P < .5$). However, it differed significantly from FL amnesics ($Z = 2.412$, $P < .05$).

Interestingly, the pattern of performance for the FL amnesics in this study was similar to the performance of the amnesic patients in Schacter et al.'s (1996c) study. That is, the FL amnesics in our study produced similar proportions of study list targets and critical lures (.24 vs. .19) ($Z = 0.730$, $P < .5$). However, the proportion of study list words recalled by the MTL/D amnesic patients was considerably lower than the proportion of critical lures intruded (.32 vs. .63) ($Z = 1.826$, $P = .068$). The performance of control subjects as a group ($N = 14$) in the present study was similar to the control subjects in Schacter et al.'s (1996c) study in that they also produced significantly more study list targets than critical lures (.49 vs. .35) ($Z = 1.978$, $P < .05$). The FL nonamnesic patients intruded a nonsignificantly smaller proportion of study list words than critical lures (.41 vs. .46), ($Z = 0.524$, $P < 1$).

The preceding analyses provide some evidence for a difference in the relation between critical lure intrusions and recall of target items in patients and controls. However, this difference, at least with respect to the MTL/D amnesic patients, is not in the predicted direction based on Schacter et al.'s (1996c) findings. MTL/D amnesic patients in this study did not intrude a significantly smaller proportion of critical lures than either control subjects or frontal patients.

Following Schacter et al. (1996c), the intrusions of critical lures were compared to the mean proportion of words recalled from the nonrecency and nonprimacy regions of the serial position curve (i.e. positions 4–11). These data are presented in Table 3. For control subjects, as a group ($N = 14$), the proportion of studied words recalled from these positions (.37) was now about equal to the proportion of lures intruded (.35). For MTL/D amnesics, the proportion of words recalled from the middle positions of the serial position curve (.23) was smaller than the proportion of critical lures produced (.63), and this difference approached significance ($Z = 1.826$, $P = .068$). For FL amnesics, the proportion of words recalled from the middle positions of the serial position curve (.12) was not significantly different from the proportion of critical lures intruded (.19) ($Z = 0.736$, $P < .5$). This suggests that the relation between recall of studied words and intrusion of critical lures differs in MTL/D amnesic patients and control subjects. The proportion of study list words recalled by FL nonamnesic patients from serial position 4–11 (.25) was significantly lower than the proportion of critical lures produced (.46) ($Z = 2.023$, $P < .05$). This suggests that FL nonamnesic patients are also more likely than control subjects to produce false recall of critical lures.

The findings by Schacter et al. (1996c) suggested that amnesics make on average many more noncritical lure intrusions than control subjects. Furthermore, the nature of these intrusions is somewhat different for the two groups. Specifically, while the two groups were equally likely to produce unrelated intrusions, amnesic patients were less likely than controls to produce intrusions related to the just-studied list, and correspondingly more likely to produce perseverations to previously studied lists. This pattern of intrusions did not emerge for the patients in the present study. Aside from one MTL/D amnesic patient (PT) who produced a large number of noncritical lure intrusions (38 in total, 4.75/list), all other MTL/D patients produced on average less than one noncritical lure intrusion per list (0.59). It is also important to note that whereas the MTL/D patients, with the exception of PT produced low levels of noncritical lure intrusions, all of the MTL/D amnesics produced at least three out of eight possible critical lure intrusions (range: 3–7). FL, amnesics produced 0.093 noncritical lure intrusions/list and FL nonamnesic patients produced 0.25 noncritical lure intrusions/list. In comparison, control subjects, as a group, produced on average 0.46 noncritical lure intrusions/list. Furthermore, with respect to the nature of these intrusions (i.e. related to the current list, unrelated to the current list, or related to a previously presented list) there were no apparent differences between controls, amnesics, and focal frontal patients in terms the type of intrusions made. Schacter et al. found that the amnesics in their study were more likely than controls to produce perseverations to previously studied lists. Considering the probable frontal lobe involvement in at least the Korsakoff's amnesics in their study, this finding is not surprising (Stuss, Craik, Sayer, Franchi, & Alexander, 1996)

Despite the fact that we did not observe significant differences between the groups in the number as well as the pattern of noncritical lure intrusions, we computed for each subject a baseline intrusion rate according to the method employed by Schacter et al. (1996c) (i.e. the proportion of critical lure intrusions as a function of the total number of intrusions). According to this adjusted measure, the baseline intrusion rate for the MTL/D patients was .32, if the patient who produced a great number of noncritical lure intrusions is included, and .39 if

Table 3. *Mean Proportion of Study List Words Produced from Nonrecency and Nonprimacy Portions of the Serial Position Curve (Positions 4–11) and Mean Proportion of Critical Lures Intruded by Patients and Controls*

Group	*Hits*	*Critical Lure Intrusions*
MTL/D amnesics ($N = 4$)	.23	.63
Controls ($N = 4$)	.40	.34
FL amnesics ($N = 4$)	.12	.19
Controls ($N = 4$)	.39	.41
FL nonamnesics ($N = 6$)	.28	.46
Controls ($N = 6$)	.33	.31

she is excluded from the analysis. The baseline intrusion rate of FL amnesic patients was .17. FL nonamnesic patients had a baseline intrusion rate of .37, and the controls had a baseline intrusion rate of .26. Although the differences between MTL/D amnesics, FL nonamnesics and control subjects is reduced, it is significant that the MTL/D amnesic patients still produced proportionately more false recall than the FL amnesics or the amnesics in the Schacter et al. study (1996c). It is important to emphasise that we would predict that the proportion of related noncritical lure intrusions rises as the proportion of critical lure intrusions rises when amnesic subjects are extracting the gist of the lists and rely almost entirely on it for recall because they lack a verbatim trace. For these reasons, we believe that a more appropriate baseline measure is to compute the proportion of critical lure intrusions as a function of the total number of unrelated intrusions. These include intrusions unrelated to the current list and intrusions representing perseverations to previously studied lists. When this is done, MTL/D amnesics have a baseline intrusion rate of .55. We included PT in the analyses because 95% of her total number of noncritical lure intrusions were related to the just-studied list. The baseline intrusion rate for FL nonamnesics is.18. FL nonamnesic patients show a baseline intrusion of .43 and controls as a group have a baseline intrusion rate of .34. This analysis also provides evidence to suggest that MTL/D amnesic patients in this study do produce higher levels of false recall than FL amnesics and control subjects and that this effect is not due to just a high intrusion rate.

If critical lure intrusions arise from associative processes operating during recall itself, then one might expect more critical lure intrusions when subjects recall many targets from a list than when they recall few targets (Roediger & McDermott, 1995). Schacter et al. (1996c) found that amnesic patients recalled more target items from lists for which they produced the critical lure than from lists for which they did not produce the critical lure. Control subjects in their experiment showed comparable levels of target recall whether or not they produced the critical lure. In the present experiment, control subjects also showed comparable levels of target recall whether they produced the critical lure (mean = 7) or not (mean = 7.6). MTL/D amnesics and FL amnesics also produced approximately the same number of target items from lists for which they produced the critical lure (mean = 4.7 for MTL/D amnesics, mean = 3.25 for FL amnesics) than from lists for which they did not produce the critical lure (mean = 4.0 for MTL/D amnesics, mean = 3.7 for FL amnesics). Although this analysis is inconclusive, it appears that controls and amnesic patients produced comparable levels of target recall regardless of whether they produced the critical lure or not. This pattern was also true of the FL nonamnesic patients, whose mean recall was 5.72 when they produced the critical lure and 6.30 when they did not.

To examine this issue further, we looked at the output position of the critical lure. It was reasoned that a relatively late output position for the critical lure would tend to indicate a role for associatively related items produced previously during the recall test. For MTL/D amnesics, the average output position for critical lures was 4.91 of 7.57 words produced for lists in which there was a critical lure intrusion. For FL amnesics, the average output position for critical lures was 3.63 of 4.5 words produced for lists in which there was a critical lure intrusion. For FL nonamnesic patients, the mean output position was 5.37 and the average number of items produced for these lists was 7.4. For controls, the average output position for critical lures was 5.52, but the average number of target items produced for these lists was 8.61. Thus, in relative terms, and in support of the finding by Schacter et al. (1996c), all three patient groups produced the critical lure later than did the control subjects. This finding appears to support the idea that for control subjects the intrusion of critical lures is less dependent on associative processes during recall than it is in amnesic and nonamnesic frontal patients.

Recognition

As already mentioned, subjects were tested on two separate occasions. On one occasion they were asked to engage in free recall prior to the recognition test and on the other they were asked to do simple arithmetic questions prior to the recognition test. As in Schacter et al.'s (1996c) study, it was found that type of task (free recall vs. arithmetic) did not significantly influence performance at recognition, so all analyses are collapsed across the free recall and arithmetic conditions.

Table 4 presents the proportion of old responses to true targets (hits), false targets (critical lures), unrelated true-target controls (distractors), and false-target controls (distractors for critical lures).

An analysis of true targets did not reveal the expected significantly higher hit rate in control subjects (.62) than in MTL/D amnesics (.56) ($Z = 0.632$, $P < .6$). There was also no significant difference in hits between FL amnesics (.56) and their controls (.68) ($Z = 1.173$, $P < .3$). FL nonamnesic patients had a hit rate of .73 which was not significantly different from their controls (.64) ($Z = 0.307$, $P < .4$). The hit rate of FL nonamnesic patients was significantly higher than MTL/D amnesics ($Z = 2.110$, $P < .04$). Due to high variability in the recognition performance of FL amnesic patients, and the limited power of the statistical analysis due to the small *N*s, the hit rate of FL amnesic patients was not significantly different from the FL nonamnesic patients ($Z = 0.830$, $P < .5$).

There was a significantly higher false alarm rate (to true-target controls) in the MTL/D amnesics (.56) than in their controls (.08) ($Z = 3.038$, $P = .001$). Similarly, FL amnesics showed significantly higher levels of false alarms (.39) than did their control subjects (.12) ($Z = 2.473$, $P < .05$). FL nonamnesics produced significantly lower levels of false alarms (.14) than either MTL/D amnesics ($Z = 2.631$, $P < .01$) or FL amnesics ($Z = 2.820$, $P < .005$), but there was no significant difference between the false alarm rate of the FL nonamnesic patients and their control subjects (.09) ($Z = 1.945$, $P < .1$). Using the standard high-threshold correction procedure, the false alarm rate was subtracted from the hit rate. Table 4 presents corrected scores for recognition accuracy. This analysis revealed that recognition accuracy in MTL/D amnesic patients was significantly lower than in control subjects ($Z = 3.048$, $P = .001$) and frontal patients ($Z = 3.223$, $P = .001$). FL amnesics also had significantly lower recognition accuracy than their controls ($Z = 2.782$, $P < .005$) and FL nonamnesic patients ($Z = 3.186$, $P = .001$). MTL/D amnesics and FL amnesics did not differ significantly in their recognition accuracy ($Z = 1.788$, $P < .09$).

False alarm rates to critical lures (nonpresented words preceded by a list of high associates, i.e. false targets) were compared to false alarm rates for their corresponding distractors (words drawn from the same pool of critical lures that were not preceded by a list of high associates, i.e. false-target controls). Although both groups of amnesic patients made more false alarms to distractors than did control subjects or FL nonamnesic patients, they did not make more false alarms to critical lures than did control subjects or FL nonamnesic patients. The proportion of old responses to critical lures for MTL/D patients (.72) did not differ from that of

Table 4. *Recognition Memory Data for True Targets, False Targets, True-Target Controls, and False-Target Controls for Patients and Control Subjects*

	Proportion of Old Responses					
Item type	*MTL/D Amnesics*	*Controls*	*FL Amnesics*	*Controls*	*FL Nonamnesics*	*Controls*
True targets	.56	.62	.56	.68	.73	.64
True-target controls	.56	.08	.39	.12	.14	.09
True − control (corrected recog)	.00	.54	.17	.56	.59	.55
False targets	.72	.70	.61	.80	.90	.67
False-target controls	.43	.16	.66	.14	.23	.10
False − controls (gist memory)	.29	.54	−.05	.66	.67	.57

their controls (.70) ($Z = 0.165$, $P < .9$). The proportion of false alarms to critical lures for FL amnesics (.61) was not significantly different from their controls (.80) ($Z = 1.186$, $P < .3$). The false alarm rate to critical lures for FL nonamnesics was .90, which was significantly higher than that of their controls (.67) ($Z = 2.128$, $P < .05$).

Because of the tendency of amnesic patients to make more false alarms to distractors, we subtracted the proportion of old responses to distractors for critical lures from the proportion of old responses to critical lures. The corrected proportion is presented in Table 4 (False – Control). This measure revealed that MTL/D amnesics produced proportionately fewer false recognition responses to critical lures than did controls ($Z = 1.064$, $P < 1$) or FL nonamnesic patients ($Z = 2.036$, $P < .05$). FL amnesics produced significantly fewer false recognition responses to critical lures than did their control subjects ($Z = 2.909$, $P < .005$) or FL nonamnesic patients ($Z = 3.326$, $P < .001$). FL nonamnesic patients did not differ from their controls in the production of false recognition responses to critical lures, ($Z = 0.934$, $P < .5$).

DISCUSSION

The primary results of this experiment can be summarised as follows: At recall, FL amnesic patients showed a lower proportion of critical lure intrusions than did control subjects. However, MTL/D and FL nonamnesic patients demonstrated a higher proportion of critical lure intrusions than control subjects. Furthermore, control subjects recalled more targets than critical lures, whereas MTL/D amnesic patients and FL nonamnesic patients produced more critical lures than targets. At recognition, both MTL/D amnesics and FL amnesics recognised a smaller proportion of studied words and produced a smaller proportion of critical lures than did either controls or FL nonamnesic patients.

It was hypothesised that abnormally high levels of false memories are related to the following three conditions: (1) impaired memory for the word lists, (2) the ability to extract and use semantic gist of the list, and (3) defective strategic monitoring processes. Although it is necessary to exercise caution in interpreting the data from this experiment due to the small number of subjects in each group, the performance of the three patient groups underscores the importance of these conditions. The first two derive from Brainerd and Reyna's "fuzzy trace" theory, which provides a useful framework for interpreting the data from this experiment (Brainerd, Reyna, & Brandes, 1995a; Brainerd, Reyna, & Kneer, 1995b; Reyna & Brainerd, 1995). They account for the phenomena of false recall and recognition by proposing that memory can be based either on a "gist trace" that preserves the general meanings and interpretations engendered by studied items or on a "verbatim trace" that preserves specific information about the exact identity of each item. Against this theoretical background, we discuss each of the three groups.

The MTL/D amnesic patients were impaired at recalling specific studied words and produced a higher proportion of critical lures than the controls at recall. Their tendency to produce the critical lure at recall was undoubtedly related to their ability to extract and retain the semantic gist of the lists. The use of gist is generally an effective strategy for amnesic patients to employ in everyday life. Since they are so impaired at retaining the specific details about a situation, they do well to focus their efforts on extracting the main theme. The performance of these patients at recognition also lends support to Brainerd et al.'s theoretical stance. Because they are severely memory-impaired, even the "gist trace" becomes degraded over time so that by the time recognition was tested they could no longer produce higher levels of false memory than controls or frontal lobe patients; in fact they performed in much the same fashion as the FL amnesics. In comparison to frontal lobe patients and control subjects, whose memory for the target items and gist is preserved, both groups of amnesics produced significantly lower levels of false recognition. They did, however, retain some gist information, as is indicated by their slight tendency to choose critical lures over other distractors. It is important to bear in mind that the recognition test was administered just 2 minutes after completion of the recall or arithmetic task that followed the final study list. It is possible that this short delay is not sufficient to cause the "gist trace" to degrade completely. Another striking finding at recognition is the very high false alarm rate to distractors for studied items (true-target controls) by the MTL/D patients. A similar, albeit less pronounced, effect is obtained by the FL amnesic patients. It is significant that the distractors for the studied items were not unrelated to each other. In fact, three items from a single nonstudied list were presented, as was the critical lure from the list. Therefore, it might be that within-test relations among words led amnesic patients to endorse these distractors. The high false alarm rate to these nonstudied distractors might itself reflect a form of gist-based false memory.

Not all amnesics can use this strategy, as was evident from the performance of the FL amnesics, who consistently produced low levels of false recall and recognition in our study. In fact the FL amnesics' performance was very similar to the performance of the amnesics in Schacter et al.'s (1996c) study. All of the amnesic patients included in these two studies have damage to memory structure, which cause their severe amnesia. The similarity in performance between the two groups supports our speculation that the absence of false memories in Schacter et al.'s patients did not result from amnesia alone but additionally involved a frontal lobe component. This is highly probable in their Korsakoff patients and likely in some of the others as well. The frontal lobe damage in these patients may also affect their ability to employ cognitive strategies effectively (Moscovitch, 1995; Moscovitch & Melo, 1997). As a result, they may have had difficulty extracting the gist of the study list or using it to guide recollection at retrieval. These strategic difficulties, when combined with poor memory, can lead to a failure to generate the type of mnemonic information that will support true or false memories[1].

The FL nonamnesic patients differ from the FL amnesics in that they have a reasonably good memory of studied words and are also able to remember the main theme of the lists. They differ from controls and MTL/D amnesics in that they are deficient in monitoring their memories effectively. If poor monitoring contributes to the production of false recall and false recognition in this paradigm, the FL nonamnesic patients should produce more false recall and false recognition than control subjects. Although the results of this study are consistent with this hypothesis, the statistical significance of our findings is limited by the small number of subjects in each group.

The tendency towards exaggerated levels of false recall and false recognition by frontal lobe patients may result from defective monitoring that allows them to generate only a vague or unfocused representation of characteristic features of the target words against which test items are matched. Items that are generally similar to previously studied ones (critical lures) are accepted as old because they match the general contextual representation and are not filtered out. This explanation is supported by two recently documented cases of patients with focal frontal lobe lesions (one with a left prefrontal cortex lesion, JW; and one with a right prefrontal cortex lesion BG), who exhibit a striking pattern of false recognition (Curran, Schacter, Norman, & Gallucio, 1997; Parkin, et al., 1996; Parkin, Ward, Bindschaedler, Powell, & Squires, this issue; Schacter et al., 1996a). Schacter, Curran et al. suggest that BG relies excessively on information about the general correspondence between a test item and previously studied words when making a recognition decision. Given previous evidence implicating the frontal lobes in memory for source or contextual information (Schacter, Harbluk, & McLachlan, 1984), these authors suggest that a source memory deficit contributes to the nature of BG's false recollection. According to this view, the right prefrontal cortex may be involved in setting up contextual representations that guide retrieval by allowing one to focus on a target episode and filter out irrelevant material. BG's deficits seem to be related to problems in generating a specific, focused representation of a study episode and filtering out

[1] Another factor that may contribute to the differences in levels of false memory in the two amnesic groups is differences in IQ (see Table 2). It may be that FL amnesics cannot extract the gist of lists because they are not as intelligent as MTL/D amnesics.

nonessential information. These observations would also hold for the FL nonamnesic patients and underscore the likelihood that monitoring processes are defective in frontal lobe patients.

It is interesting to note that BG, whose lesion primarily affected lateral regions of the right frontal lobe, was able to extract gist but could not effectively monitor related information (Schacter et al., 1996a). By comparison, Parkin et al.'s (this issue) patient, JW, who had a ruptured aneurysm of the anterior communicating artery that presumably caused a lesion to ventromedial prefrontal cortex, had the additional difficulty of extracting gist. This raises the interesting possibility that processes related to monitoring and to extracting and using gist involve different frontal mechanisms. This hypothesis is consistent with our study in which FL nonamnesic patients, who showed large numbers of false memories and normal hit rates, had lesions primarily on the lateral surface. In contrast, the FL amnesics, who showed little in the way of true or false memories, had lesions that typically included the ventromedial area. By virtue of the fact that they were amnesics, it is likely that their lesions included basal forebrain structures that are adjacent to the ventromedial frontal areas. Alternatively, it may just be the combination of amnesia and frontal lobe dysfunction as in Korsakoff's patients that are the necessary conditions for producing reduced false memories.

In summary, the present data provide important insights into the conditions that can lead to abnormally high levels of false recall and false recognition. Damage to MTL/D structures can produce false memories by forcing patients to rely on information that is semantically related to target items (gist) in the absence of memory for the items themselves. Since accurate recollection depends on the ability to distinguish between true and faulty output from the medial temporal lobe and diencephalon, an intact monitoring mechanism is essential. Damage to the frontal lobe, depending on location, can severely disrupt this mechanism and the ability to extract and work with semantic gist. Finally, our data, along with those of Schacter et al. (1996a), show that when both frontal lobe and medial temporal lobe or diencephalic structures are damaged, all of the above processes are impaired. Such patients have little or no access to information that is related to target items and the result is a reduced number of true and false memories.

REFERENCES

Anisfeld, M., & Knapp, M. (1968). Association, synonymity and directionality in false recognition. *Journal of Experimental Psychology, 77,* 171–479.

Bartlett, F.C. (1932). *Remembering.* Cambridge: Cambridge University Press.

Belli, R.F., Lindsay, D.S., Gales, M.S., & McCarthy, T.T. (1994). Memory impairment and source misattribution in postevent misinformation experiments with short retention intervals. *Memory & Cognition, 15,* 657–668.

Berlyne, N. (1972). Confabulation. *British Journal of Psychiatry, 120,* 31-39.

Brainerd, C.J., Reyna, V.F., & Brandes, E. (1995a). Are children's false memories more persistent than their true memories? *Psychological Science, 6,* 359–364.

Brainerd, C.J., Reyna, V.F., & Kneer, R. (1995b). False-recognition reversal: When similarity is distinctive. *Journal of Memory and Language, 34,* 157–185.

Burgess, P.W., & Shallice, T. (1996). Confabulation and the control of recollection. *Memory, 4*(4), 359–411.

Cermak, L.S., Butters, X., & Gerrein, J. (1973). The extent of the verbal encoding ability of Korsakoff patients. *Neuropsychologia, 11,* 85–94.

Craik, F.I.M., Morris, L.W., Morris, R.G., & Loewen, E.R. (1990). Relations between source amnesia and frontal lobe functioning in older adults. *Psychology and Aging, 5,* 148–151.

Crovitz, H.F., & Schiffman, H. (1974). Frequency of episodic memories as a function of their age. *Bulletin of the Psychonomic Society, 4,* 517–518.

Curran, T., Schacter, D.L., Norman, K.A., & Gallucio, L. (1997). False recognition after a right frontal lobe infarction: Memory for general and specific information. *Neuropsychologia, 35,* 1035–1049.

Dalla Barba, G. (1993). Confabulation: Knowledge and recollective experience. *Cognitive Neuropsychology, 10,* 1–20.

Deese, J. (1959). On the prediction of occurrence of particular verbal intrusions in immediate recall. *Journal of Experimental Psychology, 58,* 17–22.

DeLuca, J., & Cicerone, K.D. (1991). Confabulation following aneurysm of the anterior communicating artery. *Cortex, 27,* 417–423.

De Luca, J., & Diamond, B.J. (1995). Aneurysm of the anterior communicating artery: A review of neuroanatomical and neuropsychological sequelae. *Journal of Clinical and Experimental Neuropsychology, 17,* 100–121.

Johnson, M.K. (1991). Reality monitoring: Evidence from confabulation in organic brain disease patients. In G.P. Prigatano & D.L. Schacter (Eds.), *Awareness of deficit after brain injury: Clinical and theoretical issue,* pp. 176–196. New York: Oxford University Press.

Johnson, M.K., Hashtroudi, S., & Lindsay, D.S. (1993). Source monitoring. *Psychological Bulletin, 114,* 3–28.

Johnson, M.K., O'Connor, M., & Cantor, J. (1997). Confabulation, memory deficits, and frontal dysfunction. *Brain and Cognition, 34,* 189–206.

Knowlton, B.J., & Squire, L.R. (1995). Remembering and knowing: two different expressions of declarative memory. *Journal of Experimental Psychology: Learning, Memory and Cognition, 21,* 699–710.

Kopelman, M.D., Ng, N., & Van Den Brouke, O. (1997). Confabulation extending across episodic personal, and general semantic memory. *Cognitive Neuropsychology, 14*(5), 683–712.

Kroll, N.E.A., Knight, R.T., Metcalfe, J., Wolf, E.S., & Tulving, E. (1996). Cohesion failure as a source of memory illusions. *Journal of Memory and Language, 35,* 176–196.

Loftus, E.F., & Palmer, J.C. (1974). Reconstruction of automobilie destruction: An example of the interaction between language and memory. *Journal of Verbal Learning and Verbal Behavior, 13,* 585–89.

Moscovitch, M. (1989). Confabulation and the frontal systems: Strategic versus associated retrieval in neuropsychological theories of memory. In H.L. Roediger III & F.I.M. Craik (Eds.), *Varieties of memory and consciousness: Essays in honour of Endel Tulving,* (pp. 133–160). Hillsdale, NJ: Lawrence Erlbaum Associates.

Moscovitch, M. (1995). Confabulation. In D.L. Schacter, J.T. Coyle, G.D. Fischbach, M.M. Mesulam, & L.E. Sullivan (Eds.), *Memory distortion: How minds, brains, and societies reconstruct the past,* (pp. 226–254). Cambridge, MA: Harvard University Press.

Moscovitch, M., & Melo, B. (1997). Strategic retrieval and the frontal lobes: Evidence from confabulation and amnesia. *Neuropsychologia, 35,* 1017–1034.

Norman, K.A., & Schacter, D.L. (1997). False recognition in younger and older adults: Exploring the characteristics of illusory memories. *Memory and Cognition, 25,* 838–848.

Parkin, A.J., Bindschaedler, C., Harsent, L., & Metzler, C. (1996), Pathological false alarm rates following damage to the left frontal cortex. *Brain and Cognition, 32,* 14–27.

Parkin, A., Ward, J., Bindschaedler, C., Powell, G., & Squires, E.L. (this issue). False recognition following frontal lobe damage: The role of encoding factors. *Cognitive Neuropsychology, 16,* 243–265.

Reinitz, M.T., & Milberg, W. (1996). Memory conjunction errors in normal and amnesic subjects. *Journal of Memory and Language, 35,* 286–299.

Reyna, V.E., & Brainerd, C.J. (1995). Fuzzy-trace theory: An interim synthesis. *Learning and Individual Differences, 7,* 1–25.

Roediger, H.L. III, & McDermott, K.B. (1995). Creating false memories: Remembering words not presented in lists. *Journal of Experimental Psychology: Learning, Memory and Cognition, 21*(4), 803–814.

Roediger, H.L. III, & McDermott, K.B. (1996). False perceptions of false memories. *Journal of Experimental Psychology: Learning, Memory and Cognition, 22*(3), 814–816.

Schacter, D.L. (1996). Illusory memories: A cognitive neuroscience analysis. *Proceedings of the National Academy of Sciences of the United States of America, 93*(24), 13527–13533.

Schacter, D.L., Buckner, R.L., Koutstaal, W., Dale, A.M., & Rosen, B.R. (1997). Late onset of anterior prefrontal activity during true and false recognition: An event-related fMRI study. *Neuroimage, 6*(4), 259–269.

Schacter, D.L., Curran, T., Galluccio, L., Milberg, W.P., & Bates, J.F. (1996a). False recognition and the right frontal lobe: A case study. *Neuropsychologia, 34*(8), 793–808.

Schacter, D.L., Harbluk, J.L., & McLachlan, D.R. (1984). Retrieval without recollection: An experimental analysis of source amnesia. *Journal of Verbal Learning and Verbal Behaviour, 23,* 593–611.

Schacter, D.L., Koutstaal, W., Johnson, M.K., Gross, M.S., & Angell, K.E. (1997b). False recollection induced via photographs: A comparison of older and younger adults. *Psychology and Aging, 12*(2), 203–215.

Schacter, D.L., Reiman, E., Curran, T., Sheng Yun, L., Bandy, D., McDermott, K.B., & Roediger, H.L. III (1996). Neuroanatomical correlates of veridical and illusory recognition memory: Evidence from positron emission tomography. *Neuron, 17,* 267–274.

Schacter, D.L., Verfaellie, M., & Anes, M.D. (1997). Illusory memories in amnesic patients: conceptual and perceptual false recognition. *Neuropsychology, 11*(3), 331–342.

Schacter, D.L., Verfaellie, M., Anes, M.D., & Racine, C. (1998). When true recognition suppresses false recognition: Evidence from amnesic patients. *Journal of Cognitive Neuroscience, 10,* 668–679.

Schacter, D.L., Verfaellie, M., & Pradere, D. (1996). The neuropsychology of memory illusions: False recall and recognition in amnesic patients. *Journal of Memory and Language, 35,* 319–334.

Schnider, A., von Daniken, C., & Gutbrod, K. (1996). The mechanisms of spontaneous and provoked confabulation. *Brain, 119,* 1365–1375.

Shimamura, A.P., & Squire, L.R. (1987). A neuropsychological study of fact memory and source amnesia. *Journal of Experimental Psychology: Learning, Memory and Cognition, 21,* 267–287.

Stuss, D.T., Alexander, M.R., Lieberman, A., & Levine, H. (1978). An extraordinary form of confabulation. *Neurology, 28,* 1166–1172.

Stuss, D.T., Craik, F.I.M., Sayer, L., Franchi, R., & Alexander, M. (1996). Comparison of older people and patients with frontal lesions: Evidence from word list learning. *Psychology and Aging, 11,* 387–595.

Tulving, E. (1985). Varieties of consciousness and levels of awareness in memory. In A. Baddeley & L. Weiskrantz (Eds.), *Attention: Selection, awareness and control. A tribute to Donald Broadbent.* Oxford: Oxford University Press.

COGNITIVE NEUROPSYCHOLOGY, 1999, 16 (3/4/5), 361–384

VERIDICAL AND FALSE MEMORIES IN HEALTHY OLDER ADULTS AND IN DEMENTIA OF THE ALZHEIMER'S TYPE

David A. Balota, Michael J. Cortese, Janet M. Duchek, David Adams, Henry L. Roediger III, Kathleen B. McDermott, and Benjamin E. Yerys
Washington University, St. Louis, USA

Five groups of participants (young, healthy old, healthy old-old, very mild Dementia of the Alzheimer's Type, Mild Dementia of the Alzheimer's Type) studied and were tested on six 12-item lists of words selected from the DRM (Deese, 1959; Roediger & McDermott, 1995) materials. These lists of words strongly converged semantically on a nonpresented critical word. The results indicated that both veridical recall and recognition performance decreased both as a function of age of the participants and as a function of dementia severity. However, the recall and recognition of the highly related nonpresented items actually increased as a function of age, and only slightly decreased as a function of DAT. When false memory was considered as a proportion of veridical memory, there was a clear increase as a function of both age of the participants and as a function of disease severity. The results are discussed in terms of (a) age and DAT-related changes in attention and memory performance, and (b) the underlying mechanisms that produce false memories in the DRM paradigm.

INTRODUCTION

One of the most common findings in both healthy older adults and in early stages of Dementia of the Alzheimer's Type (DAT) is a breakdown in veridical episodic memory performance (see Craik & Jennings, 1992; Nebes, 1994, for reviews). The present study will explore not only veridical memory in these populations, but also memory for information that was not presented, i.e. false memories. In particular, we will explore the false memory paradigm recently developed by Roediger and McDermott (1995) based on an initial study by Deese (1959), hereafter called the DRM paradigm, in which associatively/semantically related words converge on a critical nonpresented item. For example, consider being presented with the following list of words: THREAD, PIN, EYE, SEWING, SHARP, POINT, PRICK, THIMBLE, HAYSTACK, PAIN, HURT, INJECTION. The nonpresented critical target word is NEEDLE in this list. Roediger and McDermott reported that the likelihood of recalling the nonpresented critical word NEEDLE was as high as the probability of recalling the items that were actually presented in the middle of the list (.40 in both cases). The issues addressed in the present study are the manner in which healthy ageing and

---

Requests for reprints should be addressed to David A. Balota, Department of Psychology, Washington University, St. Louis, MO 63130, USA (E-mail: dbalota@artsci.wustl.edu).

This work was supported by Grant NIA PO1 AGO3991. Thanks are extended to the clinical core at the Washington University ADRC who provided the well-specified population for this study, Martha Storandt who provided the psychometric information, and Beth Ober, Patricia Tun, and Dan Schacter for helpful comments on an earlier version of this manuscript.

DAT influence both veridical and false memories, and the mechanisms that underlie performance in the DRM paradigm.

The present study was motivated by a series of experiments that provide evidence regarding the relative integrity and disruption of specific cognitive systems (e.g. semantic memory and attentional systems) in both healthy older adults compared to younger adults, and in DAT individuals compared to age-matched healthy control individuals. We will argue that the production of false memories in older individuals and in DAT individuals may reflect a tradeoff in the integrity of these cognitive systems, which make these populations particularly sensitive to false memories. We shall now turn to a brief review of the extant literature regarding both semantic memory systems and attentional control systems in both healthy older adults and in early stage DAT individuals.

Semantic Memory Structure and Processes in Healthy Older Adults and in Early Stage DAT

In the DRM paradigm, participants are presented associatively/semantically related words that converge on a critical nonpresented target word. Of course, if there is a degradation in semantic memory in healthy older adults and/or in DAT individuals, then one might expect a decreased susceptibility to false memories. Unfortunately, the evidence regarding changes in semantic memory in both healthy older adults and in early stage DAT individuals has been somewhat controversial. For example, evidence from tasks such as verbal fluency and object naming has been taken to indicate that there is a breakdown in semantic memory structures in these populations (e.g. Albert, Heller, & Milberg, 1988; Kirshner, Webb, & Kelly, 1984; Ober, Dronkers, Koss, Delis, & Friedland, 1986; Troster, Salmon, McCullough, & Butters, 1989). However, researchers have argued that the deficits in these tasks are not simply a reflection of the integrity of semantic memory, but rather, reflect the attentional demands engaged by these tasks (see Balota, Watson, Duchek, & Ferraro, in press; Nebes, 1989; Ober & Shenaut, 1995). For example, in the verbal fluency task, the participant must generate words that begin with a specific letter and also maintain some memory of previously generated words. A breakdown in performance in this task could be due to the semantic integrity of the system, the attentional control of task goals, and/or the maintenance of previously produced words. Clearly, this task is not simply a pure measure of semantic memory structure.

In order to minimise attentional demands, researchers have turned to semantic priming tasks in which participants are asked to make simple naming or lexical decisions to targets (doctor) that follow either related (nurse) or unrelated (chair) primes. The research in the area is relatively clear: Specifically, one finds relatively intact priming effects under conditions that reflect automatic spread of activation within the memory network, whereas one finds evidence of breakdowns in both healthy older adults (Balota, Black, & Cheney, 1992) and in early stage DAT individuals (Ober & Shenaut, 1995), under conditions that reflect attentional processes. Thus, researchers have argued that the integrity of the network and automatic access to information embedded in this network are relatively intact in both healthy older adults, and in early stage DAT, and it is the attentional systems that appear to break down.

Attentional Breakdown in Healthy Ageing and in DAT Individuals

In contrast to the automatic activation of semantic pathways, recent studies indicate that there is a breakdown in processes related to inhibitory/attentional control in both healthy older adults (e.g. Duchek, Balota, & Thessing, in press; Hasher & Zacks, 1988) and in early stage DAT individuals (e.g. Spieler, Balota, & Faust, 1996; Sullivan, Faust, & Balota, 1995). It is important to note that these studies have yielded *disproportionate* breakdowns (greater than expected by overall differences in speed or accuracy), and/or qualitatively distinct patterns predicted by the inhibitory framework. For example, Spieler et al. (1996) provided evidence that there is a disproportionate breakdown in the ability to inhibit the word code when naming colours in the Stroop task in both healthy older adults, compared to young, and in DAT individuals. In addition, Balota and Duchek (1991) demonstrated that DAT individuals are more likely to keep active inappropriate meanings of ambiguous words (e.g. the BODY meaning of ORGAN) in the presence of context (e.g. MUSIC), whereas healthy older individuals appear to suppress such inappropriate interpretations (also see Faust, Balota, Duchek, Gernsbacher, & Smith, 1997). These results, coupled with the earlier cited priming studies, suggest that the activation of relevant networks is not impaired in healthy older adults or in early stages of DAT, but it is the attentional control or inhibition of partially activated pathways that appears to be compromised.

What are the implications of these observations for the DRM false memory paradigm? False memories of the critical nonpresented items in the DRM paradigm could be viewed as a situation wherein there are multiple sources of activation that need to be discriminated to make the correct response. An intact processing system should be able to discriminate between sources of activation that are directly related to what was presented compared to sources that are only indirectly related, but highly activated (see Johnson, Hashtroudi, & Lindsay, 1993, for discussion of reality and source monitoring, and Multhaup & Balota, 1997, for evidence of source deficits in DAT individuals). Based on the evidence reviewed, one might suggest that healthy older adults and DAT individuals may have difficulty controlling or inhibiting the highly activated (semantically related) nonpresented item. In this light, it is possible that a breakdown in attentional control may actually produce increased false memories. If both healthy older adults and early stage DAT individuals have intact semantic structures that produce a boost in the semantic activation for nonpresented critical items, coupled with a breakdown in attentional control systems, one might actually expect an increased likelihood of false memories in these populations. Of course, because of the group differences in memory performance, this pattern would be most likely reflected in *relative* measures in which one takes into account overall changes in veridical memory across these populations.

Norman and Schacter (1997) have recently reported evidence that healthy older adults are indeed *more* susceptible to false memories than healthy young adults (also see Tun, Wingfield, Rose, & Blanchard, 1998). Specifically, although veridical recall was lower in older adults compared to younger adults, false recall was actually higher in older adults compared to younger adults. Norman and Schacter suggested that the increased false memories in the DRM paradigm is quite consistent with age-related decreased efficiency of frontal lobe functioning. There are a number of intriguing lines of converging evidence regarding the role of frontal lobes in the creation of false memories. First Schacter, Reiman, & Curran et al. (1996b) reported evidence in a recent PET study that there is increased activation in regions of prefrontal cortex when critical nonpresented lures were presented compared to the presentation of studied words. Norman and Schacter suggested that this pattern may reflect the frontal involvement in "resisting" or opposing illusory memory for the critical lures. Obviously, this is consistent with the present view that healthy older adults and early stage DAT individuals may have some difficulty inhibiting or controlling partially activated memory representations. Second, Schacter, Curran, Galluccio, Milberg, and Bates (1996a) have recently reported evidence that an individual with a lesion in the right frontal lobe produced heightened false memories. This individual was more likely than control individuals to false alarm to information that was thematically related to the earlier studied information. Interestingly, there is a more recent study of amnesia individuals with medial temporal lobe damage which suggests that individuals with damage in this area actually are *less* likely to produce false recognition of critical words, compared to healthy controls (see Schacter, Verfaellie, & Pradere, 1996c). In this light, the false memory paradigm is ideally suited to investigate the contributions of frontal areas and medial temporal areas to the episodic memory loss in healthy ageing and in early stages of DAT. If the episodic memory loss in early stage DAT is primarily a reflection of medial temporal structures, based on the Schacter et al. arguments, one might expect relatively fewer false memories compared to healthy control individuals, whereas if there is a high degree of frontal impairment, one might actually predict relatively more false memories in these individuals, compared to healthy control individuals. Of course, the more likely case is that both structures are intimately involved in the episodic memory loss in DAT individuals.

In the present study, we will attempt to provide some leverage on the underlying neural systems of false memories by taking advantage of existing psychometric data on the healthy older adults and early stage DAT individuals. Specifically, we have recently demonstrated (Kanne, Balota, Storandt, McKeel, & Morris, 1998) that psychometric tests that (a priori) should reflect functioning of different neural systems (frontal vs. medial temporal vs. parietal) loaded on the predicted factors on an analysis of data from 407 individuals with DAT. In addition, we found that the relative factor scores were correlated with the underlying neuropathology that was observed in 41 DAT individuals who were autopsied. In the present study, we will take advantage of the heterogeneity of this subject population in the integrity of these systems to provide insights, via correlational analyses, into the different neurological systems (frontal vs. medial temporal) that might underlie veridical and false memories.

In addition to providing correlational data regarding psychometric performance, the present study may provide information regarding the underlying mechanism(s) producing false memories. Specifically, several distinct loci may play a role. For example, it is possible that during initial encoding, the nonpresented critical word may actually come to mind as the participant is studying the to-be-remembered list of words, as a result of automatic associative responses (see McDermott, 1997). If this is the case, then this may serve as a learning episode. If the underlying mechanism for this encoding episode is due to an automatic spread of activation, based on the evidence reviewed earlier, one might expect comparable effects of this mechanism in healthy aged individuals and in early stage DAT. Interestingly, there recently has been evidence that one can produce false memories under conditions in which list items are presented at a near-threshold presentation rate (i.e. 50 msec per item), thereby implicating an automatic activation process (see Robinson, 1998; Seamon, Luo, & Gallo, 1998).

It is also possible that at least some of the false recall in the DRM paradigm is occurring during retrieval. Specifically, it is possible that during the overt act of recall, participants generate associatively related words, and hence are likely to generate the critical word. For example, it is possible that participants might have difficulty discriminating between items that were initially presented during study, and items that were generated, but rejected, earlier during the recall period (i.e. a type of source error, see Johnson et al., 1993). One might a priori expect that as more items are generated during recall one might actually increase the likelihood of generating the nonpresented item. Because healthy older adults and early stage DAT individuals should recall fewer items compared to healthy younger adults, one might expect a relative decrease in false memories. However, as noted earlier, this pattern does not occur, at least not in the healthy older adults (e.g. Norman & Schacter, 1997).

In addition to the possible role of source memory during retrieval, it is also quite possible that there are gist-based representations that are driving false recall during retrieval (see, for example, Brainerd, Reyna, & Kneer, 1995). Although the notion of a gist-based representation is a bit vague, one might argue that such gist-based representations should be positively correlated with the number of related items that are stored in memory. Specifically, it would seem that the quality of the gist-based representation would at least in part depend on the quality of the list item representations that produce the gist being represented. In this way, one might expect more false memory as overt memory increases. If this were the case, then because of the expected overall decrease in memory performance in healthy older adults and in early stage DAT, one might expect fewer false memories in these individuals, which, at least with respect to healthy ageing, is inconsistent with some extant data (e.g. Norman & Schacter, 1997). We shall explore these and additional theoretical implications of the relation between veridical and false recall in the General Discussion.

The present experiment included five groups of participants. The first three groups were healthy young (mean age 20 years), healthy older (mean age 71 years), and healthy old-old adults (mean age 86 years). These three groups allowed the tracking of the influence of healthy ageing on veridical and false memories. In addition, we compared three groups of individuals that are relatively similar in age but have varying levels of dementia severity. Specifically, the healthy old (both young-old and old-old) individuals were compared to age-matched very mildly demented individuals, who in turn were compared to age-matched mildly demented individuals. Of course, it would be particularly important if the DRM paradigm was able to discriminate early stage DAT from healthy ageing.

During the experiment, each participant received 6 lists of 12 words for study. After each list was presented, participants were given a free recall task. After all lists were studied and recalled, a final overall yes/no recognition test was presented. The critical dependent measure in the present study is the probability of recalling and/or recognising the critical nonpresented item as a function of the participant's correct recall and/or recognition.

METHOD

Participants

A total of 159 participants were included in this study. They were divided into five groups. The first group was composed of 35 young adults with a mean age of 20.1 years, with a range from 17 to 33 years. The second and third groups were healthy older adults. The healthy older adults were divided into a younger and an older group. There were 37 participants in the younger old group with a mean age of 70.7 years, and a range from 60 to 79. The older old group included 24 participants with a mean age of 85.9, and a range from 80 to 96.

The remaining two groups of participants were composed of individuals with either very mild dementia or mild DAT. Thirty-seven older adults with very mild DAT and an average age of 77.9 participated, and their ages ranged from 66 to 91. Twenty-six participants with mild DAT and an average age of 78.5 participated, and their ages ranged from 56 to 90.

The young adults were students at Washington University who were either paid or received course credit in return for their participation. Older adults and DAT individuals were recruited from the participant pool at the Alzheimer's Disease Research Center (ADRC) at Washington University. These participants were screened for depression, severe hypertension, possible reversible dementias, and other disorders that could affect cognitive performance. DAT individuals were included or excluded based on the criteria set by the National Institute of Neurological and Communicative Disorders and Stroke and Alzheimer's Disease and Related Disorders Association (McKhann et al., 1984). Dementia severity was scaled according to the Washington University Clinical Dementia Rating (CDR) scale. The reliability of this scale, as well as the accuracy of the diagnosis by the research team, is well documented (e.g. Berg et al., 1998). Only those DAT individuals who were classified as having either very mild dementia or mild dementia were included as participants in this study.

Psychometric Test Performance

All the healthy older adults and the DAT individuals also participated in a 2-hour battery of psychometric tests designed to assess psychological functions including language, memory, and intelligence. Memory was assessed with the Wechsler Memory Scale (WMS; Wechsler & Stone, 1973) Associates Recall and Recognition subscales (paired-associates learning), and the Logical Memory subscale (surface-level story memory). Forward and backward digit span from the WMS were also assessed. Participants also received the Word Fluency test, on which they were required to name as many words as possible beginning with a specified letter (e.g. *P* or *S*) in a 60sec time period (Thurstone & Thurstone, 1949). Measures of general intelligence were the Information, Block Design, and

Digit Symbol subtests of the WAIS-R (Wechsler, 1955). Visual perceptual-motor performance was assessed by the Benton Copy Test and Trail Making Form A. In the Benton Copy test, participants must copy a geometric figure; in the Trail Making Form A test, participants connect numerically ordered dots that result in a specific pattern (Armitage, 1946). Participants also received the WMS Mental Control test, which evaluates the ability to produce quickly a well-rehearsed letter or digit sequence, such as the alphabet, in a specified amount of time. Finally, participants also completed the Boston Naming Test (Goodglass & Kaplan, 1983), which reflects semantic/lexical retrieval processes in naming simple line drawings.

Materials

Twelve lists of 15 words each were chosen from those used by Stadler, Roediger, and McDermott (in press). Each of these lists was created by choosing the top associates of a critical word, which was itself not part of the list. Six of these lists were adapted for use as study lists, and the other six lists were used as the source for distractor words used in the recognition phase of the experiment (see Appendix for the lists used). To create the study lists used in this experiment, the three weakest associates to the critical word were dropped from each list, creating lists of 12 words. The reduction of list length was necessary to reduce the difficulty of the task, and is actually the same length that Roediger and McDermott (1995) used in their first experiment.

The recognition test was printed on a sheet of paper, and consisted of 48 words randomly ordered in 3 columns of 16. The same order was used for all participants. The words used were the critical word and 3 of the associate words for each of 12 lists. Six of these lists were the lists studied in the first phase of the experiment; the other six served only as a source of distractors.

Procedure

Participants were tested individually. For the study, and free recall phase of the experiment, participants were instructed that they were to listen as the experimenter read a list of words slowly (at approximately 2sec per word), and that they would be asked to recall the words out loud after the experimenter finished reading the list. In order to familiarise the participants with the procedure, they were first given a practice list of six related words, which were tested for immediate recall. The participants were told to recall as many items as possible from each list and they were told to take as much time as they wished to complete their recall. After each list was finished, the participant was given an immediate free recall test. This phase of the experiment was tape recorded.

For the recognition phase of the experiment, participants were given the test sheet and instructed to circle any words that they heard presented on one of the six lists. They were additionally instructed not to spend too much time on any individual word.

RESULTS

Recall Performance

Figure 1 displays the serial recall functions as a function of group. As shown, all groups produced the standard bow-shaped serial position function, and there are clear differences across groups in overall memory performance. Specifically, one finds a large decrease in performance both as a function of healthy ageing (young is greater than the young-old, which is greater than the old-old), and DAT (the healthy old is greater than the very mild DAT, which is greater than the mild DAT). The results of a 5 (Group) by 12 (Serial Position) ANOVA yielded main effects of Group [$F(4,154) = 62.15$, $MSe = 0.15$, $P < .0001$] and Serial Position [$F(11,1694) = 80.92$, $MSe = 3.03$, $P < .0001$]. In addition, there was a reliable Group by Serial Position interaction [$F(44,1694) = 2.01$, $MSe = 0.08$, $P < .01$], which indicated that there were larger Group differences at the middle serial positions, compared to either terminal or primacy positions. For example, the difference between healthy young and mild DAT groups is 60% at Serial Position 4, whereas at Serial Position 1 and

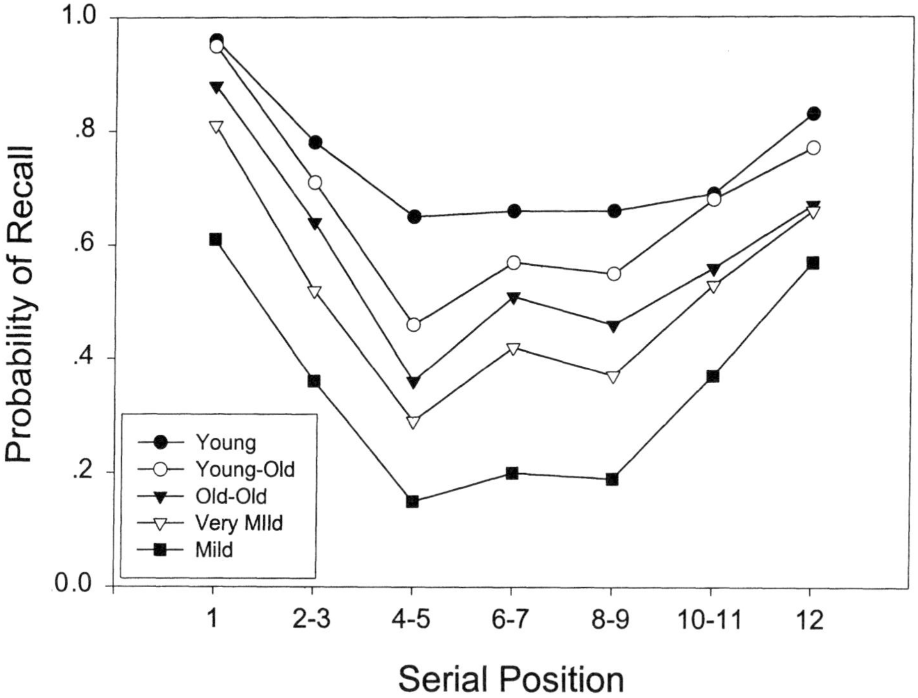

Fig. 1. *Mean proportion correct recall as a function of Serial Position and Group. The means of Serial Position 2 and 3, 4 and 5, 6 and 7, 8 and 9, 10 and 11 are presented.*

12 the differences are only 33% and 40% respectively. Of course, because of ceiling and floor effects at these serial positions, one must be cautious not to overinterpret this Group by Serial Position interaction. Overall, the results clearly indicate that the Serial Position function maintains its bowed-shape nature across groups, and there are the expected large Group differences in memory performance.

Figure 2 displays the mean proportion correct recall and the mean proportion critical intrusion rates. These results clearly indicate that there are large differences in the effects of Age and DAT on veridical recall and false recall. In order to address the influence of Age and DAT, we conducted separate ANOVAs as a function of Age and as a function of DAT. First, consider the effects of Age: There is a highly reliable drop of 26% correct in veridical recall from the healthy young adults to the old-old adults [$F(2,93) = 19.50$, $MSe = 0.011$, $P < .001$]. However, turning to the performance on the critical lure item, the results indicate that there is a small, and nonsignificant, 5% increase in recall across the groups [$F(2,93) = 1.27$, $MSe = 0.068$, $P = .29$]. There was a highly reliable interaction between Age Group and Item Type (veridical vs. critical false recall) [$F(2,93) = 6.18$, $P < .003$]. Turning to the DAT analyses, it should be noted that in this and subsequent analyses we collapsed across the young-old and the old-old groups of participants to create a single healthy older group to ensure that age was not confounded with DAT. As shown in Fig. 2, there is again a highly reliable 27% decrease in veridical recall across the healthy older group to the mild DAT group [$F(2,121) = 59.32$, $MSe = 0.014$, $P < .0001$]. However, there is only a nonsignificant 2% drop in the recall of the nonpresented critical word [$F(2,121) < 1.00$, $MSe = 0.072$]. Again, the interaction between Group and Item Type (veridical vs. critical false recall) was highly reliable [$F(2,121) = 9.71$, $MSe = 0.34$, $P < .001$]. In fact, if one considers the change across both age and DAT, one finds that

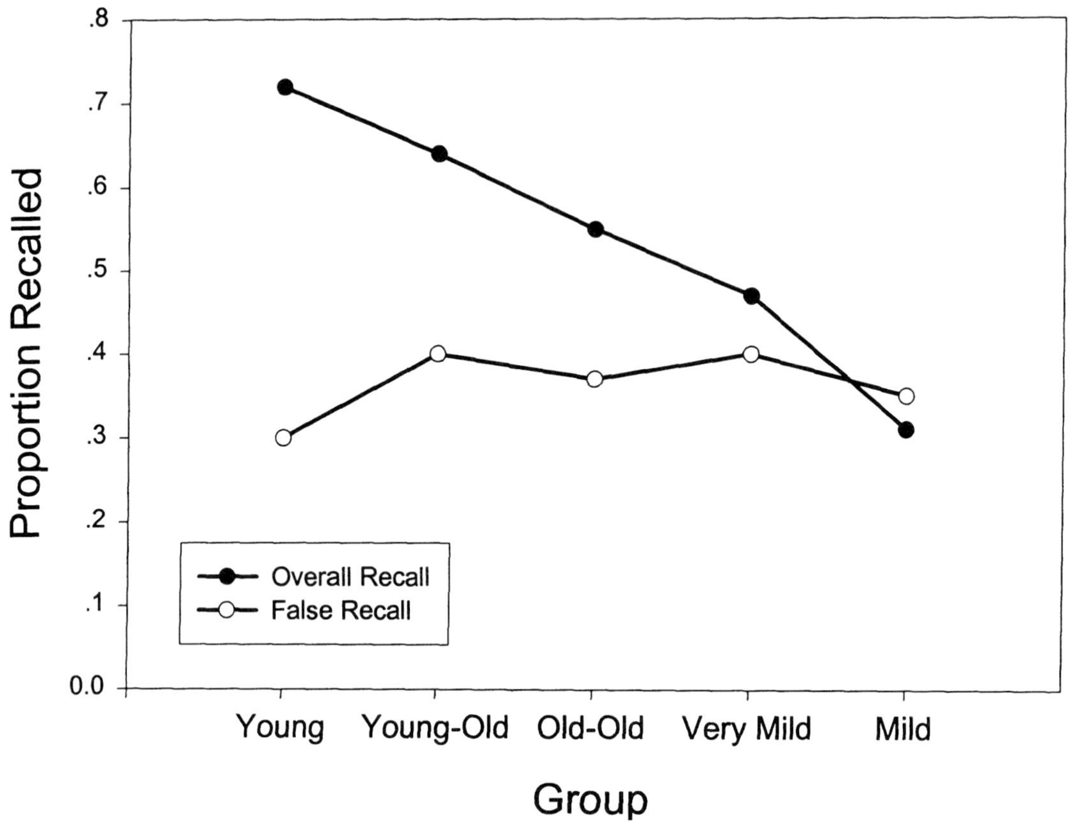

Fig. 2. *Mean proportion correct recall and mean proportion false critical recall as a function of Group.*

there is a 41% drop in veridical recall between the healthy young individuals and the mild DAT individuals [$F(4,154) = 62.15$, $MSe = 1.35$, $P < .0001$], and a nonsignificant 3% increase in recall of the nonpresented critical word [$F < 1.00$]. Of course, the interaction between Group and Item Type was highly reliable [$F(4,154) = 12.34$, $MSe = 0.48$, $P < .001$]. Clearly these results indicate that veridical recall changes dramatically across groups, whereas false recall is relatively stable.

In addition to examining critical word intrusions, we also considered intrusions of noncritical items. Because there are a number of distinct types of intrusions that may reflect different processes, we coded five different types of noncritical intrusions: (1) cross-list intrusions from previous lists; (2) cross-list critical lure intrusions (i.e. recalling a critical intrusion from a previous list); (3) semantically related, but noncritical intrusions; (4) phonologically related intrusions (most of which were rhymes); (5) "other," apparently unrelated, intrusions. The average number of intrusions per participant per list are displayed in Table 1. First, consider the cross-list intrusions. These reflect proactive interference from previous lists. The results indicate that both Age [$F(2,81) = 4.28$, $MSe = 0.047$, $P < .02$] and DAT [$F(2,116) = 11.04$, $MSe = 0.074$, $P < .0001$] affected susceptibility to proactive interference. Second, the cross-critical intrusions reflect the degree to which a highly activated critical item remained active across lists. Here there is little evidence of such intrusions in any group of participants. (Because of the low values, analyses were not conducted on this measure). The semantic intrusions reflected a semantically related word being produced on a given list. As shown in Table 1, there is an increase in semantically related intrusions as a function of Age [$F(2,81) = 5.24$,

Table 1. *Mean Number of Noncritical Intrusions per List as a Function of Group and Intrusion Type*

	Young	*Young Old*	*Old-Old*	*Very Mild*	*Mild*
Cross-list	.01	.04	.18	.21	.44
Cross-critical	.00	.00	.00	.00	.05
Semantic	.04	.15	.20	.18	.29
Phonological	.00	.00	.02	.03	.03
Other	.00	.01	.05	.08	.25
Total	.05	.20	.45	.50	1.06

*MS*e = 0.029, *P* < .01], but the effect of DAT did not reach significance [*F*(2,116) = 1.46, *MS*e = 0.087]. Also, as shown in Table 1, there were relatively few phonological intrusions in these data, which did not vary as a function of Age or DAT. (Again, because of the low values, analyses were not conducted.) Finally, the "other" intrusions reflected the output of relatively unrelated words. Although we could not conduct analyses as a function of Age because of the low levels in this category in the young adults, there was a reliable effect of DAT [*F*(2,116) = 7.75, *MS*e = 0.057, *P* < .002]. As shown here, the mild DAT individuals were likely to produce unrelated intrusions. However, further analyses of these items indicated that this was primarily produced by three participants, and when these three Mildly demented individuals were eliminated, the means were very similar across the two levels of DAT, i.e. 0.08 for the very mild DAT, and 0.11 for the mild DAT. In sum, there is clear evidence of a general tendency to produce noncritical intrusions as a function of Age and DAT status, but it is also clear that these errors are not random outputs of words, but reflected activated representations, either due to earlier list recall (proactive interference) or words that are semantically related to the current list.

One intriguing aspect of the recall data is that across groups, it appears that as overt recall decreases, the critical intrusions remain relatively stable. This is an interesting pattern because one might expect that as participants recall more items, there should be a higher incidence of critical lure intrusions. In order to address this issue, we investigated the correlation between overall recall per participant and their false recall. The correlations indicated that there was some evidence of such a relation in the healthy old-old group (*r* = .41, *P* < .05) and the very mild DAT group (*r* = .48, *P* < .01), but none of the remaining groups produced reliable correlations, i.e. young (*r* = − .20), young-old (− .06), mild DAT (+ .04). Most importantly, a correlation across all participants did not approach significance, *r* = .06. (It is worth noting here that Stadler, Roediger, & McDermott, in press, recently reported nonsignificant correlations between veridical recall and false recall across a large group of young adults and a larger set of lists.) Thus, above and beyond relatively limited correlations within specific groups, it does not appear that recalling items is a strong predictor of falsely recalling the critical nonpresented word.

We also tabulated the relative output position of both items correctly recalled and the critical intrusions. Because these analyses were based on tape recordings of the participants' verbal output, and some of the tapes were not audible (for 14 out of the 159 participants), these analyses were based on 26 young adults, 36 young-old adults, 22 old-old adults, 36 very mild DAT individuals, and 25 mild DAT individuals. There were two goals in this analysis: First, with respect to correct recall, it is possible that the present groups of participants may produce different retrieval strategies that might be reflected in the output positions. In order to address this possibility, we averaged the actual input position for each of the output positions. Of course, because there were large differences across groups, we could only do this analysis for the recall lengths of five, six, seven, and eight, in which there were sufficient number of observations per group. Moreover, to obtain stable estimates, we collapsed across the two healthy older groups and the two DAT groups. These data are displayed in Figs 3a (young), 3b (old), and 3c (DAT), as proportions of each input position that were produced in different output positions. There are three points to note from these data. First, the younger adults appear to be relatively more likely to recall the last item in the first position than the remaining two groups of participants. This pattern would be quite efficient if output of the last item would not disrupt the

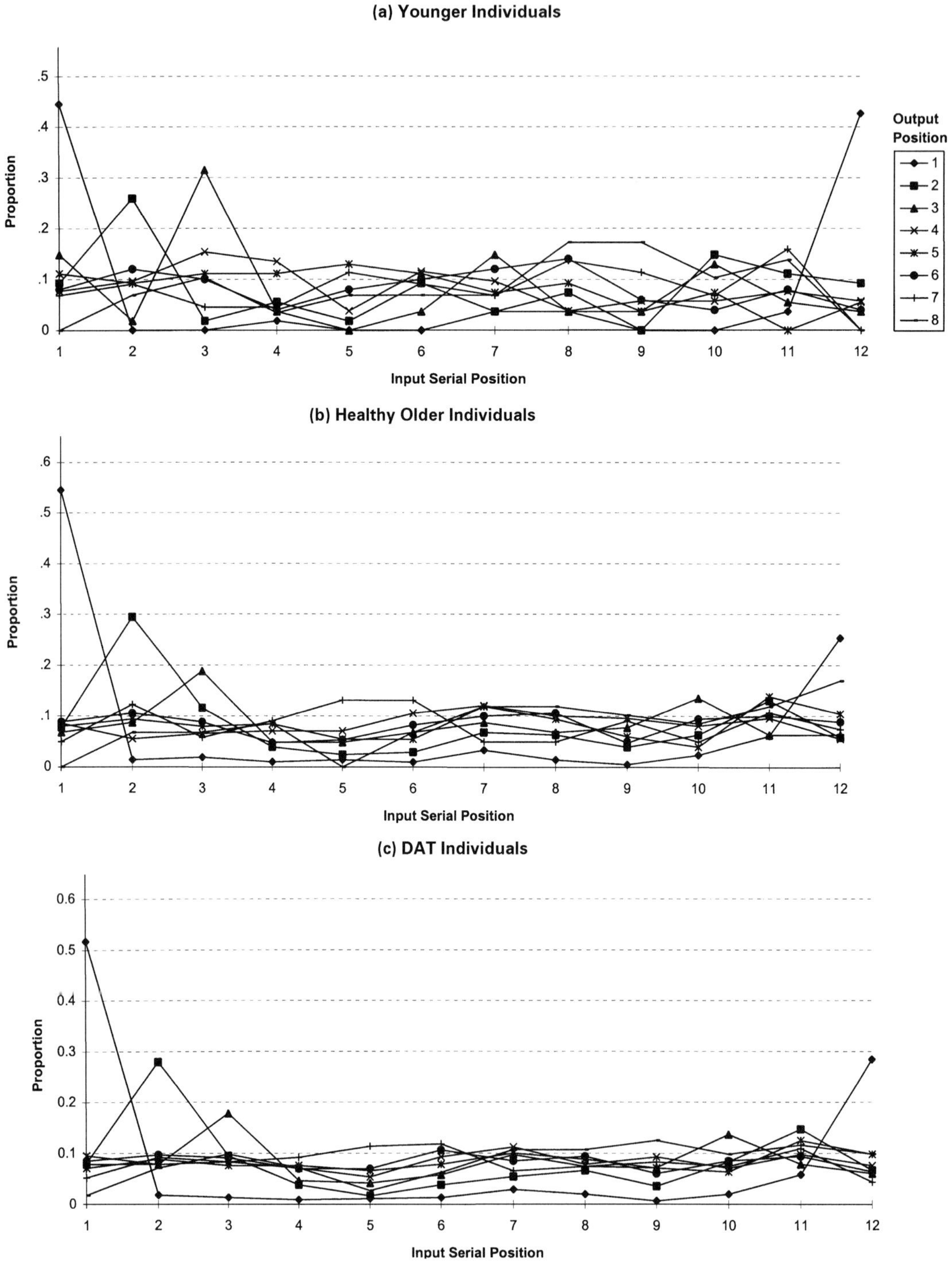

Fig. 3. *Mean proportion of each input position as a function of the output position during recall. These data are based on list recall lengths of 6, 7, and 8. The Healthy Old (Fig. 3b) is collapsed across Young-Old and Old-Old, and the DAT (Fig. 3c) is collapsed across Very Mild and Mild DAT.*

rehearsal pattern for the first few list positions, i.e. a type of memory triage. It appears that the healthy old and the DAT individuals are more likely to hold onto a rehearsal pattern that may not take advantage of the strong trace for the last presented item. In addition, as shown in Fig. 3a, one can see that for the young adults there is a consistent relation between the first three input serial positions producing high recall at the first three output positions. Turning to the healthy older adults and the DAT individuals, this pattern is only found for the first two serial positions, with a weaker effect for the third serial position being output at the third position. One possible account for this pattern is that the young adults have a three-item rehearsal set as opposed to a two-item rehearsal set in the healthy old and DAT individuals. Although the present analyses are only descriptive, it is intriguing that there are these different patterns of output when overall recall performance is equated across groups. We provide these data primarily because they provide a unique way to look at age-related and DAT-related changes in recall output and strategies.

In addition to analysing the output position of the list items as a function of input position, we also analysed the output position of the critical lure. Because there were different levels of recall for each group, we adjusted this estimate by dividing the output position of the critical nonpresented item by the total number of items recalled on that list. In this way, we provide an estimate of the relative output position of the critical lure. These proportions indicated that there was remarkable consistency in the relative output position for the critical nonpresented items. Specifically, the relative position as a function of total number of items recalled were .66 (young), .70 (young-old), .66 (old-old), .60 (very mild DAT), and .64 (mild DAT). A one-way ANOVA indicated that this effect did not approach significance [$F(4,116) = 1.36$, $MSE = 0.03$]. Thus, the *relative* output position of the critical nonpresented word was about two thirds into the recalled items, independent of group and number of items recalled. This pattern is consistent with the analyses reported by Roediger and McDermott (1995) concerning output position.

Recognition Performance

The mean percentage of hits, false alarms to noncritical items, and false alarms to critical items on the recognition test are presented in Table 2[1]. There are two points to note in this table. First, consider the effects of Age. There is relatively little change in hit rate [$F(2,93) = 0.73$, $MSe = 0.018$] and a small, yet reliable, change in the noncritical (standard) false alarm rate (4%) across Age groups [$F(2,93) = 5.33$, $MSe = 0.003$, $P < .01$]. This pattern is consistent with the observation that older adults have relatively intact recognition performance, at least compared to recall performance (see Craik & Jennings, 1994). However, a different pattern emerges from the false alarms to the critical lures. Specifically, there is a large *increase* in false alarms to the critical lures (.23) as a function of Age [$F(2,93) = 7.46$, $MSe = 0.076$, $P < .001$]. Now, consider the DAT individuals. There is dramatic .33 drop-off in hit rate in the mild DAT [$F(2,121) = 38.39$, $MSe = 0.026$, $P < .0001$], whereas the increase in the noncritical false alarm

Table 2. *Mean Proportion Hit Rate, Noncritical False Alarm Rate, and Critical Lure False Alarm Rate as a Function of Group*

	Young	*Young-Old*	*Old-Old*	*Very Mild*	*Mild*
Hits	.80	.76	.77	.68	.44
Noncritical false alarms	.02	.04	.06	.09	.14
Critical lure false alarms	.58	.80	.81	.79	.51

[1] In the present experiment, the recognition test always followed the recall test, and so this measure is somewhat contaminated by earlier recall performance. However, it should also be noted that the effect of recall on recognition is relatively inconsistent in the false memory literature (see Roediger, McDermott, & Robinson, 1998). This potential contamination is a bit more serious when there are large differences across groups in recall performance, as in the present study. Thus, one must be cautious not to overinterpret the present recognition data.

rate is relatively small (.09), albeit significant [$F(2,121) = 13.36$, $MSe = 0.006$, $P < .001$]. The lack of a large increase in false alarm rates for these participants is important because it appears that even mildly demented individuals are relatively *cautious* in making false alarms. Turning to performance on the critical lure, although the very mildly demented individuals are producing a high false alarm rate to this word, the false alarm rate decreases in the mildly demented individuals [$F(2,121) = 16.16$, $MSe = 0.055$, $P < .0001$]. However, it should be pointed out that the false alarm rate to the critical lure is quite high (.51) compared to the noncritical lures (.14), even in the mildly demented individuals.

Figure 4 displays a measure of recognition performance (hits minus noncritical false alarms) and an adjusted measure of critical false alarm performance (critical false alarms minus noncritical false alarms) as a function of Group. As shown in Fig. 4, there is a cross-over interaction in the healthy older adult groups; specifically, although accurate recognition performance remains relatively stable, false recognition of the critical lure increases across groups. Moreover, although both correct and false recognition measures decrease as a function of DAT, the difference between correct recognition and false recognition remain relatively stable across the groups. An analysis of the correct recognition measure yielded a marginally reliable main effect of Age [$F(2,93) = 2.71$, $MSe = 0.018$, $P < .07$] and a main effect of DAT [$F(2,121) = 62.56$, $MSe = 0.025$, $P < .0001$]. Turning to the critical false alarm measure, there is a main effect of Age [$F(2,93) = 5.84$, $MSe = 0.072$, $P < .01$], which indicates that there is an increase in false recognition in the older adults, and a main effect of DAT [$F(2,121) = 27.06$, $MSe = 0.052$, $P < .0001$], which indicates that there is a decrease in false recognition in the DAT individuals compared to the healthy older adults. Finally, there is a highly reliable interaction between Age and Item Type (veridical vs. false recognition [$F(2,93) = 9.71$, $MSe = 0.37$, $P < .0001$]. However, because the size

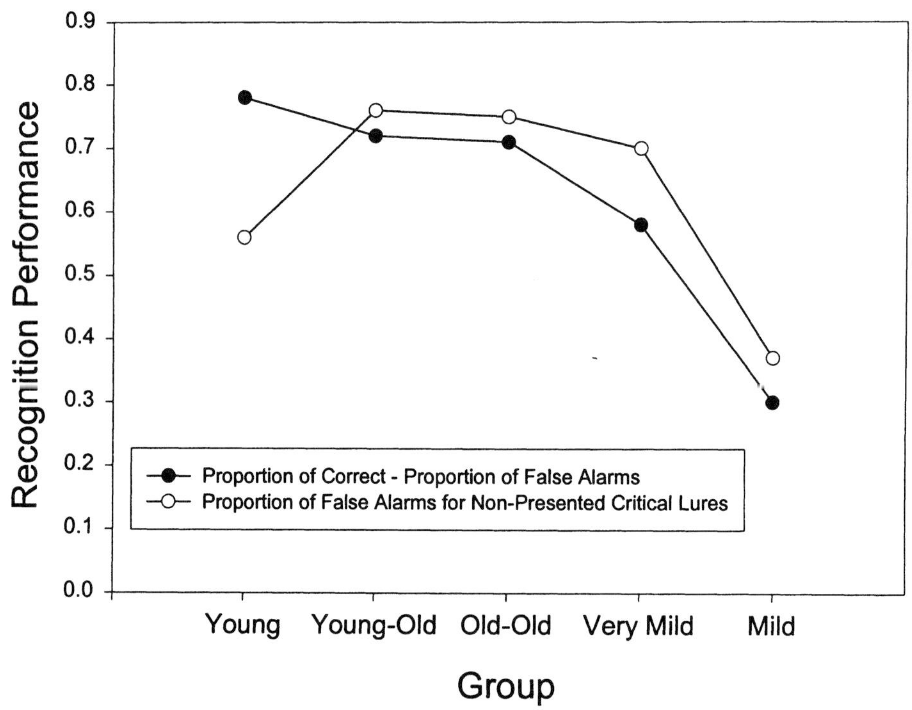

Fig. 4. *Mean recognition memory (hits minus noncritical false alarms) and false recognition (critical lures minus noncritical lures) as a function of Group.*

of the difference between veridical and false recognition did not change as a function of disease status, the interaction between DAT and Item Type did not reach significance [$F(2,121) = 1.65$, $MSe = 0.073$, $P = .20$].

Psychometric Performance

The means and standard deviations from the psychometric measures are presented in Table 3 as a function of Age and DAT. (The young adults did not receive psychometric testing.) A series of one-way ANOVAs with Group as a between-subjects factor indicated that performance on all measures decreased with increasing age and dementia severity, all $Ps < .003$. Thus, as expected, there are clear changes across groups across a wide range of cognitive measures.

The correlations between percentage correct and percentage false recall and the psychometric measures are presented in Table 4, as a function of Group. Also, as shown in this table, we have organised the psychometric tests as a function of differences in possible underlying neural systems (i.e. medial temporal, parietal, and frontal). As noted earlier, the selection of this particular grouping is based on recent work by Kanne et al. (1998). Because of the evidence suggesting a role of frontal structures in false recall, we expected that decreased frontal functioning would be associated with increased susceptibility to false recall, i.e. negative correlations. We also expected that medial temporal measures should be relatively more positively correlated with veridical recall, although there should be at least some correlations with the frontal measures. As shown in Table 4, these correlations did not support these predictions. Specifically, most psychometric measures were positively correlated with veridical recall, independent of the nature of the psychometric task. On the other hand, the pattern of correlations between the psychometric tests and false recall was much less consistent. The only groups that produced the predicted negative correlations were the healthy young-old participants and the mildly demented individuals. Unfortunately, both of these groups also produced some evidence of negative correlations with the medial temporal measures and false recall. Thus, there was relatively little support for the predicted correlations with the present psychometric tests[2].

Table 3. *Psychometric Means (SD) as a Function of Group*

	CDR 0 (Young-Old)	*CDR 0 (Old-Old)*	*CDR 0.5 (Very Mild DAT)*	*CDR 1 (Mild DAT)*
WAIS Information	23.8 (2.9)	20.6 (3.8)	17.6 (5.6)	12.0 (4.2)
Boston Naming	57.6 (3.0)	51.8 (8.7)	49.1 (11.8)	37.7 (12.6)
Logical Memory	10.3 (2.6)	8.2 (3.2)	6.2 (3.8)	2.6 (1.5)
Associate Memory	15.1 (3.5)	12.3 (3.7)	11.4 (3.8)	7.5 (1.8)
Benton Copy	9.8 (0.7)	9.4 (0.8)	9.1 (1.3)	8.2 (2.1)
Trailmaking A[a]	38.0 (11.6)	45.2 (11.8)	45.3 (23.4)	78.3 (32.2)
Block Design	35.3 (7.4)	29.0 (6.7)	24.1 (7.5)	16.2 (8.2)
Digit Symbol	50.6 (9.8)	38.0 (9.6)	39.7 (12.6)	23.3 (9.1)
Digit Span	12.1 (2.2)	11.1 (2.6)	10.5 (2.2)	9.4 (1.9)
Word Fluency	31.2 (11.2)	26.9 (10.3)	25.6 (12.2)	19.8 (9.0)
Mental Control	8.0 (1.3)	7.5 (1.8)	7.1 (1.9)	6.2 (2.1)

[a]Represents time in seconds.

[2] In addition to the correlations within groups displayed in Table 4, we also conducted overall correlations independent of group. Moreover, we also conducted correlations in which we converted each psychometric score to a z-score and then obtained a relative measure of each set of scores (i.e. mean of frontal, mean of medial temporal, and mean of parietal scores) divided by overall z-scores across all tasks. None of these individual correlations produced the predicted pattern of correlations between frontal measures and false recall.

Table 4. *Correlations between Percentage Correct and Percentage False Recall and Psychometric Measures by Group*

	CDR 0 (Young-Old)	*CR 0 (Old-Old)*	*CDR 0.5 (Very Mild DAT)*	*CDR 1 (Mild DAT)*
Percentage Correct Recall				
Medial Temporal				
WAIS Information	.12	.55*	.71	.31
Boston Naming	.14	.47*	.69*	.35
Logical Memory	.13	.60*	.68*	.69*
Associate Memory	.24	.75*	.50*	.51*
Parietal				
Benton Copy	.39*	.29	.23	−.02
Trailmaking A	−.15	−.50*	−.48*	.16
Block Design	.23	.62*	.44*	.18
Digit Symbol	.37*	.62*	.73*	.02
Frontal				
Digit Span	.27	.44*	.40*	.38
Word Fluency	.46*	.72*	.57*	.27
Mental Control	.11	.21	.50*	−.01
Percentage False Recall				
Medial Temporal				
WAIS Information	−.65	.32	.26	−.24
Boston Naming	−.42*	.25	.28	−.47*
Logical Memory	−.20	.08	.23	−.10
Associate Memory	−.15	.28	.15	.20
Parietal				
Benton Copy	.15	.49*	.17	−.23
Trailmaking A	.00	−.14	−.40*	.24
Block Design	.16	.48*	.28	−.36
Digit Symbol	.14	.53*	.38*	−.25
Frontal				
Digit Span	−.07	.08	.11	−.46*
Word Fluency	.04	.17	.60*	−.05
Mental Control	−.19	.21	.38*	−.20

*$P < .05$

GENERAL DISCUSSION

The results of the present experiment are clear. Both healthy ageing and DAT produced large changes in veridical recall performance. However, there was relatively little influence of either age or DAT on false recall performance. A similar pattern was found in recognition performance (although see Footnote 1). We shall now turn to a discussion of the implications of these results for the understanding of the memory changes that occur in both healthy older adults and in DAT individuals, and the mechanisms that may underlie false memories in the DRM paradigm.

Age Differences in False Memory Performance

The results from the young adults and the young-old adults nicely replicate the findings of Norman and Schacter (1997) and Tun et al. (1998) with the DRM materials. Moreover, the addition of the old-old adults extends this pattern to a group of individuals in their mid 80s. Specifically, in the present study, veridical recall decreased as a function of age, whereas false recall and recognition increased as a function of age (although the effect in recall was not reliable). The fact that this pattern has been replicated in three different laboratories clearly solidifies the robustness of this finding. Interestingly, even under conditions in which there is not a reliable increase in the false recall or recognition performance, if one considers false memory relative to the overall veridical memory, there is evidence of an age-related change in the *relative* presence of false memory performance in healthy older adults, compared to healthy young adults (see McEvoy & Nelson, 1998). It is important to note here that this pattern does not appear to be limited to the DRM materials, because older adults have shown increased susceptibility to memory distortions and illusions across a wide set of experimental paradigms (e.g. Bartlett, Strater, & Fulton, 1991; Cohen & Falkner, 1989; Dywan & Jacoby, 1990; Jacoby, this issue, in press; Kensinger & Schacter, this issue; Koutstaal & Schacter, 1997; Rankin & Kausler, 1979; Schacter, Israel, & Racine, 1999).

The more intriguing question regarding these data concerns the underlying mechanisms. There have been a number of such mechanisms recently proposed in the literature. For example, Norman and Schacter (1997) have suggested that, compared to younger adults, older adults might have less specific detail regarding perceptual characteristics of the list items. Hence, older adults may be more susceptible to confusing correctly recalled items with highly activated critical nonpresented items, thereby producing a type of source misattribution error (Johnson et al., 1993). Younger adults presumably have more perceptual information available to make the appropriate source attribution. This possibility is consistent with the work of Hashtroudi, Johnson, and Chrosniak (1990), who found that confusions in perceptual details appear to increase the likelihood of source errors in older adults, compared to younger adults. Tun et al. (1998) have suggested that there is an age-related increase in gist-based processing. Specifically, as individuals age, and the item-specific information decreases, there is an increased reliance on other sources, such as overall gist. Because the critical items in the DRM materials are highly activated by gist-based information, this would clearly produce the observed pattern. This view is also consistent with the work by Reder, Wible, and Martin (1986), who argued that older adults are more likely to rely on "plausibility" in making their judgements regarding previously presented sentences, whereas younger adults were more likely to recall item-specific information. Reder et al. suggested that this may be due to differences in attentional resources across groups, i.e. older adults have fewer resources, and it is less demanding to retrieve plausibility information than item-specific-information. Similarly, Rabinowitz, Craik, and Ackerman (1982) have noted that older adults are more likely to encode generic information than younger adults. All of these theoretical perspectives suggest that older adults are more likely to rely on overall list relations than on item-specific information.

Why might older adults rely more heavily on relations across items than on deindividuating information for specifically encoded items? We have suggested that this pattern may not simply be a reflection of memory specific changes in older adults, but rather may be reflective of attentional control changes. Specifically, with the DRM materials, the participant needs to discriminate between two types of information: (a) highly activated semantic convergence on a given nonpresented representation and (b) activated item-specific information due to initial encoding. As shown in Fig. 5, one could envisage these two sources competing for correct output during an episodic memory task. An efficient attentional control system needs to be able to discriminate between these two sources of information, i.e. accentuating (as indicated by the plus sign) the item-specific recollection, and inhibiting (as indicated via the minus sign) the pathway that produces high availability due to the spreading activation across items that converge on critical nonpresented words. In this light, there appears to be an analogy to the Stroop task, wherein the participant must select between a strong word processing pathway and a weaker, but task-relevant, colour naming pathway. One might argue that the critical nonpresented item is like the word pathway in Stroop, wherein the participant must control the tendency to respond with the highly activated representation. As noted earlier, there is clear evidence that there are age-related effects in both the Stroop task, along with other non-memory tasks such as in

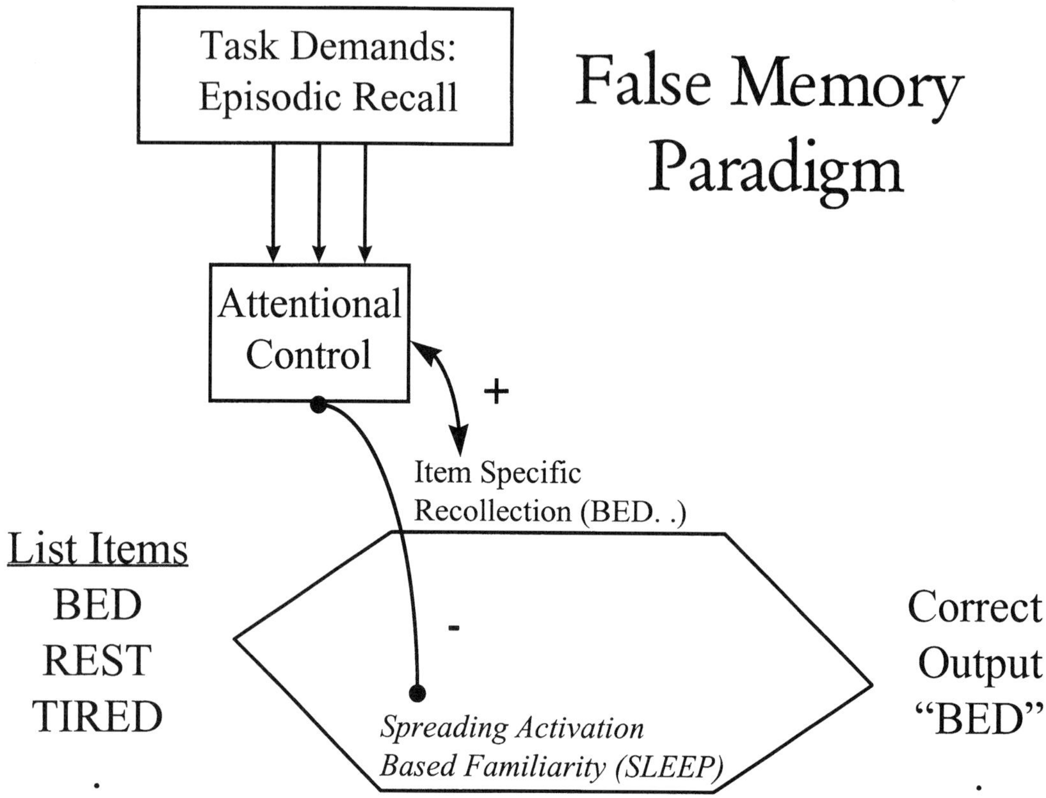

Fig. 5. *An attentional control framework for interpreting performance in the DRM recall paradigm. Deficits as a function of Age and DAT might be expected in the attentional control module.*

picture word interference paradigms (e.g. Duchek, Balota, Faust, & Ferraro, 1995), and the speeded naming of low-frequency exception words (e.g. Balota & Ferraro, 1993). Before further discussion of this framework, we shall turn to a discussion of the results from Alzheimer's Disease individuals.

Veridical and False Recall in DAT

The results from the DAT individuals appear to be in large part an extension of the changes we find in healthy older adults. Specifically, veridical recall continued to decrease across levels of dementia; however, the false recall remained relatively stable (see Fig. 2). Turning to the recognition data (see Fig. 4) there is a similar pattern, with the exception of the mildly demented individuals, in whom there is a decrease in both veridical recognition and false recognition. However, it is important to note that both the very mild and the mildly demented individuals produced a higher probability of false recognition than of correct recognition. Overall, these results indicate that relative to veridical memory, the DAT individuals are even more susceptible to false memories than are healthy older adults.

The DAT individuals not only falsely recalled the critical nonpresented items at disproportionately high levels relative to their overall recall performance but, as shown in Table 1, they were also more likely to produce cross-list intrusions (reflecting an increased susceptibility to proactive interference) and semantically related intrusions. Hence, one must entertain the possibility that the increase in false memories in the DAT individuals simply reflects a criterion shift in these participants. However, if this were the case, then one might expect a relatively high false alarm rate on the recognition test. Interestingly, however, both the very mild and mild DAT individuals produced relatively low false alarm rates to noncritical lures, .09 and .14 respectively. Thus, at least in the recognition test, the DAT individuals were resistant to respond "yes" to a lure stimulus. Of course, this cautiousness in responding primarily applies to the noncritical lures, because the critical lures produced a false alarm rate o f .51[3]. Thus, although there is an overall increase in cross-list intrusions and semantically related intrusions, we believe these errors reflect relatively high activation for competing sources that need to be controlled via attentional systems. In this light, we do not believe that the present results are simply a reflection of a criterion shift in the DAT individuals.

As in the healthy older adults, there is also evidence that DAT individuals produce breakdowns in attentional control processes that, as suggested earlier (and in Fig. 5), may lead to a relative increase in false recall. For example, DAT individuals are more likely to produce failures to resist highly activated, but competing, representations. The Stroop task again nicely documents this problem. Specifically, DAT individuals are more likely to produce the incongruent word responses under colour naming instructions, compared to healthy age-matched controls (Spieler et al., 1996). Thus, if there is a further breakdown in the attentional control system that controls highly activated pathways in DAT individuals, then (based on the framework displayed in Fig. 5), one might expect a further increase in false memories in these participants. Of course, this assumes that there is intact spreading activation for the critical nonpresented item. As noted earlier, the evidence from the semantic priming literature indicates that the automatic activation process is relatively intact in both healthy ageing and in early stage DAT individuals (Balota & Duchek, 1991; Duchek & Balota, 1993; Nebes, 1989; Shenaut & Ober, 1996). Thus, there should be activation for the critical nonpresented item that competes for output against contextualised item-specific information[4].

Although we have been discussing the present healthy ageing and DAT results within the attentional control framework displayed in Fig. 5, there is an important alternative account that must be discussed. Specifically, it is possible that one does not need to invoke changes in attentional control systems, but rather that these results simply reflect an imbalance in the strength of the two sources of information. There is already considerable extant literature that both healthy older adults and to a greater extent DAT individuals produce large decrements in episodic memory performance. This, of course, was also reflected in the present recall performance. Within the framework displayed in Fig. 5, this would be viewed as suggesting that the item-specific recollection pathway is impaired in these groups of participants. Also, as noted, there is considerable evidence that the automatic spreading activation is relatively intact in both healthy older adults and in early stage DAT. Thus, the spreading activation-based pathway in Fig. 5 should be relatively intact. The present results do not demand a change in attentional control systems, but rather may simply reflect changes in the balance of the strength of the two underlying

[3] It is also worth noting here that if one adjusts the false recall data by the overall intrusion rate, then one would also need to adjust the veridical recall for the intrusion rate, because a simple shift in output criterion is likely to reflect both correct recall and false recall. Of course, if one makes the same adjustment for both false recall and veridical recall, then this will not have any effect on the important observation in Fig. 2 that veridical and false recall change in a dramatically different manner across groups.

[4] It is worth noting that the present discussion focuses on group-related changes in attentional control processes at retrieval in producing the relative increase in false memories across groups. However, it is important to note that these group-related differences in attention would also change the nature of the encoded traces across groups. In fact, one might expect decreased semantic elaborative encoding across the participant groups due to changes in attentional control systems at encoding across the participant groups. Interestingly, there is evidence that deeper, more elaborative encoding processes actually increase rather than decrease false recall (Thaper, McDermott, & Fong, 1998; Toglia, Neuschatz, & Goodwin, 1999). Because the older adults and DAT individuals may be expected to engage in less elaborative processing, the present results might actually *underestimate* the relative increase in false memories to veridical memories in these groups.

processing pathways, i.e. the item-specific recollection pathway decreases in strength across groups, whereas, the spreading activation-based pathway remains relatively stable across groups. Therefore, because of the potential competition between the two pathways, memory performance is more driven by the spreading activation-based pathway, as the recollection-based pathway decreases as a function of both healthy ageing and DAT.

In order to address this alternative account of the present results, and also to shed some light on past false memory studies, we attempted to equate the strength of the recollection-based pathway across our participants. Thus, we attempted to match participants on both mean performance (and range) across groups on their veridical recall. If indeed there is an attentional control problem in controlling the spreading activation-based pathway as a function of age and DAT, then one should find a relative increase in false recall performance across groups of participants who are matched on veridical recall. These data are shown in Fig. 6, and clearly support this prediction. Specifically, if one equates veridical recall across groups by matching participants, the false recall performance actually increases for these same participants. This increase in false recall was reliable in the comparison of the healthy young vs. old [$t(59) = 2.27$, $P < .05$]; however, because of the decreased power (due to selective matching) this comparison did not reach significance in the comparison of the healthy old vs. very mild DAT or in the comparison of the very mild vs. mild DAT individuals. However, when one includes these later two comparisons in an overall ANOVA (with no participant represented twice in the analyses), there is a marginally reliable increase [$F(1,78) = 3.61$, $P < .06$]. In addition to these analyses, and in order to avoid the problem with differential subject selection, we also conducted a regression analysis in which we predicted false recall after veridical recall was partialled out. This analysis indicated that participant group reliably predicted false recall after we had partialled out the variance due to veridical recall [$t(156) = 2.23$, $P < .05$]. Thus, these results indicate that the increased susceptibility to false recall is not simply a reflection of a decrease in the item-specific recollection-based pathway, because there is an overall increase in false recall even when participants were equated on veridical recall. Rather, these results are more consistent with the notion that there is a change across groups in attentional control of relevant processing pathways.

Potential Neurological Underpinnings for False Memories

What might be the neural underpinnings for the breakdowns in attentional control systems in healthy older adults and in early stage DAT individuals? There has been some suggestion in the literature that older adults have more difficulty in tasks that reflect frontal functioning rather than medial temporal or parietal functioning (e.g. Craik, Morris, Morris, & Loewen, 1990; Moscovitch & Winocur, 1995; Shimamura & Jurica, 1994). There is also evidence that there is an increased influence of age on volumetric measures of frontal areas of the brain (e.g. West, 1996, for a review), and recent neuropathological studies of DAT (Morris et al., 1996) indicate a relatively high presence of plaques in frontal areas. As reviewed in the Introduction, false recognition and confabulation effects have been shown to increase in individuals with frontal damage (e.g. Schacter et al., 1996a). In addition, tasks that involve selection from a number of activated pathways, such as the Stroop and Wisconsin Card Sorting tasks, appear to load more on frontal systems (e.g. Dempster, 1992). All of these observations converge on the notion that breakdowns in frontal systems may be related to the observed relative increase in false memories. Although this account is clearly tempting, an analysis of the selected psychometric tests did not provide much support for this prediction. Specifically, although medial temporal measures were nicely correlated with veridical recall, there was relatively little correlation between the frontal measures and false recall. Unfortunately, as discussed earlier, the false recall measures were relatively uncorrelated with most measures of either memory or attention. Of course, it is quite possible that the selected set of psychometric tasks to measure frontal functioning (which were limited in scope due to the longitudinal

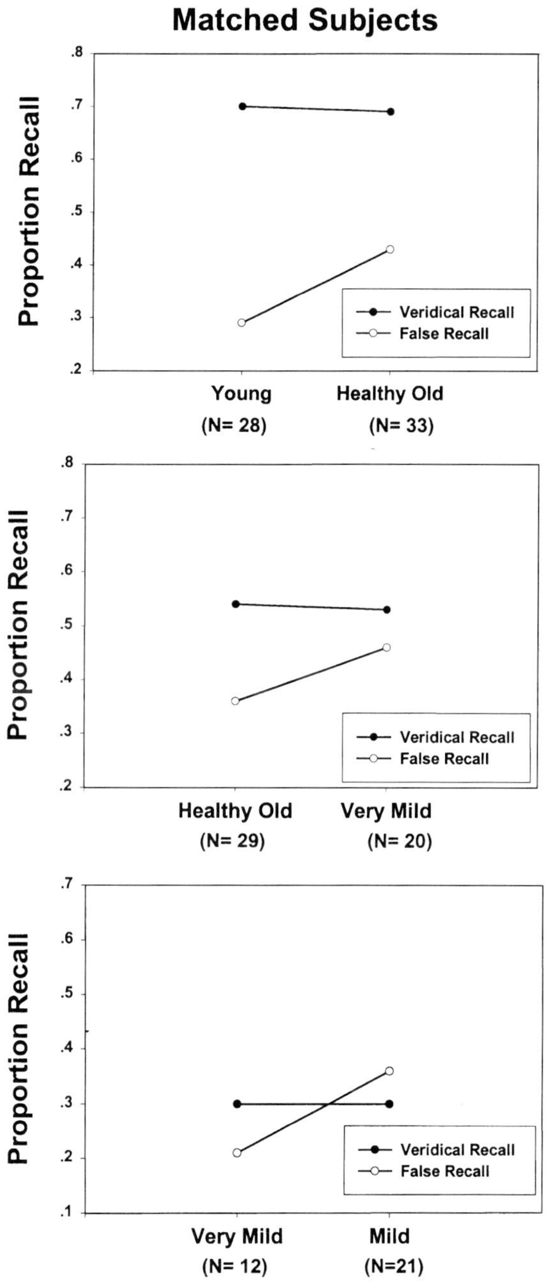

Fig. 6. *Matched subjects as a function of Age (top panel), Age and Very Mild DAT (middle panel), and Very Mild and Mild DAT (bottom panel). The number of participants in each group are in parentheses.*

studies in which these subjects are participating) did not capture the critical operations, which still could be mediated by frontal systems. Thus, it would be quite useful to use the psychometric tasks that Glisky, Polster, and Routhieaux (1995) have recently used to determine if one could predict false recall performance in the DRM paradigm via frontal functioning as evidenced from a more targeted neuropsychological battery. In this light, it should be noted that Henkel, Johnson, and De Leonardis (1998) recently provided evidence that false memories were predicted by both frontal and medial temporal psychometric measures. Clearly further work is needed to examine the contribution of frontal systems in the production of false memories in the DRM paradigm across healthy ageing and DAT.

Implications of the Present Results for Understanding the Mechanisms Underlying False Recall and Recognition

The present results not only have implications for understanding age-related and dementia-related changes in memory performance, but these results also have implications for understanding the mechanisms that might underlie false memories in the DRM paradigm. Following Deese (1959) and Roediger and McDermott (1995), we have suggested that false memories may reflect a type of automatic implicit association that occurs during list presentation. The underlying mechanism for this might be a spread of activation within a semantic network, which converges on a nonpresented critical representation. This activation is likely to summate across the related words until some critical threshold is reached. In fact, Balota and Paul (1996) have demonstrated that automatic semantic priming effects are additive across multiple related words in both lexical decision and naming tasks. Recent work by Robinson (1998) and Seamon et al. (1998) has indicated that conscious processing of the list words is not a necessary condition for producing false memories. For example, Robinson found evidence for robust false recall and recognition under presentation conditions that greatly minimised conscious processing (50msec per word with a backward masking stimulus). Under these conditions, participants were not consciously generating the nonpresented items at encoding and so this does not appear to be the primary locus of the false memories. Finally, it is noteworthy that Stadler, McDermott, Roediger, Miller, and Cowan (1999) have recently found that divided attention tasks disrupt veridical recall more than false recall. These studies all appear to converge on the notion that the conscious generation of the critical nonpresented item during list presentation is not a necessary condition to produce false recall.

What are the implications of the present results for the notion that retrieval is the locus of false recall? One might argue that in the process of generating words at retrieval, the participant actually generates the critical item because of the previously generated related words. Once the critical item is generated, it is likely to be output because of the high activation due to the convergence of the semantic associates. However, the present results also produce some constraints on this interpretation. That is, one of the most striking aspects of the present data is that although veridical recall decreases by nearly 50% across the present groups of participants, false recall is invariant across these same groups. This is important because it suggests that the overt act of recalling associates does not produce the false recalls.

CONCLUSIONS

The present results clearly indicate that the relative incidence of false memories to veridical memories increases as a function of both age and DAT. We have argued that part of this effect may be due to breakdowns in attentional control systems that select among activated pathways due to spreading activation and item-specific information due to memory encoding. Clearly, this pattern of results can be informative regarding age-related and DAT-related changes in memory performance and also can provide insight to basic memory mechanisms that produce false memories in healthy young adults. Of course, one might also ask whether there may be ways of increasing the functioning of the attentional control system in both healthy older adults and in DAT individuals. For example, Multhaup (1995) has shown that older adults are less likely to fall prey to illusions of fame when provided with a more exhaustive set of response alternatives at retrieval. It is also possible that older adults may benefit more than younger adults if there is a warning signal that indicates the presence of such highly related distractors, or possibly if they are given more time during the retrieval task. Given the potential negative consequences of false memories, it is important not only to understand this phenomenon but also consider how to limit it in populations that appear to be particularly susceptible (see Schacter et al., 1998, for further discussion of these issues).

REFERENCES

Albert, M.S., Heller, H.S., & Milberg, W. (1988). Changes in naming ability with age. *Psychology and Aging, 3,* 173–178.

Armitage, S.G. (1946). An analysis of certain psychological tests used for the evaluation of the brain injury. *Psychology Monographs, 60,* (Whole No. 277).

Balota, D.A., Black, S., & Cheney, M. (1992). Automatic and attentional processes in young and old adults: A re-evaluation of the two-process model of semantic priming. *Journal of Experimental Psychology: Human Perception and Performance, 18,* 485–502.

Balota, D.A., & Duchek, J.M. (1991). Semantic priming effects, lexical repetition effects, and contextual disambiguation effects in healthy aged individuals and individuals with senile dementia of the Alzheimer's type. *Brain and Language, 40,* 181–201.

Balota, D.A., & Ferraro, F.R. (1993). A dissociation of frequency and regularity effects in pronunciation performance across young adults, older adults, and individuals with senile dementia of the Alzheimer type. *Journal of Memory and Language, 32,* 573–592.

Balota, D.A., & Paul, S.T. (1996). Summation of activation: Evidence from multiple primes that converge and diverge within semantic memory. *Journal of Experimental Psychology: Learning, Memory, and Cognition, 22,* 336–345.

Balota, D.A., Watson, J.M., Duchek, J.M., & Ferraro, R.F. (in press). Cross-modal priming with ambiguous and unambiguous words in young, healthy older adults, and in individuals with Dementia of the Alzheimer's Type: Explorations of semantic memory. *Journal of International Neuropsychological Society.*

Bartlett, J.C., Strater, L., & Fulton, A. (1991). False recency and false fame of faces in young adulthood and old age. *Memory and Cognition, 19,* 177–188.

Berg, L., McKeel, D.W. Jr., Miller, J.P., Storandt, M., Rubin, E.H., Morris, J.C., Baty, J., Coats, M., Norton, J., Goate, A.M., Price, J.L., Gearing, M., Mirra, S.S., & Saunders, A.M. (1998). Clinicopathologic studies in cognitively healthy aging and Alzheimer's disease: Relation of histologic markers to dementia severity. *Archives of Neurology, 55,* 326–335.

Brainerd, C.J., Reyna, V.F., & Kneer, R. (1995). False-recognition reversal: When similarity is distinctive. *Journal of Memory and Language, 34,* 157–185.

Cohen, G., & Faulkner, D. (1986). Memory for proper names: Age differences in retrieval. *British Journal of Developmental Psychology, 4,* 187–197.

Craik, F.I.M., & Jennings, J.M. (1992). Human memory. In F.I.M. Craik & T.A. Salthouse (Eds.), *Handbook of aging and cognition* (pp. 451–110). Hillsdale, NJ: Lawrence Erlbaum Associates Inc.

Craik, F.I.M., Morris, L.W., Morris, R.G., & Loewen, E.R. (1990). Relations between source amnesia and frontal lobe functioning in older adults. *Psychology and Aging, 5,* 148–151.

Deese, J. (1959). On the prediction of occurrence of particular verbal intrusions in immediate recall. *Journal of Experimental Psychology, 58,* 17–22.

Dempster, F.N. (1992). The rise and fall of the inhibitory mechanism: Toward a unified theory of cognitive development and aging. *Developmental Review, 12,* 45–75.

Duchek, J.M., & Balota, D.A. (1993). Sparing of activation processes in older adults. In J. Cerella & W. Hoyer (Eds.), *Adult information processing: Limits on loss* (pp. 383–406).

Duchek, J.M., Balota, D.A., Faust, M.E., & Ferraro, F.R. (1995). Inhibitory processes in young and older adults in a picture-word task. *Aging and Concern, 2,* 156–167.

Duchek, J.M., Balota, D.A., & Thessing, V.C. (in press). Inhibition of visual and conceptual information during reading in healthy aging and Alzheimer's disease. *Neuropsychology, Aging, and Cognition.*

Dywan, J., & Jacoby, L.L. (1990). Effects of aging on source monitoring: Differences in susceptibility to false fame. *Psychology and Aging, 5, 379*–387.

Faust, M.E., Balota, D.A., Duchek, J.M., Gernsbacher, M.A., & Smith, S. (1997). Inhibitory control during sentence comprehension in individuals with Dementia of the Alzheimer Type. *Brain and Language, 57,* 225–253.

Glisky, E.L., Polster, M.R., & Routhieaux, B.C. (1995). Double dissociation between item and source memory. *Psychology and Aging, 9,* 229–235.

Goodglass, H., & Kaplan, E. (1983). *Boston Naming Test.* Philadelphia, PA: Lea & Febiger.

Hasher, L., & Zacks, R.T. (1988). Working memory, comprehension, and aging: A review and a new view. In G.H. Bower (Ed.), *The psychology of learning and motivation* (pp. 193–225). San Diego, CA: Academic Press.

Hashtroudi, S., Johnson, M.K., & Chrosniak, L.D. (1990). Aging and qualitative characteristics of memories for perceived and imagined complex events. *Psychology and Aging, 5,* 119–126.

Henkel, L.A., Johnson, M.K., & De Leonardis, D.M. (1998). Aging and source monitoring: Cognitive processes and neuropsychological correlates. *Journal of Experimental Psychology: General, 127,* 251–269.

Jacoby, L.L. (this issue). Deceiving the elderly: Effects of accessibility bias in cued recall performance. *Cognitive Neuropsychology, 16,* 417–436.

Jacoby, L.L. (in press). Ironic effects of repetition: Measuring age-related differences in memory. *Journal of Experimental Psychology, Learning, Memory and Cognition.*

Johnson, M.K., Hashtroudi, S., & Lindsay, D.S. (1993). Source monitoring. *Psychological Bulletin, 114,* 3–28.

Kanne, S.M., Balota, D.A., Storandt, M., McKeel, D.W., & Morris, J.C. (1998). Relating anatomy to function in Alzheimer's disease: Neuropsychological profiles predict regional neuropathology five years later. *Neurology, 5,* 979–985.

Kensinger, E.A., & Schacter, D.L. (this issue). When true memories suppress false memories: Effects of aging. *Cognitive Neuropsychology, 16,* 399–415.

Kirshner, H.S., Webb, W.G., & Kelly, M.P. (1984). The naming disorder of dementia. *Neuropsychologia, 22,* 23–30.

Koutstaal, W., & Schacter, D.L. (1997). Gist-based false recognition of pictures in older and younger adults. *Journal of Memory and Language, 37,* 555–583.

McDermott, K.B. (1997). Priming on perceptual implicit memory tests can be achieved through presentation of associates. *Psychonomic Bulletin and Review, 4,* 582–586.

McEvoy, C.L., & Nelson, D.L. (1998). *False memories in young and older adults: The view from an associative model of memory.* Paper presented at the 1998 Cognitive Aging Conference, Atlanta, Georgia.

McKhann, G., Drachman, D., Folstein, M., Katzman, R., Price, D., & Stadlan, E.M. (1984). Clinical diagnosis of Alzheimer's disease: Report of the NINCDS-ADRDA work group under the auspices of the Department of Health and Human Services Task Force on Alzheimer's disease. *Neurology, 34,* 934–939.

Morris, J.C., Storandt, M., McKeel, D.W. Jr, Rubin, E.H., Price, J.L., Grant, E.A., & Berg, L. (1996). Cerebral amyloid deposition and diffuse plaques in "normal" aging: Evidence for presymptomatic and very mild Alzheimer's Disease. *Neurology, 46,* 707–719.

Moscovitch, M., & Winocur, G. (1995). Frontal lobes, memory, and aging. In J. Grafman, K.J. Holyoak, & F. Boller (Eds.), *Structure and functions of the human prefrontal cortex* (Annals of the New York Academy of Sciences, Vol. 769, pp. 119–150). New York: New York Academy of Sciences.

Multhaup, K.S. (1995). Aging, source, and decision criteria: When false fame errors do and do not occur. *Psychology and Aging, 10,* 492–497.

Multhaup, K.S., & Balota, D.A. (1997). Generation effects and source memory in healthy older adults and individuals with dementia of the Alzheimer type. *Neuropsychology, 11,* 382–391,

Nebes, R.D. (1989). Semantic memory in Alzheimer's disease. *Psychological Bulletin, 106,* 377–394.

Nebes, R.D. (1994). Cognitive dysfunction in Alzheimer's disease. In F.I.M. Craik & T.A. Salthouse (Eds.), *The handbook of aging and cognition* (pp. 373–446). Hillsdale, NJ: Lawrence Erlbaum Associates Inc.

Norman, K.A., & Schacter, D.L. (1997). False recognition in younger and older adults. Exploring the characteristics of illusory memories. *Memory and Cognition, 25,* 838–848.

Ober, B.A., Dronkers, N.F., Koss, E., Delis, D.C., & Friedland, R.P. (1986). Retrieval from semantic memory in Alzheimer-type dementia. *Journal of Clinical and Experimental Neuropsychology, 8, 75–92.*

Ober, B.A., & Shenaut, G.K. (1995). Semantic priming in Alzheimer's disease. Meta-analysis and theoretical evaluation. In P.A. Allen & T.R. Bashore (Eds.), *Age difference in word and language processing* (pp. 247–271). Amsterdam: Elsevier.

Rabinowitz, J.C., Craik, F.I.M., & Ackerman, B.P. (1982). A processing resource account of age differences in recall. *Canadian Journal of Psychology, 36,* 325–344.

Rankin, J.S., & Kausler, D.H. (1979). Adult age differences in false recognition. *Journal of Gerontology, 34,* 58–65.

Reder, L.M., Wible, C., & Martin, J. (1986). Different memory changes with age: Exact retrieval versus plausible inference. *Journal of Experimental Psychology: Learning, Memory, and Cognition, 12,* 72–81.

Robinson, K.J. (1998). *The automatic mechanisms of false memory.* Unpublished Masters thesis.

Roediger, H.L., & McDermott, K.B. (1995). Creating false memories: Remembering words not presented in list. *Journal of Experimental Psychology: Learning, Memory, and Cognition, 21,* 803–814.

Schacter, D.L., Curran, T., Galliccio, L., Milberg, W.P., & Bates, J.F. (1996a). False recognition and the right frontal lobe. *Neuropsychologia, 34,* 793–808.

Schacter, D.L., Israel, L., & Racine, C. (1999). Suppressing false recognition in younger and older adults: The distinctive heuristic. *Journal of Memory and Language, 40,* 1–24.

Schacter, D.L., Reiman, E., Curran, T., Yun, L.S., Bandy, D., McDermott, K.B., & Roediger, H.L. III (1996b). Neuroanatomical correlates of veridical and illusory recognition memory revealed by PET. *Neuron, 17,* 267–274.

Schacter, D.L., Verfaeillie, M., & Pradere, D. (1996c). The neuropsychology of memory illusions: False recall and recognition in amnesic patients. *Journal of Memory and Language, 35,* 319–334.

Seamon, J.G., Luo, C.R., & Gallo, D.A. (1998). Creating false memories of words with or without recognition of list items: Evidence for nonconscious processes. *Psychological Science, 9,* 20–26.

Shenaut, G.K., & Ober, B.A. (1996). Methodological control of semantic priming in Alzheimer's disease. *Psychology and Aging, 11,* 443–448.

Shimamura, A.P., & Jurica, P.J. (1994). Memory interference effects and aging: Findings from a test of frontal lobe function. *Neuropsychology, 8,* 408–412.

Spieler, D.H., Balota, D.A., & Faust, M.E. (1996). Stroop performance in younger adults, healthy older adults and individuals with senile dementia of the Alzheimer's type. *Journal of Experimental Psychology: Human Perception and Performance, 22,* 461–479.

Stadler, M.A., McDermott, K.B., Roediger, H.L., Miller, E.C., & Cowan, N. (1999). *Effects of attention on false recognition.* Unpublished data.

Stadler, M.A., Roediger, H.L., & McDermott, K.B. (in press). Normed materials for creating false memories: Remembering words not presented in lists. *Memory and Cognition.*

Sullivan, M.P., Faust, M.E., & Balota, D.A. (1995). Identity negative priming in older adults and individuals with dementia of the Alzheimer type. *Neuropsychology, 9,* 537–555.

Thapar, A., McDermott, K.B., & Fong, C.T. (1997). *Effects of level of processing and retention interval on false recall.* Poster presented at the 38th Psychonomics Society Conference in Philadelphia, PA.

Thurstone, L.E., & Thurstone, T.G. (1949). *Examiner manual for the SRT Primary Mental Abilities.* Chicago, IL: Science Research Associates.

Toglia, M.P., Neuschatz, J.S., & Goodwin, K.A. (1999). Recall accuracy and illusory memories: When more is less. *Memory, 7,* 233–256.

Troster, A.I., Salmon, D.P., McCullough, D., & Butters, N. (1989). A comparison of category fluency deficits associated with Alzheimer's and Huntington's disease. *Brain and Language, 37,* 500–513.

Tun, P.A., Wingfield, A., Rosen, M.J., & Blanchard, L. (1998). Response latencies for false memories: Gist-based processes in normal aging. *Psychology and Aging, 13,* 230–241.

Wechsler, D. (1955). *WAIS Manual.* New York: Psychological Corporation.

Wechsler, D., & Stone, C.P. (1973). *Manual: Wechsler Memory Scale,* New York: Psychological Corporation.

West, R.L. (1996). An application of prefrontal cortex function theory to cognitive aging. *Psychological Bulletin, 120,* 272–292.

APPENDIX A

Lists Used During Study and Free Recall

List 1: door, glass, pane, shade, ledge, sill, house, open, curtain, frame, view, breeze (critical word WINDOW)
List 2: bed, rest, awake, tired, dream, wake, snooze, blanket, doze, slumber, snore, nap (critical word SLEEP)
List 3: nose, breath, sniff, aroma, hear, see, nostril, whiff, scent, reek, stench, fragrance (critical word SMELL)
List 4: nurse, sick, lawyer, medicine, health, hospital, dentist, physician, ill, patient, office, stethoscope (critical word DOCTOR)
List 5: sour, candy, sugar, bitter, good, taste, tooth, nice, honey, soda, chocolate, heart (critical word SWEET)
List 6: table, sit, legs, seat, couch, desk, recliner, sofa, wood, cushion, swivel, stool (critical word CHAIR)

Words Used for Recognition

house, smoke, lawyer, window, trash, waste, rough, curtain, taste, refuse, wood, smell, soft, aroma, gravel, needle, soda, chocolate, pillow, snooze, billow, eye, cushion, chair, rugged, anger, blanket, point, pollution, cotton, thimble, fear, swivel, snore, sweet, feather, rage, sweep, ill, see, frame, office, wrath, sand, doctor, cigar, sleep, fragrance

COGNITIVE NEUROPSYCHOLOGY, 1999, 16 (3/4/5), 385–398

CONFABULATION, EXECUTIVE FUNCTIONS, AND SOURCE MEMORY IN ALZHEIMER'S DISEASE

Gianfranco Dalla Barba
INSERM, Paris and Hôpital Henri Mondor, Créteil, France

Zahia Nedjam
INSERM, Paris, France

Bruno Dubois
INSERM and Hôpital de la Salpêtrière, Paris, France

Most current views consider confabulation strictly related to the dysfunction of frontally based processes subserving the control of retrieval from long-term memory. This study addresses the relationship between confabulation, source memory, and executive functions in 17 Alzheimer disease (AD) patients and 18 normal controls. The following tasks were used: Six tasks tapping executive functions; a task in which subjects had to discriminate the origin of a given information, i.e. visual perception or imagination; a modified version of the Confabulation Battery (Dalla Barba, 1993a) tapping episodic memory, general semantic memory and personal plans; and a modified version of the Crovitz test, in which, in response to a cue word, subjects had to produce a personal memory, a general semantic memory, or a personal plan.

AD patients were clearly impaired on tests of executive functions, and showed poor monitoring abilities for the source of information. AD patients confabulated when they were required to retrieve a personal episode and also, although less frequently, when they were required to make a personal plan. Correlation studies showed that AD patients' confabulation did not correlate with their performance on executive tasks or with their ability to discriminate the origin of information. It is suggested that confabulation reflects a pathological awareness of personal temporality.

INTRODUCTION

The term confabulation refers to a particular memory disturbance, observed in some brain-damaged patients, which consists of both actions and verbal statements that are unintentionally incongruous to history, background, and present situation (Dalla Barba, 1993a). Although confabulation has often been reported in Korsakoff's syndrome (Bonhoeffer, 1904; Dalla Barba, Cipolotti, & Denes, 1990; Kopelman, Ng, & Van Den Brouke, 1997; Mercer, Wapner, Gardner, & Benson, 1977; Talland, 1961), it is also observed in other pathological conditions, including rupture of the anterior or posterior communicating artery, subarachnoid haemorrhage, encephalitis, head injury, Binswanger's encephalopathy, psychotic disorders (Baddeley & Wilson, 1986; Berlyne, 1972; Conway & Tacchi, 1996; Dalla Barba, 1993a, 1993b; Dalla Barba, Cappelletti, Signorini, & Denes, 1997; Delbecq-Derouesné, Beauvois, & Shallice, 1990; Johnson, O'Connor, & Cantor,

Requests for reprints should be addressed to Gianfranco Dalla Barba MD, PhD, U.324 INSERM, Centre Paul Broca, 2ter rue d'Alésia, 75014 Paris, France (Tel: 33 1 40 78 92 17; Fax: 33 1 45 89 68 48; E-mail: dallabarba@broca.inserm.fr).

1997; Kapur & Coughlan, 1980; Kopelman, 1987; Luria, 1976; Mercer et al., 1977; Moscovitch, 1989; Moscovitch & Melo, 1997), and also on some occasions in normal subjects (e.g. Burgess & Shallice, 1996; Kopelman, 1987). Alzheimer's patients may demonstrate intrusions—confabulatory-like behaviours that consist of the production of extra-study material in learning tasks (Butters, Granholm, Salmon, & Grant, 1987; Dalla Barba, Parlato, Iavarone, & Boller, 1995). However, the presence of overt confabulation in this pathological condition has been reported only anecdotally.

Confabulation has been associated with dysfunction of frontally based cognitive processes subserving the control of retrieval from long-term memory. The disruption of control functions, resulting from damage to the frontal lobe and related structures, prevents the active process of retrieval of information and the evaluation of its output (Baddeley & Wilson, 1986; Moscovitch, 1989, 1995; Moscovitch & Melo, 1997). In a similar vein Johnson (1991) argues that confabulation is a disorder resulting from a failure of "reality monitoring" or source monitoring (i.e. deciding whether a memory is based upon something that actually happened or whether it is imagined). In a study based on the analysis of healthy volunteers' autobiographical recollections of recent events, Burgess and Shallice (1996) argue that errors in recall made by normal subjects and those made by confabulators may be the result of disruption of different components of control processes. These are considered part of the Supervisory System (Norman & Shallice, 1980), which is held to be a function of the frontal cortex.

Some data, however, are in contradiction with the frontal/executive model of confabulation. In fact, some patients show confabulation in the absence of executive deficits and frontal pathology (Dalla Barba, 1993a; Dalla Barba et al., 1990). In addition, patients may have executive deficits and frontal pathology without confabulation (e.g. Johnson et al., 1997). Therefore the relation between confabulation and frontal/executive functions, including source monitoring abilities, remains an open question. Experiments 1 and 2 will address this question. The frontal/executive model of confabulation implies that structural damage in the frontal lobe disrupts retrieval or post-retrieval processes and that deficits should emerge in any domain of memory, provided that the tasks devised to assess different memory domains are equated in terms of retrieval or post-retrieval control demands. However, this idea is contradicted by the observation that some patients may show confabulation restricted to the episodic/autobiographical aspect of memory (Dalla Barba, 1993a, 1993b; Dalla Barba et al., 1990, 1997) Experiments 3 and 4 will address the question of domain-specific aspects of confabulation.

In a recent paper, Dalla Barba and co-workers (Dalla Barba et al., 1997) argued that confabulation is often associated with impaired discrimination of temporal and spatial stimuli (Dalla Barba, 1993a, 1993b; Dalla Barba et al., 1990). Confabulating patients may also make erroneous judgements when they are required to plan their future (Dalla Barba, 1993a). The relation between confabulation and personal temporality will be addressed in Experiments 3 and 4.

In summary: the following questions will be addressed in this study: (1) What is the relationship between executive functions and confabulation? (2) What is the relation between confabulation and source monitoring abilities? (3) Does memory-domain specific confabulation really exist? (4) What is the relationship between confabulation in personal past and personal future?

METHODS

Subjects

Seventeen patients with Alzheimer's disease (AD) (11 women and 6 men), together with 18 normal controls (10 women and 8 men) entered the study. The diagnosis of probable AD was made according to the criteria suggested by McKhann and his associates (McKhann et al., 1984). A number of laboratory tests (e.g. CT brain scan, urinanalysis, folate levels) were performed to rule out various viral, metabolic, or traumatic causes of dementia. Patients with a history of severe head injury, alcoholism, or serious psychiatric illness were excluded from this group. Patients with a score of five or greater on the Hachinski scale (Hachinski et al., 1975) were excluded to reduce the possibility of including ischemic vascular dementia.

Controls were either spouses of patients or other individuals who volunteered to participate in the research projects of our laboratory. Informed consent was obtained from all subjects participating in the study.

Table 1 shows the demographic data of the two groups, and the performance of AD patients on the Mini Mental State Examination (Folstein, Folstein, & McHugh, 1975). Analysis of variance (ANOVA) revealed that the groups did not differ significantly in terms of mean age and years of education.

Experiment 1: Executive Functions

Six tests considered sensitive to frontal dysfunction were performed: the Modified Card Sorting Test (MCST; Nelson, 1976); a verbal fluency test that involves generating as many words as possible starting with the letters F, P, and L in 1 minute; a verbal fluency test that involves generating as many words as possible from the categories of animals, fruits, and vegetables in 1 minute; the Cognitive Estimation Test (Shallice & Evans, 1978), a sequencing test that involves drawing two graphic sequences of figures of length 2 and 3 (i.e. cross, circle; and cross, circle and triangle) (Luria, 1966), and the Stroop test (Stroop, 1935). Subjects' performance on these tests is presented in Table 2. Multiple t-tests revealed that AD patients were significantly impaired (all P at least .0005) relative to normal control subjects on all executive tasks.

Table 1. *Demographic and Clinical Data*

	AD Patients	*Normal Control*
	Mean (SD)	*Mean (SD)*
Age in years	74.7 (5.0)	73.3 (5.9)
Education in years	8.5 (4.0)	6.4 (2.7)
Gender (M/F)	6/11	8.10
MMSE	19.1 (2.1)	

Table 2. *Subjects' Performance on Tests Considered Sensitive to Executive Dysfunction*

	AD Patients	*Normal Controls*
	Mean (SD)	*Mean (SD)*
Modified Card Sorting Test		
Categories achieved	2.7 (1.6)	5.4 (1.4)
Error score	42.9 (18.3)	6.6 (1.8)
Verbal Fluency		
Letters FPL, each 60sec (total retrieved)	21.1 (8.4)	32.6 (9.1)
Categories animals, fruits, vegetables, each 60sec (total retrieved)	24.2 (7.6)	41.1 (10.4)
Cognitive Estimates		
Error score	8.7 (4.6)	3.9 (2.5)
Luria's Graphic Sequences		
Total correct	20.6 (10.5)	80.9 (17.3)
Stroop Test		
Interference score	11.0 (8.1)	< 5th centile

Experiment 2: Source Monitoring

Source monitoring performance was measured following a procedure used elsewhere (Dalla Barba et al., 1997). The first task was devised as a baseline control task. In the study phase 16 coloured drawings of common objects were presented one after the other, for 3sec each, to AD patients and controls. Immediately following presentation of the items, subjects were presented with a list of 32 printed words, half of which were names of the objects seen in the study phase and the other half of which were distracters (i.e. names of common objects not presented for the study). Subjects had to indicate the words corresponding to the objects seen in the study phase.

In the second task, performed immediately after the previous task, a set of 32 coloured drawings of common objects corresponding to medium- to high-frequency words (Content, Mousty, & Radeau, 1990) of 4 to 8 letters in length was selected and divided randomly into 2 sets of 16 items. In the study phase, within each group, half of the subjects were first presented with one of the two sets of drawings. They were then read a list of 16 words corresponding to the set of drawings they were not presented with, and for each word they were asked to imagine the corresponding object. Subjects' imaging abilities were monitored by asking them preliminary questions such as "Is the red of a strawberry deeper than the red of a cherry?" There was no evidence that AD patients failed to engage in imagery. Immediately after this they were presented with a list of 32 printed words, where half of the words were names of the objects seen and the other half were names of the objects they had imagined. For each word subjects were asked to say whether that word was the name of an object they had seen or of one they had imagined in the study phase. Table 3 reports subjects' performance on the recognition and the source monitoring tasks together with the percentage of "seen" and "imagined" responses (regardless whether correct of not) of the two groups. The percentage or correct responses for "seen" and "imagined" responses was equivalent within AD patients and controls (58% vs. 59%, and 87% vs. 89%, respectively). Recognition scores were computed by applying a correction procedure in which the frequency of incorrect acceptance of new items as old (false alarm rate) is subtracted from the frequency of correct recognition of old items (hit rate). *T*-tests performed on recognition and monitoring scores revealed a significant difference among groups, $t(1,33) = -9.0$, $P < .0001$ and $t(1,33) = -10.0$, $P < .0001$, respectively. The rates of "seen" and "imagined" responses were entered in a 2 × 2 ANOVA with Group (AD patients vs. controls) as between-subjects factor, and Type of Response ("seen" vs. "imagined") as within-group factor. Results indicated a main effect of Group [$F(1,33) = 8.0$, $P < .01$], an effect of Type of Response [$F(1,1) = 13.7$, $P < .001$], and a Group by Type of Response interaction [$F(1,33) = 11.2$, $P < .005$]. Post hoc comparisons (Scheffé's *F* corrected for multiple nonindependent comparisons) showed that AD patients produced significantly more "seen" than "imagined" responses ($P < .0001$), whereas this was not the case for controls.

EXAMINATION OF CONFABULATION

Experiment 3: Modified Confabulation Battery

According to the observation that confabulators often confabulate on tasks of spatial and temporal orientation, as well as when they are questioned about their personal future, it has been proposed (Dalla Barba, 1993a; Dalla Barba et al., 1997) that confabulation is not only a disturbance of memory but also involves all subjectively experienced temporality extending to the personal present and to the personal future. In Experiment 3, we selected 10 episodic memory questions concerning personal past and 10 questions concerning general semantic memory (i.e. knowledge of past and current famous people and events) from the Confabulation Battery (Dalla Barba, 1993a).

In addition, we constructed 10 questions concerning subjects' personal future. Episodic memory questions and questions concerning the future were matched for proximity to the moment when the questions were asked. This Modified Confabulation Battery (MCB) was administered in a randomised form to AD patients and controls. Answers were scored as "correct," "wrong," or "confabulation," according to whether or not they were consis-

Table 3. *AD Patients' and Normal Controls' Performance on Recognition and Source Monitoring Tasks*

	Recognition	*Source Monitoring*		
	Correct	*Correct*	*"Seen"*	*"Imagined"*
	Mean (SD)	*Mean (SD)*	*Mean (SD)*	*Mean (SD)*
AD patients	46.5 (20.9)	55.7 (10.6)	66.4 (16.2)	33.6 (16.2)
Normal controls	95.4 (9.40)	87.5 (7.8)	50.6 (9.5)	49.4 (9.3)

tent with information (collected from relatives) concerning the subjects' past, present situation, and probable future activities.

Any possible answer to questions about the future can be considered a confabulation, since by definition the future is only "probable" and there is in principle no "correct" answer to questions about the future. Yet, answers concerning the personal future can be confabulatory when there is a significant discrepancy with a predicted future action. For example, in response to the question "What are you going to do in a few minutes?," some patients answered "I will go back to work" even though none of them were working at the time of the study. The MCB and some examples of confabulatory reports are presented in Appendix A.

The results of the MCB are reported in Table 4. Where a response was not either correct or a confabulation, it was an omission error. These data were entered in a 2 × 3 × 2 ANOVA with Group (AD patients vs. controls) as between-subjects factor, and Test (episodic vs. semantic vs. "future") and Type of Response (correct vs. confabulation) as within-group factors. Results indicated a main effect for Group [$F(1,33) = 51.3$, $P < .0001$], for Test [$F(1,2) = 13.3$, $P < .0001$], and for Type of Response [$F(1,1) = 526.6$, $P < .0001$]. There was also a Group by Test interaction [$F(1,2) = 5.1$, $P < .01$]; a Group by Type of Response Interaction [$F(1,1) = 90.7$, $P < .0001$]; and a Group by Test by Response interaction [$F(1,2,1) = 4.7$, $P < .01$].

Post hoc analysis (Scheffé's F corrected for multiple nonindependent comparisons) revealed that AD patients produced significantly fewer correct responses than controls in any test condition (all $P < .001$). No significant differences emerged comparing correct responses in the different tests within each group of subjects. As far as confabulation was concerned, AD patients produced significantly more confabulations in the episodic test than in the semantic test ($P < .01$).

Correlation coefficients were calculated between confabulations in the MCB and the performance on executive tests and the source monitoring task. The only significant correlations were observed between confabulation in the "future" test, the number of categories achieved on the MCST (Rho = .56, $P < .01$), and the score on Luria's graphic sequences (Rho = .49, $P < .05$). Quite paradoxically, these results suggest that good performance on these two executive tests is positively correlated with the tendency to confabulate in the future.

Experiment 4: Modified Crovitz Test

According to Moscovitch (1989, 1995; Moscovitch & Melo, 1997), confabulation is a consequence of a deficit of strategic retrieval and should affect episodic and semantic memory equally if both episodic and semantic memory tasks require the involvement of the strategic retrieval process. In order to equate the strategic retrieval demands of semantic and episodic memory tasks, Moscovitch (1995, Moscovitch & Melo, 1997) devised a semantic, historical version of the classic word-cue test technique developed by Galton (1879) and more recently revised by Crovitz and Shiffman (1974). Moscovitch (1995; Moscovitch & Melo, 1997) found that patients with damage to the ventromedial portion of the frontal lobe confabulated on both the episodic and the semantic versions of the test.

Table 4. *AD Patients' and Normal Controls' Performance on the Modified Confabulation Battery*

	AD		*Normal Controls*	
	% of Correct Responses	*% of Confabulation*	*% of Correct Responses*	*% of Confabulation*
	Mean (SD)	*Mean (SD)*	*Mean (SD)*	*Mean (SD)*
Episodic	51.9 (12.8)	22.2 (15.3)	96.6 (5.9)	0
Semantic	47.7 (25.5)	8.2 (20.6)	91.6 (10.4)	0
Future	51.1 (20.2)	10.5 (11.9)	77.2 (13.6)	0

We used the same procedure in order to ascertain whether AD patients would show an equal tendency to confabulate in both versions of the test. In the episodic version of the test, subjects were presented with eight cue words and asked to produce a specific detailed account of an autobiographical event related to that word. In the semantic version of the test the procedure was identical to that used in the episodic version, except that this time subjects in response to the cue word had to describe in detail a historical event that occurred before they were born.

In addition to the episodic and the semantic versions of the test, a "future" version of the test was administered. In this task the same eight cue words used in the episodic version of the test were given to AD patients and to controls (see Appendix B). For each word, subjects were asked to produce a specific, detailed account of a personal plan related to that word. Responses on this Modified Crovitz Test (MCT) were scored on a 0–2 scale, with two points for a detailed description of the event, one point for a less detailed description, and 0 points for a general statement or if nothing was provided. All responses were scored by two independent raters. Agreement between them was 87%.

Memories for semantic, personal past, and personal future cue words were verified for confabulations by using historical sources for the semantic test and questioning close relatives for the episodic and the future versions of the test. The results of the MCT are reported in Table 5. Where a response was not either correct or a confabulation, it was an omission error. These data were entered in a 2 × 3 × 2 ANOVA with Group (AD patients vs. controls) as between-subjects factor, Test episodic vs. semantic vs. "future"), and Type of Response (correct vs. confabulation) as within-group factors. Results indicated a main effect for group, [$F(1,33) = 61.3$, $P < .0001$], for Test [$F(1,2) = 18.2$, $P < .0001$], and for Type of Response [$F(1,1) = 444.9$, $P < .0001$]. There was also a Group by Test interaction [$F(1,2) = 3.9$, $P < .05$]; a Group by Type of Response interaction [$F(1,1) = 67.6$, $P < .0001$]; and a Type of Response by Test interaction [$F(1,2) = 12.2$, $P < .0001$].

Post hoc analysis (Scheffé's *F* corrected for multiple nonindependent comparisons) revealed that AD patients produced significantly fewer correct responses than controls in any test condition (all $P < .0001$). No significant differences emerged comparing correct responses in the different tests within the AD patients group, whereas controls produced significantly fewer correct responses in the "future" test than in the episodic and semantic tests. As far as confabulation were concerned, no significant difference emerged between the episodic and the "future" test.

Correlation coefficients were calculated between confabulations in the MCT and the performance on executive tests and the source monitoring task. The same pattern of results as in the MCB emerge from this analysis. In fact, significant positive correlations were observed between confabulation in the "future" test, the number of categories achieved on the MCST (Rho = .47, $P < .05$), and the score on Luria's graphic sequences (Rho = .448, $P < .05$).

A further correlation study showed that confabulation in the episodic test of the MCT as significantly correlated with confabulation in the "future" test of the MCT (Rho = .49, $P < .05$) and with confabulation in the episodic test of the MCB (Rho = .55, $P < .05$). Confabulation in the "future" test of the MCT was significantly correlated with confabulation in the episodic test of the MCB (Rho = .52, $P < .05$), and with confabulation in the "future" test of the MCB (Rho = 55, $P < .05$). Confabulation in the semantic test of the MCB did not correlate significantly with confabulation in any other test.

Confabulation on the MCB and MCT did not correlate with Mini Mental State Examination scores, nor with patients' performance on the Logical Memory subtest and the Paired Associate subtest of the Wechsler Memory Scale.

DISCUSSION

Experimental data revealed that AD patients were clearly impaired on tests of executive functions and in their monitoring abilities for the source of infor-

Table 5. *AD Patients' and Normal Controls' Performance on the Modified Crovitz Test*

	AD		*Normal Controls*				
	Correct Responses		*Confabulation*		*Correct Responses*		*Confabulation*
	Mean % (SD)	*Mean Score (SD)*	*Mean % (SD)*	*Mean Score (SD)*	*Mean % (SD)*	*Mean Score (SD)*	*Mean*
Episodic	48.3 (27.5)	0.96 (0.4)	14.5 (21.7)	0.94 (1.0)	90.6 (13.8)	1.68 (0.3)	0
Semantic	48.2 (24.7)	0.63 (0.3)	0		94.1 (9.1)	1.2 (0.2)	0
Future	34.3 (19.0)	0.59 (0.3)	6.5 (9.9)	0.62 (0.89)	65.6 (15.3)	1.5 (0.3)	0

mation. In addition, in the source monitoring task, where their performance was almost at the level of chance, they demonstrated a clear bias to attribute the source of information to visual perception rather than mental imagery. Other findings indicated that AD patients confabulated when they were required to retrieve a personal episode and, although less frequently, when they were required to make a personal plan. In one test, the MCB, they also produced confabulation on responses to semantic memory questions. Frequency of confabulation in the "future" tests positively correlated with performance on the MCST and with scores on Luria's graphic sequences. Finally, within- and across-test comparisons revealed that confabulation in episodic and "future" tests were positively and significantly correlated, whereas there were no significant relationship between these and confabulation in the semantic test of the MCB.

Confabulation in AD

As a group, our AD patients could be considered "mild confabulators." The percentage of confabulation produced by our patients was lower than that observed in previous studies (e.g. Dalla Barba, 1993a, 1993b, 1997, 1998) concerning single cases with florid confabulatory syndromes.

It could be argued that the relatively low incidence of confabulatory reports in our AD patients limits our ability to make inferences about the nature and the underlying mechanisms of confabulation in this patient group. Florid confabulatory tendencies are usually associated with severe cognitive deficits, whereas our patients were only mildly impaired. However, we believe that confabulation in our AD patients provides valuable information on the nature of this phenomenon for at least two reasons. First, our patients demonstrated confabulation in the MCB and MCT, whereas control subjects did not produce a single confabulation in those tasks. This suggests that confabulation in AD patients does not reflect the exaggeration of a normal tendency to produce false memories, but rather a distinct phenomenon. Second, there was a clear difference between the number of confabulations produced in episodic and future tasks and general semantic tasks; this dissociation shows that confabulation in our patients was task-specific. Taken together, these arguments allow us to examine our data in the framework of a possible hypothesis on the origin of confabulation.

Confabulation and Executive Functions

A goal of this study was to elucidate the relationship between confabulation and executive functions. Various authors (cited earlier) have argued that executive dysfunction is a prerequisite for confabulation because such a dysfunction would negatively impact upon retrieval or post-retrieval processes, lowering the threshold for acceptance of any candidate memory. The present results demonstrate that AD patients were impaired on tests of executive abilities. However, confabulatory tendencies did not correlate with performance on any of the six executive tests employed in this study. In fact, there was a paradoxical positive correlation between confabulation (in the "future" tests of the MCB and the MCT) and executive functions performance on the MCST and on Luria's graphic sequences.

In a recent study of confabulation, Kopelman and colleagues (1997) conclude that their findings are consistent with the idea that an executive dysfunction is a "common, perhaps necessary precursor to confabulation, but some more specific factor must account for confabulation in episodic memory." This position, in our opinion, actually reflects a realistic account of confabulation.

Based on our data, we cannot exclude the possibility that frontal/executive dysfunction and confabulation are related. However, as the data only show evidence of a positive statistical correlation between the two conditions, a relation of causality is doubtful.

Confabulation and Source Monitoring

The current investigation is relevant to models of source monitoring. In a series of papers Johnson and colleagues (Johnson, 1988, 1991; Johnson, Foley, Suengas, & Raye, 1988; Johnson & Raye, 1981) proposed that discriminating of the origin of information was the result of deficits in *reality monitoring*. Reality monitoring operates on the basis of qualitative characteristics of information (e.g. amount of perceptual detail, supporting memories) in combination with judgement processes that use this information as evidence as to whether something was real or imagined. According to this model, confabulation is considered the result of a failure of reality monitoring (Johnson, 1991).

This interpretation of confabulation is consistent with the idea that confabulation is a form of source amnesia (Moscovitch, 1989; Schacter, Harbluk, & McLachlan, 1984) combined with misattribution of temporal and spatial context (Schacter, 1987; Shimamura, Janowsky, & Squire, 1987). However, in a more recent paper, Johnson and co-workers (Johnson et al., 1997), demonstrated that "reality monitoring," or source monitoring, was equally disrupted in a confabulatory patient and in nonconfabulating patients with frontal lobe damage. The latter findings lead Johnson and colleagues to propose that a reality monitoring or source monitoring deficit may occur with confabulation but that it is not the only factor involved in' the genesis of confabulation. Our present findings are in agreement with Johnson et al.'s conclusions. Our AD patients demonstrated markedly impaired source monitoring abilities, but their poor performance on source monitoring tasks did not correlate with confabulatory tendencies.

Domain-specific Confabulation

Confabulation may be domain-specific, affecting only one aspect of memory. Episodic/autobiographical confabulations were seen in a previous study where two patients confabulated in response to questions about personal episodes, orientation in time and place, and, to a much lesser extent, personal semantic memory (Dalla Barba, 1993a; Dalla Barba et al., 1990). In another study, Dalla Barba (1993b) described a patient in whom confabulation extended beyond episodic memory, affecting semantic memory. In this patient a considerable amount of confabulation, both in episodic and semantic memory, was semantically incoherent or bizarre. Accordingly, Dalla Barba argued that when the semantic system is preserved confabulations are semantically appropriate, whereas they become anomalous (or bizarre) when memory impairment also affects the semantic system. It appears that the content of confabulation is determined by the presence or absence of a semantic deficit. In other words, semantic deficits determine the content of confabulation, not its presence or absence in different domains of memory.

Moscovitch's (1989, 1995; Moscovitch & Melo, 1997) hypothesis of confabulation as a consequence of a deficit of strategic retrieval is meant to apply equally to all domains of memory. In other words, confabulation should equally affect episodic and semantic memory if both episodic and semantic memory tasks require the involvement of the strategic retrieval process. Moscovitch (1995, p. 16) argued that a "reason for the greater prevalence of confabulation about episodic memory is that retrieval of episodic memories in the laboratory and in real life are likely to make greater demands on strategic processes than retrieval of semantic memories." Moscovitch (1995) further argued that Dalla Barba and co-workers' patients (Dalla Barba, 1993a; Dalla Barba et al., 1990) showed confabulation in episodic memory but not in semantic memory because the tests used to assess episodic memory made greater demands on strategic retrieval processes than did those used to assess semantic memory. Accordingly, and in order to attempt to equate the strategic retrieval demands of semantic and episodic memory, Moscovitch (1995, Moscovitch & Melo, 1997) devised the semantic, historical version of the Crovitz test and found that patients with damage to the ventromedial portion of the frontal lobe confabulated on both the episodic and the semantic versions of the test. In a recent paper, Dalla Barba and colleagues (1997) described a patient, GA, who developed an amnesic-confabulatory syndrome, following a subarachnoid haemorrhage and ischaemia due to rupture of the anterior communicating artery and subsequent vasospasm. GA was studied with the same techniques used in this study, i.e. the MCB and the MCT. It was found that confabulation was virtually absent in semantic tasks, whereas it was florid in episodic/autobiographical tasks. This suggests that confabulation can affect a specific domain of memory even when tests of episodic and semantic memory are equated for the amount of strategic retrieval required. The findings of this study are similar to the findings in GA's case, with the exception that confabulation was observed (though in minor degree) on semantic questions of the MCB. Taken together, these results further support the idea that the dissociation between confabulation in episodic autobiographical memory and semantic memory is a real entity and not the result of a methodological artefact. Confabulation in episodic and semantic memory can be associated as it has repeatedly been reported (Dalla Barba, 1993b; Kopelman et al., 1997; Moscovitch, 1995; Moscovitch & Melo, 1997), but the fact that they can be dissociated suggests that confabulation in episodic and semantic memory probably reflect different underlying disorders (see following for further discussion on this point.)

Confabulation and Temporality

The findings of this study indicate that AD patients confabulate when they are required to make a personal plan. Results indicated a significant correlation between confabulation in the past and future. It has been suggested that confabulation reflects a disturbance of chronological memory, so that real memories are confused in temporal context (Korsakoff, 1889; Schnider, Von Däniken, & Gutbrod, 1996; Talland, 1961; Van der Horst, 1956; Victor, Adams, & Collins, 1971). This interpretation, however, is challenged by the fact that many amnesic and nonamnesic patients have disordered chronology, yet do not confabulate (Milner & Petrides, 1984; Nichelli, 1993; Stuss, Alexander, Lieberman, & Levine, 1978; Vriezen & Moscovitch, 1990). Accordingly, it does not seem that confabulation in the past and in the future can simple be traced back to a disorder of time-order memory. One possibility is that confabulation in our AD patients, and in GA, does not affect memory *stricto sensu*, but involves, although to different degrees, all the subjectively experienced temporality, extending from the past to the future. Subjective experienced temporality has been considered as a function of Temporal Consciousness in Dalla Barba et al.'s model. This model, schematically represented in Fig. 1 (see Dalla Barba et al., 1997, for details), is based on the following assumptions.

Assumption 1. Events produce atemporal and aspecific modifications in the Long Term Storage System (LTSS). These modifications, represented in Fig. 1 as X, Y, and Z are atemporal in the sense that they do not contain any information concerning time. They are aspecific in the sense that they do not contain any information specifying that they are representing episodes, meanings, rules, procedures, algorithms, etc.

Assumption 2. The modifications in the LTSS can be more or less stable and more or less vulnerable depending on variables such as attention at encoding, emotional value of encoded and stored event, depth of encoding, rehearsal and repeated experience of the same event or similar events.

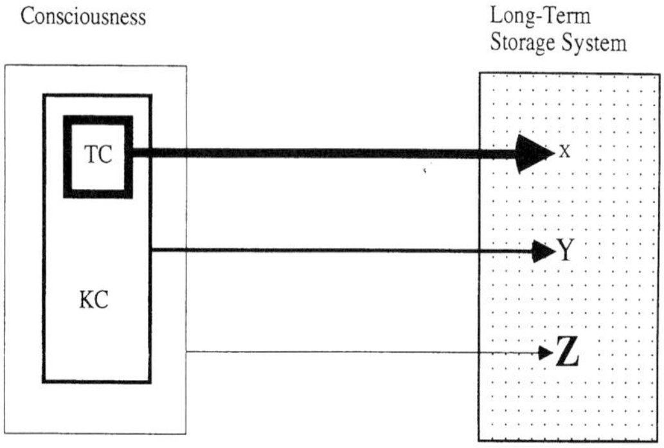

Fig.1 . *A hypothesis concerning the relation between memory, consciousness and temporality. TC = temporal consciousness; KC = knowledge consciousness; x, y and z = aspecific modifications of the Long-Term Storage System, varying from less (x) to more stable (z).*

Assumption 3. Different types of consciousness exist, each representing an original and irreducible way of addressing the object. Different types of consciousness include, among others, temporal consciousness (TC) and knowing consciousness (KC). TC means to become aware of something as part of a personal past, present- or future. KC means to become aware of something as a meaning or as an element of impersonal knowledge or information.

Assumption 4. TC can, and usually does, interact with the less stable and more vulnerable modifications of the LTSS in order to remember the past, be oriented in the present, and plan the future.

According to this model, confabulation in episodic memory (e.g. Dalla Barba, 1993a; Dalla Barba et al., 1990), in orientation in time and place, and in personal future planning tasks (Dalla Barba et al., 1997; the present study), is the result of a condition in which TC is still intact but can not use less stable modifications of the LTSS but only more stable ones, in order to remember the personal past and plan the personal future. In other terms, this is a condition in which TC is still working but is no longer able to accomplish its usual task, i.e. to operate a sort of fine-grain search in the LTSS and use less stable modifications in order to set up a personal temporal workspace. What TC does instead in this condition is to use more stable modifications of the LTSS, with the result being that habits or personal semantic information are considered in a personal temporal framework. When asked what they have done the previous day or what they are going to do the following day, confabulating patients of this type typically answer with memories and plans that they usually have in their daily life. Although admitted to the hospital, they will say, for example, that the previous day they went out shopping and that the following day they will be visiting some friends, acts that presumably were part of their routine life. Examples of confabulations of this type are reported in Appendix A.

It could be argued that some confabulators are well oriented in time and that others are disoriented but do not confabulate in orientation tasks (De Luca & Cicerone, 1991). In addition, patients who confabulate, like our AD patients for example, do not confabulate answering to any question. Indeed our AD patients produced considerably more correct and "I don't know" answers than confabulatory answers in the episodic and "future" tests of the MCB and of the MCT. Finally, AD patients produced roughly half the amount of confabulation in the "future" tests compared to the episodic tests of the MCB and MCT. Taken together it seems that these observations are not predicted by the model we have described. However, the hypothesis proposed in the model is not meant to apply equally to all conditions according to an "all-or-nothing" mechanism. In other words, there is no contradiction in assuming that TC (but see also Tulving's "retrieval mode" Tulving, 1983) can sometimes use the correct information in the LTSS (for correct responses) can sometimes not use this information, (as in "I don't know" responses), and sometimes uses the wrong information (as in confabulatory answers). This pattern of behaviour is what is usually observed in normal subjects. The point is, why in some pathological conditions does TC show an abnormal tendency to use wrong information and to generate confabulations? The model predicts that in some conditions TC is biased to use the wrong information (more stable modifications, in the model) when it can not access the correct information. This model does not predict the conditions in which correct responses (i.e. less stable modifications), confabulations (i.e. more stable modifications), or omissions (i.e. "I don't know" responses) are produced. However, indirect evidence suggests that the relevance of information to one's biography may be a crucial factor. It is known (Dalla Barba, 1993a; Dalla Barba et al., 1990), and it was actually the case in this study, that patients confabulate much more on tasks of autobiographical/episodic recall than on tasks of nonautobiographical/episodic recall, such as the recall of short stories. It is possible, therefore, that in autobiographical/episodic tasks the ratio between omissions and confabulations is a function of the relevance of the to-be-remembered information to one's biography.

The fact that some patients confabulate in episodic memory while being oriented in time, or that they confabulate less in the future than in the past, is also not in contradiction with the hypothesis summarised in the model. TC reflects the synthesis of the subordinate structures of temporality, that is, past, present, and future, but these structures are not identical. In that case, no distinction could be made between past, present, and future. So, as these structures are not identical, it might well be the case that both correct responses and confabulation are differently distributed in episodic, orientation, and "future" tasks. What the hypothesis predicts, however, is that the performance in each "temporal" task (i.e. episodic, orientation, and "future") should be correlated more strictly with each other temporal task than with nontemporal tasks (e.g. semantic memory tasks). As far as episodic and "future" tasks are concerned, this prediction is confirmed by the results of this study.

According to our model (see also Dalla Barba et al., 1997), confabulation in semantic memory tasks reflect a condition in which KC is no longer able to use the more stable modifications of the LTSS. In this condition, patients confabulate in tasks tapping knowledge of public and historical facts and knowledge of famous people (Kopelman et al., 1997: Moscovitch, 1995; Moscovitch & Melo, 1997), but they do not confabulate in tasks that require the use of the more stable modifications of the LTSS, such as word definition tasks. Patients who confabulate in word definition tasks (e.g. Dalla Barba, 1993b) also produce confabulations in episodic memory tasks that are described as fantastic (Berlyne, 1972), implausible (Baddeley & Wilson, 1986), incoherent (Kopelman, 1987), or semantically anomalous (Dalla Barba, 1993a). According to the model, this type of confabulation reflects a condition in which the modifications in the LTSS are degraded so that the material used by TC and KC is *per se* incoherent. Therefore, in this condition the content of confabulation in episodic and semantic memory tasks is semantically anomalous and confabulation takes a bizarre and fantastic form.

REFERENCES

Baddeley, A., & Wilson, B. (1986). Amnesia, autobiographical memory and confabulation. In D.C. Rubin (Ed.), *Autobiographical memory* (pp. 225–252). Cambridge: Cambridge University Press.

Berlyne, N. (1972). Confabulation. *British Journal of Psychiatry*, *120*, 31–39.

Bonhoeffer, K. (1904). Der Korsakowsche Symptomenkoplex in seinen Beziehungen zu den verschiedenen Krankheitsformen. *Allgemeine Zeitung Psychiatric*, *61*, 744–752.

Burgess, P.W., & Shallice, T.E. (1996). Confabulation and the control of recollection. *Memory*, *4*, 359–411.

Butters, N., Granholm, E., Salmon, D.P., & Grant, I. (1987). Episodic and semantic memory: a comparison of amnesic and demented patients. *Journal of Clinical and Experimental Neuropsychology*, *9*, 479–497.

Content, A., Mousty, P., & Radeau, M. (1990). Brulex, une base de données lexicales informatisée pour le français écrit et parlé. *L'année Psychologique*, *90*, 551–566.

Conway, M.A., & Tacchi, P.C. (1996). Motivated confabulation. *Neurocase*, *2*, 325–339.

Crovitz, H.F., & Shiffman, H. (1974). Frequency of episodic memories as function of their ages. *Bulletin of the Psychonomic Society*, *4*, 517-518

Dalla Barba, G. (1993a). Confabulation: knowledge and recollective experience. *Cognitive Neuropsychology*, *10*(1), 1–20.

Dalla Barba, G. (1993b). Different patterns of confabulation. *Cortex*, *29*, 567–581.

Dalla Barba, G., Cappelletti, Y.J., Signorini, M., & Denes, G. (1997). Confabulation: Remembering "another" past, planning "another" future. *Neurocase*, *3*, 425–436.

Dalla Barba, G., Cipolotti, L., & Denes, G. (1990). Autobiographical memory loss and confabulation in Korsakoff's syndrome: A case report. *Cortex*, *26*, 525–534.

Dalla Barba, G., Mantovan, M.C., Cappelletti, Y.J., & Depes, G. (1998). Temporal gradient in confabulation. *Cortex*, *34*, 417–426.

Dalla Barba, G., Parlato, V., Iavarone, A., & Boller, F (1995). Anosognosia, intrusions and "frontal" functions in Alzheimer's disease and depression. *Neuropsychologia*, *33*(2), 247–259.

Delbecq-Derouesné, L, Beauvois, M.F., & Shallice, T. (1990). Preserved recall versus impaired recognition. *Brain*, *113*, 1045–1154.

Folstein, M.F., Folstein, S.E., & McHugh, P.R. (1975). "Mini Mental State": A practical method for grading the cognitive state of patients for the clinician. *Journal of Psychiatric Research*, *12*, 189–198.

Galton, F. (1879). Psychometric experiments. *Brain*. *2*, 149–162.

Hachinski, V.C., Iliff, L.D., Zilhka, E., Du Boulay, G.H., McAllister, V.L., Marshall, J., Russell, R.W.R., & Symon, L. (1975). Cerebral blood flow in dementia. *Archives of Neurology*, *32*, 632–637.

Johnson, M. (1988). Discriminating the origin of information. In F. Oltmanns & B. Mahers (Eds.), *Delusional beliefs* (pp. 34–65). New York: John Wiley.

Johnson, M.K. (1991). Reality monitoring: Evidence from confabulation in organic brain disease patients. In G.P. Prigatano & D.L. Schacter (Eds.), *Awareness of deficit after brain injury*. New York: Oxford University Press.

Johnson, M.K., Foley, M. A., Suengas, A.G., & Raye, C.L. (1988). Phenomenal characteristics of memories for perceived and imagined autobiographical events. *Journal of Experimental Psychology: General*, *117*(4), 371–376.

Johnson, M.K., O'Connor, M., & Cantor, J. (1997). Confabulation, memory deficits, and frontal dysfunction. *Brain and Cognition*, *34*, 189–206.

Johnson, M.K., & Raye, C.L. (1981). Reality monitoring. *Psychological Review*, *88*, 67–85.

Kapur, N., & Coughlan, A.K. (1980). Confabulation after frontal lobe dysfunction. *Journal of Neurology, Neurosurgery and Psychiatry*, *43*, 461–463.

Kopelman, M.D. (1987). Two types of confabulation. *Journal of Neurology, Neurosurgery and Psychiatry*, *50*, 1482–1487.

Kopelman, M.D., Ng, N., & Van Den Brouke, O. (1997). Confabulation extending across episodic, personal and general semantic memory. *Cognitive Neuropsychology*, *14*(5), 683–712.

Korsakoff, S.S. (1889). Etude médico-psychologique sur une forme des maladies de la mémoire. *Revue Philosophique*, *28*, 501–530.

Luria, A.R. (1966). *Higher cortical functions in man*. London: Tavistock.

Luria, A.R. (1976). *The neuropsychology of memory*. New York: John Wiley.

McKhann, G., Drachman, D., Folstein, M., Katzman, R., Price, D., & Stadlan, E.M. (1984). Clinical diagnosis of Alzheimer's disease: Report of the NINCDS-ADRDA Work Group under the auspices of the Department of Health and Human Services Task Force on Alzheimer's Disease. *Neurology*, *34*, 939–944.

Mercer, B., Wapner, W., Gardner, H., & Benson, F. (1977). A study of confabulation. *Archives of Neurology*, *14*, 429–433.

Milner, B., & Petrides, M. (1984). Behavioural effects of frontal lobe lesions in man. *Trends in Neuroscience*, *7*, 403–407.

Moscovitch, M. (1989). Confabulation and the frontal system: Strategic versus associative retrieval in neuropsychological theories of memory. In H.L. Roedinger & F.I. Craik (Eds.), *Varieties of memory and consciousness: Essay in honor of Endel Tulving*. Hillsdale, NJ: Lawrence Erlbaum. Associates Inc.

Moscovitch, M. (1995). Confabulation. In D.L. Schacter (Ed.), *Memory distortion*, (pp. 226–251). Cambridge, MA: Harvard University Press.

Moscovitch, M., & Melo, B. (1997). Strategic retrieval and the frontal lobes: Evidence from confabulation and amnesia. *Neuropsychologia*, *35*(7), 1017–1034.

Nelson, H.E. (1976). A modified card sorting test sensitive to frontal defects. *Cortex*, *12*, 313–324.

Nichelli, P. (1993). Human temporal information processing. In F. Boller & Grafman (Eds.), *Handbok of neuropsychology*. Amsterdam: Elsevier.

Norman, D.A., & Shallice, T. (1980). Attention to action: Willed and automatic control of behavior. Technical 99:Center for Human Information Processing Reprinted, 1986, revued, in R.J. Davidson, G.E. Schwarz, & D. Shapiro Eds.), *Consciousness and self-regulation. Advances in research and theory*, Vol.4. New York: Plenum Press.

Schacter, D.L. (1987). Memory, amnesia and frontal lobe dysfunction. *Psychology*, *17*, 21–36.

Schacter, D.L., Harbluk, J.L., & McLachlan, D.R. (1984). Retrieval without recollection: An experi-

mental analysis of source amnesia. *Journal of Verbal Learning and Verbal Behaviour*, *23*, 593–611.
Schnider, A., von Däniken, C., & Gutbrod, K. (1996). The mechanisms of spontaneous and provoked confabulations. *Brain*, *119*, 1365–1375.
Shallice, T., & Evans, M. (1978). The involvement of the frontal lobe in cognitive estimation. *Cortex*, *14*, 294–303.
Shimamura, A.P., Janowsky, J.S., & Squire, L.R. (1987). What is the role of frontal lobe damage in memory disorders? In H.D. Levin, H.M. Eisemberg, & A. L. Benton (Eds.), *Frontal lobe functioning and dysfunctioning*, (pp. 173–195). New York: Oxford University Press.
Stroop J.R. (1935). Studies of interference in serial verbal reactions. *Journal of Experimental Psychology*, *18*, 643–662.
Stuss, D.T., Alexander, M.P., Lieberman, A., & Levine, H. (1978). An extraordinary form of confabulation. *Neurology*, *28*, 1166–1172.
Talland, G.A. (1961). Confabulation in the Wernicke-Korsakoff sindrome. *Journal of Nervous and Mental Disease*, *132*, 361–381.
Tulving, E. (1983). *Elements of episodic memory*. Oxford: Oxford University Press.
Van der Horst, L. (1956). Le sens de la temporalisation pour la mémoire et pour l'orientation. *Evolution Psychiatrique*, *1*, 189–205.
Victor, M., Adams, R.D., & Collins, G.H. (1970). *The Wernicke-Korsakoff Syndrome*. Philadelphia, PA: Davis.
Vriezen, E.R., & Moscovitch, M. (1990). Memory for temporal order and conditional associative-learning in patients with Parkinson's disease. *Neuropsychologia*, *28*, 1283–1293.

APPENDIX A

The Modified Confabulation Battery

Episodic

1. What did you do a few minutes ago?
2. Who did you see this morning?
3. What did you eat for dinner yesterday?
4. What did you do yesterday?
5. What did you do the day before yesterday?
6. How did you spend last Christmas?
7. Do you remember the last time you went to see a doctor?
8. Do you remember the last time you went to visit a friend or a relative?
9. Do you remember the last time you went to a restaurant?
10. Do you remember the last time you took vacation?

Semantic

1. When did World War I start?
2. When did World War II start?
3. What happened to President Kennedy?
4. What happened to the Pope a few years ago?
5. What happened to Princess Grace of Monaco?
6. What happened in Paris in May 1968?
7. What happened to Coluche?
8. What happened in rue des Rosiers a few years ago?
9. What happened in rue Copernic a few years ago?
10. What happened in the Saint Michel Subway station some time ago?

APPENDIX A (CONT.)

Future	
1.	What are you going to do in a few minutes?
2.	Who are you going to see this evening?
3.	What are you going to eat this evening?
4.	What are you going to do tomorrow?
5.	What are you going to do the day after tomorrow?
6.	How will you spend next Christmas?
7.	When will be the next time you visit a doctor?
8.	When will be the next time you visit a friend?
9.	When will be the next time you go to a restaurant?
10.	When will be the next time you go on vacation?

Examples of Confabulatory Reports

"What did you do last Christmas?"
"I was with my daughter and her in-laws in Paris"
This is what the patient had done for years. However, he had spent his last Christmas with his son in the countryside.
"What did you do yesterday?"
"I cleaned up my office and then I watered the flowers in the garden"
This is what the patient did as a routine but in fact he was watching television, his main occupation since his disease.
"What are you going to do tomorrow?"
"Tomorrow I'm going to see a pupil for a cello lesson"
The patient was a musician and used to give cello lessons at home. He had not done that for 2 years.
"When will be the next time you go on vacation?"
"I will be going to the Pyrénées with my wife next July"
This is what the patient and his wife used to do for vacations, but they hadn't done that for 3 years and they didn't plan to do it for the next summer.

APPENDIX B

B. The List of Words Used in the Modified Crovitz Test

Episodic/"Future"	Semantic
Train	Assassination
Mountain	Attack
Letter	Discovery
Money	Train
Cinema	War
Restaurant	President
Hospital	Revolution
Market	King

COGNITIVE NEUROPSYCHOLOGY, 1999, 16 (3/4/5), 399–415

WHEN TRUE MEMORIES SUPPRESS FALSE MEMORIES: EFFECTS OF AGEING

Elizabeth A. Kensinger and Daniel L. Schacter
Harvard University, Cambridge, USA

After studying a list of words that are all associated to a nonpresented target word, people often falsely recall or recognise the nonpresented target. Previous studies have shown that such false memories are greatly reduced when study lists are presented and tested several times compared to a single study/test trial. We report that older adults, who are sometimes more susceptible to memory distortions than are young adults, failed to exhibit any reduction in false recall or false recognition after five study/test trials compared to a single trial. By contrast, younger adults showed robust suppression of false memories after five study/test trials compared to a single trial. These results are consistent with the idea that older adults rely on memory for the general features or gist of studied materials, but tend not to encode or to retrieve specific details of individual items.

INTRODUCTION

Numerous studies of ageing memory have documented that older adults exhibit lower levels of veridical recall and recognition of recently studied information than do younger adults (for reviews, see Craik, Anderson, Kerr, & Li, 1995; Light, 1991). But a growing body of evidence converges on the conclusion that, compared to younger adults, older adults sometimes show equal or greater levels of false recall and false recognition of items not previously studied. Early studies by Smith (1975) and Rankin and Kausler (1979) investigated false recognition using a procedure in which subjects make old/new decisions about previously studied words, new words that are related to a previously studied associate (related lures), and new words that are not related to previously studied words (unrelated lures). Both Smith and Rankin and Kausler reported higher levels of false recognition in older adults than in younger adults, although the overall magnitude of the false recognition effect was small (see also Isingrini, Fontaine, Taconnat, & Duportal, 1995).

More recent research has shown that larger false recognition effects can be obtained when subjects study numerous items that are conceptually or perceptually similar to a novel test item (Hintzman, 1988; Shiffrin, Huber, & Marinelli, 1995). Particularly striking demonstrations of robust false recognition and false recall have been reported by Roediger and McDermott (1995). They revived and modified a procedure, described initially by Deese (1959), in which subjects are initially exposed to lists of semantic associates (e.g., *candy, sour, sugar, bitter, good, taste,* and so forth) that all

---

Requests for reprints should be addressed to Daniel L. Schacter, Department of Psychology, Harvard University, 33 Kirkland St., Cambridge, MA 02138, USA.

Supported by grant AGO8441 from the National Institute on Aging and a grant from the Human Frontiers Science Program. These experiments were conducted by the first author under the supervision of the second author as part of a senior honours thesis at Harvard College. We thank Carrie Racine for assistance with the research, and thank Marc Hauser, Larry Jacoby, Wilma Koutstaal, Michelle Leichtman, Kathleen McDermott, and Anthony Wagner for helpful comments and discussion.

converge on a nonpresented theme word or "false target" (e.g. *sweet*). Deese found that subjects frequently introduced the false target on a recall test. Roediger and McDermott replicated Deese's findings concerning false recall and extended them to false recognition, showing exceptionally high levels of false alarms (e.g. 80%) to the theme word.

In studies of ageing memory using the Deese/Roediger-McDermott paradigm, Norman and Schacter (1997) and Tun, Wingfield, Rosen, and Blanchard (1998) reported that older adults are relatively more susceptible to false recall and false recognition than are younger adults: Older adults showed lower levels of veridical recall or recognition than did younger adults, together with either equivalent or higher levels of false recall or false recognition.

Even more striking age differences in false recognition have been reported by Koutstaal and Schacter (1997). In their paradigm, younger and older adults studied detailed coloured pictures from various categories. When given a recognition test after a 3-day delay, older adults showed considerably higher levels of false recognition to nonpresented pictures from studied categories than did younger adults. The age differences were most pronounced when subjects studied large numbers of pictures (18) from a given category, with older adults showing approximately twice as many false alarms (60–70%) as younger adults (e.g. 25–35%).

Why are older adults sometimes more susceptible to robust false recall and recognition than are younger adults? Although a variety of factors are likely to play some role (for review and discussion, see Schacter, Koutstaal, & Norman, 1997c), one probable contributor to the observed effects involves age-related deficits in the ability to recall specific details of previously studied items, together with increased reliance on memory for general features of studied items—what has been termed gist (Brainerd, Reyna, & Kneer, 1995; Reyna & Brainerd, 1995) or general similarity information (Hintzman & Curran, 1994). Several investigators have argued that false recall and recognition in the Deese/Roediger-McDermott paradigm depends, at least in part, on memory for the semantic gist of studied items (cf. Brainerd & Reyna, 1998; Payne, Elie, Blackwell, & Neuschatz, 1996; Schacter, Norman, & Koutstaal, 1998a; Schacter, Verfaellie, & Pradere, 1996b). Similarly, Koutstaal and Schacter (1997) hypothesised that false alarms to nonpresented categorised pictures reflects reliance on gist or general similarity information. Previous studies have shown that older adults have difficulties recollecting specific details of previously studied information (e.g. Glisky, Polster, & Routhieaux, 1995; McIntyre & Craik, 1987; Schacter, Osowiecki, Kaszniak, Kihlstrom, & Valdiserri, 1994), relying instead on encoding of generic features of target materials (Rabinowitz, Craik, & Ackerman, 1982).

Schacter et al. (1997c; see also Reyna & Brainerd, 1995; Schacter et al. 1998a) noted that impaired recollection of item-specific information, together with preserved retention of general similarity or gist information, should lead to a relatively greater susceptibility to robust false recall and recognition in older than in younger adults. This hypothesis is supported by findings from Norman and Schacter (1997), who probed qualitative features of true and false memories with the memory characteristics questionnaire (MCQ) developed by Johnson, Foley, Suengas, and Raye (1988). Elderly adults showed less discrimination between studied items and related lure words than did younger adults on MCQ categories concerned with perceptual and contextual features of remembered items. If the elderly have less access to item-specific information than do younger adults, then it follows that they would have less ability to discriminate presented items from nonpresented items based on that information.

Two recent studies have shown that increasing the availability of item specific information by repeatedly presenting lists of semantic associates can produce significant reductions in levels of false recall and false recognition. McDermott (1996) found that college students showed increased veridical recall rates and decreased false recall rates across five study/test trials: the proportion of items correctly recalled nearly doubled across trials, and the proportion of items falsely recalled was reduced by nearly one-half. In a study comparing true and false recognition in anmesic patients and normal controls, Schacter, Verfaellie, Anes, and Racine (1998b) observed across-trial patterns in the control group that were similar to those reported by McDermott, with true recognition increasing and false recognition decreasing across trials. However, amnesic patients failed to show any evidence of decreasing false recognition with increasing study/test trials; in fact, there were trends for increasing false recognition across trials in the amnesic group.

The overall pattern of results from McDermott (1996) and Schacter et al. (1998b) suggests that when healthy volunteers show increasing recollection of the items that actually appear on a particular list, they are also better able to remember which items did not appear, thereby reducing levels of false memories. As access to item-specific information builds across trials, subjects may rely less on gist or general similarity information and instead depend increasingly on their ability to remember information about specific items on the list. By contrast, Schacter et al. (1998b) suggested that amnesic patients retain little or no item-specific information that can be used to suppress the strengthening influence of gist information with increasing repetitions.

In the present experiments, we examine whether repeated presentation and testing of lists of semantic associates reduces false recall and recognition in older adults. We assume that repetition of associate lists increases the accessibility of *both* gist *and* item-specific information. We thus expect that, with repeated trials, elderly adults will increase their veridical recall and recognition rates because veridical memories can be enhanced both by gist and item-specific information. If, however, increasing levels of veridical recall and recognition across trials in elderly adults depend more on gist and less on item-specific information than in younger adults, then older adults should be less able than younger adults to use item-specific information to suppress false recognition across trials. By this view, older adults should show smaller repetition-related decreases in false recall and false recognition than younger adults. In the present study, we examine this possibility using false recall (Experiment 1) and false recognition (Experiment 2).

EXPERIMENT 1

In Experiment 1 we used the false recall paradigm reported previously by McDermott (1996). Elderly and young adults were presented with a 45-word list, consisting of three 15-word associate sets that were each related to a nonpresented related lure or false target (e.g. *table, sit, legs, seat, couch, desk, recliner, sofa, wood, cushion, swivel, stool, sitting, rocking, bench* for the false target *chair*). Study lists were presented in a blocked format, with all items of an associate set presented together. All subjects studied the same list five times, and after each list presentation completed a free recall test.

Method

Subjects

Twenty-nine Harvard Summer School students and Harvard undergraduates and 25 elderly subjects from the Boston/Cambridge area participated in the experiment. Elderly subjects were recruited via posters and fliers and were individually screened so as to exclude those with a history of alcoholism or substance abuse, any present or past treatment for a psychiatric illness, current treatment with psychoactive medications, drug toxicity, primary brain degenerative disorders, and brain damage sustained earlier from a known cause. Young subjects were recruited through sign-up sheets posted at Harvard University and were screened for current treatment with psychoactive medications. All subjects were native English speakers and had normal or corrected to normal vision and normal hearing. Each subject was paid $10/hour for his/her participation. The data from 5 young adults and 1 elderly adult who did not follow the testing procedures correctly were eliminated, and the data for the remaining 24 young adults (ages 17–25; mean age = 19.9; range of education = 11–17 years; mean years of education = 13.4) and 24 elderly adults (ages 60–75; mean age = 67.4; range of education = 12–19 years; mean years of education = 14.8) were included.

Materials and Design

Six of the 15-word associate sets used by Roediger and McDermott (1995) were used. These sets were divided into two 45-word lists, consisting of three 15 word associate sets per list (as in McDermott, 1996). Each subject listened to the 45-word list over a headset; words were presented in the same order for all 5 trials. All words of an associate set were presented together, with words in each set always presented in order of decreasing associative relatedness to the false target (i.e. most strongly to least strongly associated). Subjects listened to lists associated with either the false targets *chair, fruit,* and *mountain*, or with the false targets *cold, needle,* and *sleep*.

Subjects in each age group were randomly assigned to one of the two 45-word lists. The 15-word associate sets within these 45-word lists were presented in 3 separate orders (sets 1, 2, 3; sets 2, 3, 1; sets 3, 1, 2) to eliminate the possibility of presentation order effects. For each 45-word list, 4 subjects from each age group were assigned to each of these orders. Each of the five 45-word list presentations was followed by a free recall test.

Procedure

Subjects were tested individually. They were informed that they would be hearing a list of words presented a total of five times, and that after each presentation of the words they would be asked to recall as many words as possible. Study list words were recorded by a female speaker and were presented auditorily at a rate of one word every 2 seconds. The three lists were presented as one long list, without a break between them. After study list presentation, subjects were told to write down all of the words they could remember from the list, and to try to include only those that they were confident appeared on the list. Four minutes were provided for this free recall test. The same study-test sequence was repeated on each of the five trials.

Two scoring systems were used: In the lenient scoring system, small alterations such as "sleepy" or "fruits" for the words "sleep" and "fruit" were counted as true or false recalls for presented words and related lures, respectively; in the strict scoring system, these words were not scored as true or false recalls.

Results

Mean proportions of studied items (true targets) and related lures (false targets) were recorded for each trial. There were only slight differences between the lenient and strict scoring systems, and there were no substantial differences in statistical analyses between the two systems, so all results are reported using the lenient scoring system. Intrusions of items other than the false targets were virtually non-existent for both age groups (1 % or less of total responses) and so are not reported.

Veridical Recall

As Fig. 1 shows, younger adults recalled more true targets than did older adults on the first trial, both groups showed an increase in veridical recall across the five trials, and the magnitude of the increase was greater in younger than older adults (increasing from a difference of .11 in the first trial to a difference of .25 in the fifth trial). An overall ANOVA performed on the veridical recall rates with Age as a between-subjects variable and Trial as a within-subjects variable confirms these patterns, showing a significant effect of Age [$F(1,46) = 36.49$, $MSe = 0.064$ $P < .0001$], Trial [$F(4,184) = 257.17$, $MSe = 0.005$, $P < .0001$], and a Trial × Age interaction [$F(4,184) = 10.95$, $MSe = 0.005$, $P < .0001$]. Separate ANOVAs show significant effects of Trial on veridical recall for both elderly adults [$F(1,115) = 24.31$, $MSe = 0.017$, $P < .0001$] and young adults [$F(1,115) = 56.98$, $MSe = 0.017$, $P < .0001$], and a focused contrast shows that the young adults remembered significantly more true targets on Trial 1 as compared to the elderly adults [$F(1,23) = 11.67$, $MSe = 0.009$, $P < .003$].

False Recall

On Trial 1, older and younger adults showed the same rate of false recall (.38). For the young, this false recall rate was approximately equal to their rate of veridical recall (.37). However, older adults intruded a marginally greater proportion of false targets compared to the true targets they correctly recalled [.28; $F(1,23) = 2.64$, $MSe = 0.04$, $P < .13$].

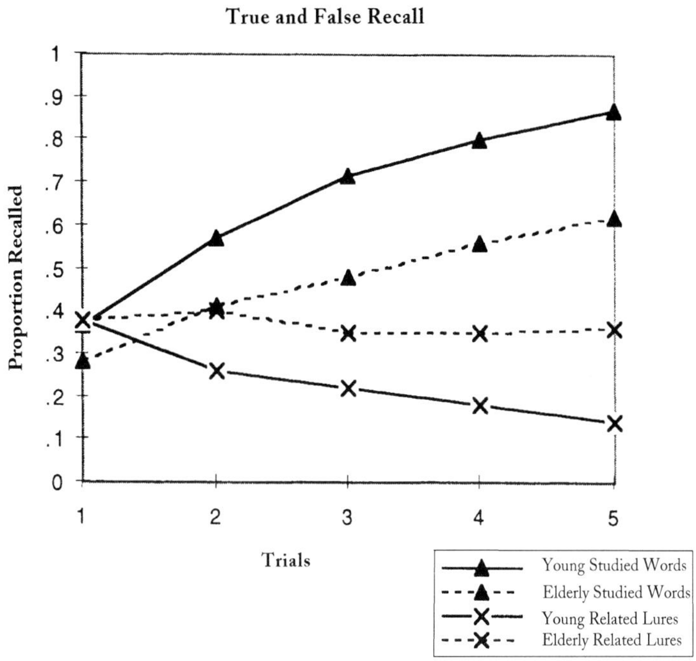

Fig. 1. *Proportion of studied words and related lures recalled as a function of study/test trials in Experiment 1. Both the young and elderly adults increased their veridical recall across the trials, although the elderly adults showed a more modest increase than did the young adults. The young adults reduced their false recall across the trials, whereas the elderly adults did not show any such reduction.*

As Fig. 1 shows, although older and younger adults began with identical false recall rates, the young adults sharply reduced their false recall responses across trials, from .38 on Trial 1 to .14 on Trial 5. In contrast, however, elderly adults continued to intrude similar proportions of false targets across the five trials, with no indication of any across-trials reductions. An overall ANOVA shows an effect of Age that approaches significance [$F(1,46) = 3.10$, $MSe = 2.97$, $P < .09$], an effect of Trial [$F(4,184) = 3.38$, $MSe = 0.34$, $P < .02$] and a Trial × Age interaction that approaches significance [$F(4,184) = 2.11$, $MSe = 0.34$, $P < .09$]. Separate ANOVAs that were performed for younger and older groups indicate a significant effect of Trial on false recall rates for young adult [$F(4,115) = 2.43$, $MSe = 0.73$, $P = .05$] but no such effect for the elderly adults [$F < 1$]. A focused contrast reveals that, by the fifth trial elderly adults showed significantly higher false recall rates than did young adults [$F(1,23) = 8.36$, $MSe = 0.638$, $P < .009$.

DISCUSSION

The results of Experiment 1 replicate the findings of McDermott (1996), with young adults showing a significant reduction in false recall across trials. Such a reduction suggests that the young adults are able to acquire increasing amounts of item-specific information across trials, and to use that information to suppress some of their false recollection responses. in contrast, the elderly adults did not show any reduction in false recall across trials, thereby suggesting that they may be less capable of using item-specific information to distinguish between presented words and related, but nonpresented, false targets.

Impaired acquisition of item-specific information not only contributes to impaired suppression of false recall, but could also be responsible for the elderly adults' smaller across-trial increases in veridical recall. Whereas young adults presumably rely on both gist and item-specific information to increase veridical recall across the trials, elderly adults may rely more on gist information, leading to more modest increases in veridical recall compared to younger adults.

Results from Trial 1 revealed patterns similar to those reported previously by Norman and Schacter (1997) and Tun et al. (1998), who reported that younger adults recalled more studied items than did older adults, whereas older adults produced as many (Tun et al.) or more (Norman & Schacter) related lures than did younger adults. Although the observed Trial 1 effects did not attain statistical significance, this is probably attributable to the small number of observations per subject for the false recall analysis: There were only three false targets that could possibly be intruded. The relatively small number of observations may also be why the Age × Trial interaction in false recall achieved only marginal levels of significance. To increase the numbers of observations, and to explore the generality of the age-related effects we did observe, Experiment 2 examines across trial suppression of false recognition in older and younger adults.

EXPERIMENT 2

In Experiment 2, we used a recognition paradigm similar to the one described by Schacter et al. (1998b). Subjects initially heard a 90-word list (consisting of six 15 word associate sets) and were then given an old/new recognition test of previously studied words (true targets), related lures (false targets), and unrelated lures (target controls); as in Experiment 1, there were a total of 5 study/test trials. We hypothesised that young and elderly adults would show the same general trends as in Experiment 1: An increase in veridical recognition across trials for both the young and elderly adults—possibly with a more pronounced increase for the young adults—together with a greater decrease in false recognition across trials for the young adults than for the elderly adults.

Method

Subjects

Twenty-two Harvard Summer School students and Harvard undergraduates and 21 elderly adults from the Boston/Cambridge area participated in the experiment. All participants were recruited, screened, and reimbursed in the same manner as described in Experiment 1. The data from two undergraduates and one elderly adult who did not conform to testing procedures were eliminated. Data were analysed for the remaining 20 undergraduates (ages 17–25; mean age = 19.3; range of education = 11–18 years; mean years of education = 13.6) and 20 elderly adults (ages 60–75; mean = 68.2; range of education = 12–20 years; mean years of education = 14.6). None of the subjects participated in both Experiments 1 and 2.

Materials and Design

Twelve of the Roediger and McDermott (1995) 15-word associate sets were used in this experiment. The sets were divided to form two 90-word lists, each consisting of 6 associate sets. Each participant listened to the same 90-word list, with the words presented in the same order, a total of 5 times. All words of an associate set were presented together. Subjects either listened to lists associated to the false targets *chair, fruit, mountain, window, soft,* and *rough,* or to lists associated with the false targets *cold, needle, sleep, sweet, music,* and *thief.* These lists included the three associate sets used in the previous recall experiment; the three added sets were chosen from those that produced the highest rates of false recognition in a previous norming study (ranging from .69–.84 false recognition; see Stadler, Roediger, & McDermott, in press). Lists also were designed to avoid overlap in the themes of multiple associate sets (e.g the *doctor* set was not used because many of its words could also be associated with the words in the *needle* set).

Subjects in each age group were randomly assigned to the two 90-word lists. The 15-word associate sets within these 90-word lists were presented in 2 different orders. The words were presented at a rate of 1 word/2 seconds, as in

Experiment 1, in decreasing order of association (most- to least-highly associated).

Each 90-word list presentation was followed by a 36-word recognition test in which words were shown, in a different random order for each subject, on a computer screen (Chicago font; 48-point). This recognition test included 18 true targets (words #1, #8, and #10 from the 6 presented Roediger & McDermott 1995, associate sets), 6 false targets, and 12 unrelated lures consisting of 6 words from nonpresented associate sets (word #6 on each of 6 lists; true target controls) and 6 words that were false targets for the 6 nonpresented lists (false target controls). Results indicated slightly more false alarms to false target controls (.14) than to true target controls [.11; $F = 2.9$, $P = .087$], and no interactions between Type of Unrelated Lure and Age, Trial, or Age × Trial [Fs < 1]. Thus, for purposes of analysis we combined the true target controls and false target controls into a single unrelated lure category.

Each of the five recognition tests used a different set of unrelated lures; words were taken from unused Roediger and McDermott (1995) lists and from lists created by Stadler et al. (in press). The order of the recognition tests was counterbalanced across subjects.

Procedure

Subjects were tested individually. They were informed that they would be hearing a list of words a total of five times and that they would be asked to take a recognition test after each of these five presentations of the list. During study list presentation, words were presented auditorily at a rate of 1 word per 2 seconds, as in Experiment 1. Also as in Experiment 1, study list words were presented as a single list with no breaks between the various associate sets. Immediately following list presentation, subjects were given instructions for the recognition test. They were informed that some words might appear on multiple recognition tests and other words might appear on only one test. They were instructed to make their old/new recognition judgements based only on whether or not the word had been auditorily presented, not on whether or not it had appeared on a previous recognition test. There was no time limit for the recognition test; each word remained on the screen until the participant made his or her response, at which point the next word appeared on the screen.

Results

Figure 2 displays the proportions of "old" responses to true targets, false targets, and unrelated lures as a function of trials. Table 1 displays the results of signal detection analyses that we used to provide estimates of sensitivity and bias as a function of the main experimental manipulations. We consider the overall analyses of recognition first and then turn to the signal detection analyses.

Veridical Recognition

As shown in Fig. 2, younger adults correctly recognised a greater proportion of true targets on the first trial than did elderly adults, as confirmed by a focused contrast performed on Trial 1 hit rates in younger and older adults [$F(1,19) = 7.78$, MSe = 0.056, $P < .0.1$]. However, by the second trial, there were no significant differences between the hit rates of young and elderly adults, probably because performance in both groups increased to near-ceiling levels. An ANOVA revealed a significant effect of Trial [$F(4,152) = 34.43$, MSe = 0.009, $P < .0001$], no interaction effect of Age [$F(1,38) < 1$], and a nonsignificant Trial × Age interaction [$F(4,152) = 1.79$, $MSe = 0.009$, $P > .13$].

Analyses of corrected recognition scores that were obtained by subtracting false alarms rates to unrelated lures from hit rates to true targets reveal that elderly adults showed less accurate recognition than did young adults across trials, perhaps because ceiling effects in the hit rate data are now removed. An overall ANOVA indicates main effects of Age [$F(1,38) = 4.08$, $MSe = 0.155$, $P = .05$]. Trial [$F(4,152) = 17.57$, $MSe = 0.036$, $P < .0001$], and a nonsignificant Trial × Age interaction [$F(4,152) < 1$]. Separate ANOVAs indicate that both young and elderly adults significantly increased their corrected recognition scores across trials (for young, [$F(4,95) = 7.05$, $MSe = 0.054$, $P < .0001$; for elderly, $F(4,95) = 5.96$, $MSe = 0.066$, $P = .0003$],

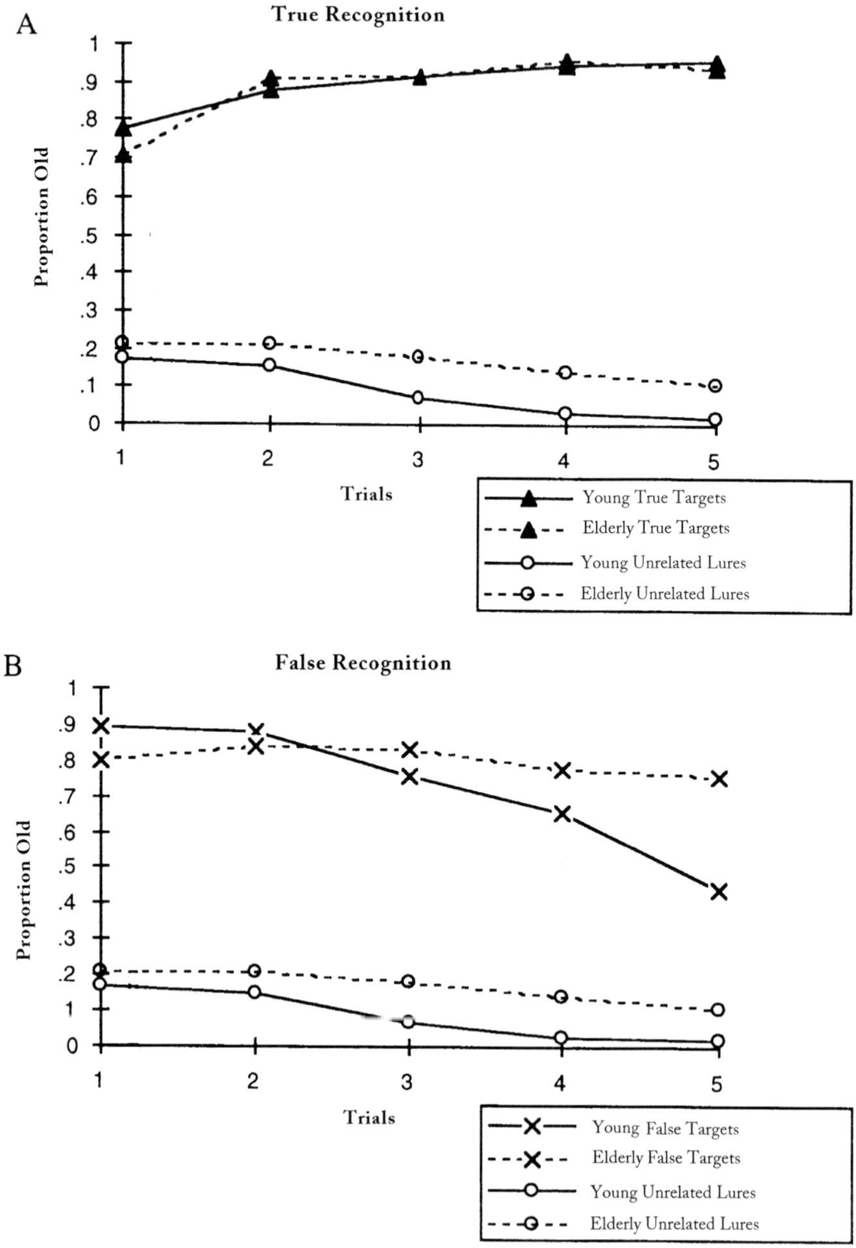

Fig. 2. *Proportions of old responses to true targets (Panel A), false targets (Panel B), and unrelated lures (Panels A and B) in young and elderly adults as a function of study/test trial in Experiment 2. Both the young and elderly adults showed an increase in true recognition across trials, whereas only the young adults demonstrated a reduction in false recognition across trials.*

Table 1. *Signal Detection Analyses of Sensitivity (A') and Bias (B''_D) as a Function of Study/Test Trials in Young and Elderly Adults*

Hits compared to Unrelated False Alarms (Item-specific Memory)

	Young Adults		*Elderly Adults*	
Trial	*A'*	B''_D	*A'*	B''_D
1	.843	.215	.805	.213
2	.872	−.029	.886	−.082
3	.939	−.033	.903	−.178
4	.963	−.055	.93	−.118
5	.968	−.037	.941	−.065

Hits compared to Related False Alarms (Item-specific Memory)

	Young Adults		*Elderly Adults*	
Trial	*A'*	B''_D	*A'*	B''_D
1	.529	−.81	.571	−.599
2	.623	−.895	.541	−.906
3	.679	−.911	.585	−.93
4	.751	−.912	.707	−.916
5	.836	−.795	.695	−.924

Related False Alarms compared to Novel False Alarms (Gist Memory)

	Young Adults		*Elderly Adults*	
Trial	*A'*	B''_D	*A'*	B''_D
1	.898	.039	.815	.099
2	.886	.168	.821	.118
3	.885	.419	.849	.199
4	.878	.693	.842	.344
5	.808	.871	.885	.422

although young adults maintained higher corrected recognition rates than did elderly adults across all trials.

False recognition

On Trial 1, both groups of subjects made similar proportions of "old" responses to false targets, although there was a trend for fewer false recognition responses in the older adults. However, a focused contrast indicates no significant difference between the false recognition rates of the young and elderly adults [$F(1,19) = 1.23$, $MSe = 0.056$, $P > .28$].

However, although younger and older adults were reasonably well equated on Trial 1 with regard to their overall false recognition rates, young adults showed a significant decrease in false recognition rates across trials [$F(4,95) = 13.99$, $MSe = 0.048$, $P < .0001$], whereas elderly adults did not [$F(4,95) < 1$]. An overall ANOVA with Age as a between-subjects variable and Trial as a within-subjects variable indicates no effect of Age [$F(1,38) = 2.19$, $MSe = 0.158$, $P > .14$], a significant effect of Trial [$F(4,152) = 19.93$, $MSe = 0.02$, $P < .0001$], and most importantly, a significant Trial × Age interaction [$F(4,152) = 13.39$, $MSe = 0.02$, $P < .0001$].

When recognition scores were corrected for the general tendency to call an item "old" by subtracting "old" responses to unrelated lures from "old" responses to false targets, the same pattern was observed, with decreasing false recognition rates across trials for young adults [$F(4,95) = 4.12$, $MSe = 0.08$, $P < .005$], and no change across trials for elderly adults [$F < 1$]. An overall ANOVA performed on these corrected false recognition rates shows no effect of Age [$F(1,38) < 1$], or Trial [$F(4,152) = 1.90$, $MSe = 0.05$, $P > .11$]. along with a significant Trial × Age interaction [$F(4,152) = 5.63$, $MSe = 0.05$, $P < .0004$].

It should also be noted that both younger and older adults showed across-trial trends in false recognition of true and false target controls. Both age groups showed significant reductions in their false recognition responses to unrelated lures across the trials, and the degree of this decrease was approximately equal for the two age groups. An ANOVA performed on the combined data from true and false target controls showed no effect of Age [$F(1,38) < 1$], an effect of Trial [$F(4,152) = 6.58$, $MSe = 0.022$, $P < .0001$], and no Trial × Age interaction [$F(4,152) < 1$].

Signal Detection Analyses

To determine whether the patterns of effects described above are attributable to changes in sensitivity or response bias, signal detection analyses were conducted, following the procedures used by Koutstaal and Schacter (1997) and Schacter et al. (1998b). A' is used as an estimate of sensitivity and B''_D is used as an estimate of response bias (see Donaldson, 1993; Snodgrass & Corwin, 1988).

Values of A' can range between 0 and 1.00. Higher values indicate greater sensitivity, with .50 indicating chance performance. B"$_D$ can range between − 1.00 and + 1.00, with − 1.00 signifying extremely liberal responding, and + 1.00 signifying extremely conservative responding. Because measures of A' and B"$_D$ are undefined with hit rates of 0 or 1, the data were first transformed, as recommended by Snodgrass and Corwin, by setting $P(x) = (x + .5)/N + 1$ rather than $P(x) = x/N$. When subjects showed below-chance sensitivity (A' < .5, signifying that hits < false alarms), modified formulas given by Aaronsen and Watts (1987) were used. It should be noted that signal detection analysis is based on different underlying assumptions than is the foregoing corrected recognition analysis (for discussion, see Snodgrass & Corwin). Thus, the signal detection analyses reported next provide a different perspective on our data than do the corrected recognition analyses, rather than simply providing additional information.

Three different types of signal detection analyses were performed. The first analysis compares "old" responses to true targets (hits) and to true target controls (unrelated lure false alarms), providing measures of item-specific true recognition that we call A' unrelated and B"$_D$ unrelated. The second analysis compares "old" responses to true targets with "old" responses to false targets (related false alarms), providing different measures of item-specific true recognition that assess participants' abilities to distinguish between true targets and false targets. We call these measures A' related and B"$_D$ related. The third set of analyses compares "old" responses to false targets with "old" responses to false target controls. These measures provide an index of subjects' willingness to rely on gist information, despite any counterveiling influences of item-specific memory; we call them A' gist and B"$_D$ gist. Table 1 displays A' and B"$_D$ values for each of these three comparisons.

Hits Compared to Unrelated False Alarms (Item-specific Memory). As Table 1 shows, A' unrelated did not differ significantly between the elderly and young adult groups (perhaps because of ceiling effects), but did increase across trials. An ANOVA shows a nonsignificant effect of Age [$F(1,38) < 1$], a significant effect of Trial [$F(4,152) = 13.56$, $MSe = .01$, $P < .0001$], and no Trial × Age interaction, [$F(4,152) < 1$], B"$_D$ also did not differ significantly between the two age groups. An ANOVA indicates no significant effect of Age [$F < 1$], along with a significant effect of Trial [$F(4,152) = 3.9$, $MSe = 0.18$, $P < .005$], and no Trial × Age interaction [$F < 1$]. Across trials, young and elderly adults appear to have been using similar criteria for their decisions, and both became modestly more liberal in their responding across the trials.

Hits Compared to Related False Alarms (Item-specific Memory). A' related values indicate that on the first trial, both young and elderly adults had little ability to distinguish studied words from related lures, with A' values hovering near the chance level of .50 (.53 for young adults and .57 for elderly adults; Table 1). A' related generally increased for both groups across trials, although somewhat more steeply in the young group, reaching .84 for the young adults and .70 for the elderly adults by the fifth trial. An overall ANOVA shows no effect of Age [$F(1,38) = 2.35$, $MSe = 0.06$, $P > .13$], an effect of Trial [$F(4,152) = 14.39$, $MSe = 0.02$, $P < .0001$], and a nonsignificant Trial × Age interaction [$F(4,152) = 1.87$, $MSe = 0.02$, $P > .11$.

Values of B"$_D$ related show that when "old" responses to false targets are treated as false alarms, there is generally increasingly liberal responding across trials for both young and elderly adults. The elderly actually show a stronger trend of increasingly liberal responding; on Trial 1, they responded slightly more conservatively than the young but by Trial 5 were responding more liberally than the young. An ANOVA supports these observations, showing no significant effect of Age [$F(1,38) < 1$], along with a significant effect of Trial, [$F(4,152) = 7.69$, $MSe = 0.04$, $P < .0001$, and a significant Trial × Age interaction [$F(4,152) = 3.6$, $MSe = 0.04$, $P < .008$].

Related False Alarms Compared to Unrelated False Alarms (Gist Memory). In this analysis, we treat false alarms to related lures as a form of memory for the "gist" of previously studied items. A' gist values indicate that whereas young adults were more sensitive to gist influences on the first trial (.89) than were the elderly (.82), this trend reversed across trials, with the elderly showing higher levels of A' gist on the last trial (.89) than did the young (.81). An ANOVA supports this observation, showing no effect of Age [$F(1,38) < 1$] or Trial, [$F(4,152) < 1$] together with a significant Trial × Age interaction [$F(4,152) = 4.53$, $MSe = 0.01$, $P > .002$]. Thus, even though older adults were somewhat better able to distinguish between studied words and related lures with repetition (as indicated by the preceding analysis of A' related), they were nonetheless more willing than younger adults to rely on gist information as repetitions increased.

B''_D gist values increased across trials for both younger and older adults, indicating a trend for increasingly conservative responding, but the trend was more pronounced in younger than older adults, with the young showing much more conservative responding by the last trial (.87) than did the elderly (.42). Consistent with these observations, an overall ANOVA shows no effect for Age [$F(1,38) = 1.99$, $MSe = 1.02$, $P > .16$], along with a significant effect of Trial, [$F(4,152) = 16.55$, $MSe = 0.14$, $P < .0001$], and a significant Trial × Age interaction, [$F(4,152) = 4.03$, $MSe = 0.14$, $P < .02$]. Thus, across trials young adults tightened their retrieval criteria to a greater extent than did elderly adults.

Discussion

Experiment 2 extended the major results of Experiment 1 from recall to recognition. As expected, both older and younger adults showed significantly increased veridical recognition across trials. However, whereas in Experiment 1 young adults increased veridical recall to a greater extent than did elderly adult, Experiment 2 there were equivalent increases in veridical recognition for the two age groups (although the young adults had somewhat higher rates of correct recognition across all trials). This difference might indicate that item-specific memory is more beneficial for free recall than recognition: Access to general semantic information may not always be adequate for free recall of a word, so that readier access to item-specific information may result in a more rapid build-up of veridical recall across trials. By contrast, detailed item-specific information may be less important for recognition, where gist information may be sufficient for determining that a word on the recognition test had been presented at study.

Consistent with our major hypothesis, the trends for false recognition paralleled those in Experiment 1: Young adults reduced false recognition responses across trials whereas elderly adults did not. The young adults showed a decrease from an initial false recognition rate of .89 to a rate of .44 on the fifth trial; in contrast, elderly adults began with a rate of .80 and ended with a rate of .76. These trends remained when corrected false recognition scores were used, with young adults showing a decrease in corrected false recognition scores from .72 (Trial 1) to .42 (Trial 5), and the elderly showing a nonsignificant increase in corrected false recognition from .59 (Trial 1) to .65 (Trial 5).

The signal detection data suggest that a reduction in gist influences at least partially accounts for the observed suppression of false recognition in young adults. Across trials, the young adults showed decreasing influence of gist memory, as indicated by the gist A' measure, whereas the elderly actually show increased levels of gist A' across trials. Thus, younger adults were able to use increasing item specific information to counteract or oppose (Dywan & Jacoby, 1990) the corresponding build-up of gist influences, whereas elderly adults were largely unable to do so, instead responding mainly on the basis of gist information. The idea that older adults rely heavily on the increasing influence of gist representations also helps to explain why the elderly were able to decrease their false recognition responses to unrelated lures across trials to the same extent as the young adults. Whereas increasing gist information does not help older adults to rule out related lure words as presented items, it does help them to conclude that entirely unrelated items were not presented, thus leading to the decreases in false recognition to unrelated lure words.

In addition to increasing reliance on gist information, two of the three signal detection analyses (B_D'' related and B''_D gist) revealed that across trials, older adults used increasingly liberal response criteria compared to younger adults. Thus, changes in both sensitivity and bias are implicated in the pattern of across trials age differences we observed.

The results of Trial 1 in Experiment 2 were somewhat unexpected, with the elderly adults showing a trend for lower overall rates of false recognition than the young adults. Although these effects were not statistically significant, whereas Trial 1 analyses of true recognition did reveal significant age effects, this is probably because there were more observations in the true recognition data (18 items per subject) than in the false recognition data (6 items per subject). It is possible that the trend for reduced Trial 1 false recognition in older adults is attributable to the fact that there were no breaks between the study lists, in contrast to previous experiments that showed similar or greater levels of false recognition in older than younger adults (Norman & Schacter, 1997; Tun et al., 1998). Instead, all six associate sets were presented together to form one continuous 90-word list. With so many words presented at a rapid rate, elderly adults initially may have been less able to encode as much gist (or item-specific) information as the young adults, leading them to show trends for reduced false recognition and significantly reduced veridical recognition on the first trial. This analysis might also apply to some extent in Experiment 1, where older adults and younger adults showed similar levels of false recall, even though some previous evidence indicates higher levels of false recall in older than younger adults (Norman & Schacter, 1997; but see Tun et al., 1998, for data similar to ours).

GENERAL DISCUSSION

The results of our experiments support the hypothesis that elderly adults are more reliant on gist influences than are younger adults, and that elderly adults have more difficulty than younger adults using item-specific information to reduce false recognition. Both experiments showed clearly that elderly adults continued to make similar levels of false recall and false recognition responses across trials, whereas younger adults showed sharp reductions in both types of false memories. In Experiment 2, signal detection analyses suggested that the elderly adults' increased susceptibility to false memories stems from a combination of increased sensitivity to gist information and more lenient retrieval criteria.

The observation that repetition of target items has different effects on false memories in younger and older adults complements recent work by Jacoby (1999; see also, Jacoby, this issue) showing a related phenomenon. When instructed to respond "yes" to words they had heard earlier, and "no" to words they had seen earlier, false alarms to previously read words in younger adults decreased as a function of prior study list repetitions. By contrast, false alarms to previously read words increased as a function of study list repetitions in older adults. Thus, older adults fail to use recollection of item-specific information that accrues from repetition as a basis for rejecting previously studied lure words in Jacoby's (1999) procedure, and failed to use such information as a basis for rejecting nonstudied but related lure words in our paradigm.

Our results are also broadly similar to those reported previously by Schacter et al. (1998b), who used a similar multi-trial paradigm to examine false recognition suppression in amnesic patients and matched control subjects. Schacter et al. found that across repeated study/test trials, patients with amnesic syndromes resulting from damage to the medial temporal lobes (i.e, anoxia, encephalitis) showed flat or fluctuating levels of false recognition; Korsakoff amnesic patients actually showed increased false recognition across trials. While both types of patients also showed some across-trial increases in veridical recognition, Schacter et al. attributed those increases to strengthening gist representations rather than to a build-up of item-specific information. Schacter et al. suggested that both amnesic subgroups had difficulty remembering item-specific information, thus accounting for their failures to suppress false recognition, and that the Korsakoff patients in addition had problems with strategic monitoring and control processes that may result from frontal lobe damage (for review and discussion, see Schacter, 1987;

Shimamura, 1995). Therefore, as the Korsakoff patients strengthened gist representations across trials, but without a corresponding increase in item-specific information and with impaired retrieval monitoring processes, they showed significantly increased false recognition rates.

Previous studies of ageing memory have implicated both medial temporal and frontal regions in age-related memory changes (e.g., Glisky et al., 1995; Grady et al., 1995; Henkel, Johnson, & De Leonardis, 1998; Moscovitch & Winocur, 1992; Schacter, Savage, Alpert, Rauch, & Alpert, 1996a). Although we have no direct information concerning possible brain system correlates of the effects we observed, future studies using neuroimaging techniques, which have already proven helpful in the analysis of false recognition (e.g. Schacter, Buckner, Koutstaal, Dale, & Rosen, 1997a), could provide relevant information. Note also that when viewed in light of the performance of Korsakoff amnesics—who showed significant across-trial increases in false recognition—the fact that older adults are able to maintain constant levels of false recognition across trials, rather than showing increases, indicates that they are capable of some degree of false recognition suppression, although considerably less than that shown by younger adults.

Although we have emphasised that impaired suppression of false recognition reflects age-related increases in reliance on gist information (cf., Reyna & Brainerd, 1995), older adults' failures to reduce their false recall and recognition responses may also stem, at least in part, from a deficit in source memory. Source memory confusions may contribute to false recognition of semantic associates in either of two different ways. First, participants may generate a related lure word during study list presentation, and later have difficulty determining whether they actually heard the word or only thought about it. Second, because subjects were given multiple test trials as well as multiple study trials, false targets were that were produced on an earlier free recall test (Experiment 1), or that appeared on a prior recognition test (Experiment 2), may be misattributed to a study list. Given their difficulties on source memory tasks (e.g. Bartlett, Strater, & Fulton, 1991; Dywan & Jacoby, 1990; Henkel et al., 1998; McIntyre & Craik, 1987; Multhaup, 1995; Schacter et al. 1994; for review, see Spencer & Raz, 1995), elderly adults may be more susceptible to source confusions arising during study list presentation, or might be more susceptible to test-induced source confusions, having more difficulty than younger adults in determining whether a false target was written on a previous recall test, encountered visually on a previous recognition test, or actually heard during study list presentation (see Schacter et al., 1998b, for a discussion of similar issues with amnesic patients).

The first possibility (study list-induced source confusions) is difficult to address experimentally, although relevant evidence has been presented (cf. Koutstaal & Schacter, 1997; Mather, Henkel, & Johnson, 1997; McDermott, 1997; Norman & Schacter, 1997). The second possibility (test-induced source confusions) can be addressed by further experiments in which the number of study list presentations is varied without any intervening recall or recognition tests. If elderly adults are still unable to suppress their false responses under such conditions, then test-induced source memory confusion can be ruled out as a major contributor to the effects observed here. If, on the other hand, the elderly are able to suppress false recall or recognition under such conditions, then a role for test-induced source memory deficits would be implicated.

However, even if the latter outcome were obtained, and test-induced source confusions are a contributor to elderly adults' failure to reduce false recall and recognition across trials, such an outcome would still be broadly consistent with our hypothesis that elderly adults are relatively impaired in memory for item-specific as compared to gist information. If the elderly adults encode less item-specific information, and are more reliant on general features of the studied items, then presumably they are less able to determine whether a word was heard at study or seen at test (either on a computer screen or on their own recall sheet; cf. Schacter, Koutstaal, Johnson, Gross, & Angell, 1997b).

Our findings contrast sharply with two other recent sets of studies from our laboratory in which older adults have shown normal suppression of false recognition. Using the categorised pictures paradigm that previously produced large age-related increases in false recognition of novel pictures (Koutstaal & Schacter, 1997), Koutstaal, Schacter, Galluccio, and Stofer (in press) reported that false recognition was reduced significantly in both younger and older adults when subjects were given, at the time of study, distinctive verbal elaborators that emphasised unique aspects of each picture. Schacter, Israel, and Racine (1999) compared false recognition of Deese/Roediger-McDermott lists in an encoding condition where subjects hear and see study list words with an encoding condition in which subjects hear study list words and see a picture corresponding to each word. Both younger and older adults showed a significant reduction in false recognition of semantic associates after pictorial encoding compared to word encoding.

Why did older adults show normal suppression of false recognition in the studies of Koutstaal et al. (in press) and Schacter et al. (1999), and no suppression at all in our experiments? The source monitoring problems alluded to earlier may be relevant, because our paradigm allowed for a form of study/test source confusion that was not operative in the paradigms used by Koutstaal et al. and Schacter et al. Additional and possibly related clues are provided by a second experiment from Schacter et al. (1999). In the experiment that produced false recognition suppression after pictorial encoding in both younger and older adults, Schacter et al. manipulated picture versus word encoding on a between-groups basis. Likewise, in the Koutstaal et al. experiment with categorised pictures, the presence or absence of distinctive elaborators was manipulated between groups. By contrast, when Schacter et al. manipulated word versus picture encoding within-groups (i.e. for each participant, some word lists were studied with pictures and others as only words), neither younger nor older adults showed any suppression of false recognition after picture encoding compared to word encoding. Schacter et al. thus argued that false recognition suppression after picture encoding in the between-groups paradigm involves a global shift in responding produced by reliance on what they call a "distinctiveness heuristic": A mode of responding based on subjects' metamemorial awareness that recognition of studied items should be accompanied by recollection of distinctive details (i.e. pictorial information). After studying lists of words that are all accompanied by pictures, subjects require access to distinctive information before they are willing to call an item "old." The same sort of reasoning may apply to the between-groups suppression of false recognition observed by Koutstaal et al. (in press). By contrast, when some lists are studied with pictures and others with words, application of such a global heuristic cannot produce differential suppression of false recognition after picture encoding versus word encoding.

The foregoing observations raise the possibility that older adults can show normal suppression of false recognition when suppression is driven by a global shift in responding, such as the distinctiveness heuristic described by Schacter et al. (1999). Applying these ideas to the present experiments, false recognition suppression in our paradigm may involve mechanisms other than the distinctiveness heuristic or some similar global shift in responding. We have argued that across trial suppression of false recall and recognition depends on the build-up of item-specific information about studied lists: Younger subjects recollect more details of items that were presented with increasing repetitions, thereby allowing them to better determine which items did not appear on each study list; elderly adults are less able to do so. If this line of reasoning is correct, then it should be possible to demonstrate false recognition suppression in our paradigm, at least in younger adults, under conditions that are conceptually analogous to the within-group manipulation of picture vs. word encoding used by Schacter et al. (1999): Subjects study some lists five times, and other lists just once; after studying all lists, they are tested for true and false recognition. Under these conditions, false recognition suppression in the five repetition condition compared to the single repetition condition cannot be produced by a general shift in responding; it must involve access to specific items on specific lists. We would expect younger but not older adults to exhibit such effects.

On the other hand, it is logically possible that the suppression effect we observed in younger adults does reflect a general shift in responding, perhaps involving mechanisms analogous to a distinctiveness heuristic. But, in addition (as discussed earlier), the inclusion of false targets on recognition tests creates source monitoring problems that prevent older adults from usefully invoking the relevant heuristic. By this view, older adults might indeed show significant false recognition suppression under conditions in which one group of older adults receives a single exposure to the study lists prior to a recognition test and a separate group receives multiple study exposures before the recognition test. A global shift in responding could underlie whatever suppression effects occur under such conditions, and there would be no study/test source confusions that could prevent older adults from successfully using the relevant heuristic.

However, because the encoding conditions used in our experiments are rather impoverished, involving simple auditory presentation of word lists, any global suppression effects based on a distinctiveness heuristic are likely to be small. Unlike the picture encoding condition used by Schacter et al. (1999), repeated auditory presentation of word lists may not lead subjects to demand increasingly distinctive recollections before calling items "old". Perhaps by enriching the study context (e.g. having distinct sources present study words), it would be possible to create a situation in which repeated presentation of study lists leads subjects to demand increasingly distinctive recollections and thereby produces a global suppression effect. If our analysis of the suppression effects exhibited by older adults in the Koutstaal et al. (in press) and Schacter et al. (1999) studies is correct, then we would expect to observe significant suppression effects in older adults under such conditions.

Because we have invoked the phrase "false recognition suppression" throughout this article, it is perhaps worth noting that the term can be used in at least two different ways: (1) a theoretically neutral sense that is roughly equivalent to "false recognition reduction", simply describing the fact that false recognition rates are lower in one experimental condition than in another, and (2) a theoretically more loaded sense that refers to a process that actively counters or opposes gist-based false recognition influences that, if unchecked, would produce false recognition. Although we have used the term in both senses, we do not yet have direct evidence for the operation of an active suppression process. For instance, repetition of studied items might result in lower false recognition rates because repetition produces more differentiated representations of studied words, which in turn bear less similarity to nonstudied associates than do words that were studied only once (for discussion, see McClelland & Chappell, 1998; Schacter et al., 1998a). From this perspective, no active suppression may be necessary to produce reduced rates of false recall or recognition after repetition. Further experiments are needed to determine whether active suppression is involved in the repetition effects reported here.

In summary, we have found that older adults fail to exhibit suppression of false recall and recognition under conditions in which younger adults show robust suppression effects. Although the exact mechanisms underlying these age-related impairments remain to be elucidated, we believe that further exploration of the effects we have documented should provide useful insights into important but poorly understood aspects of cognitive ageing.

REFERENCES

Aaronsen, D., & Watts, B. (1987). Extensions of Grier's computational formulas for A" and B" to below-chance performance. *Psychological Bulletin, 102,* 439–442.

Bartlett, J.C., Strater, L., & Fulton, A. (1991). False recency and false fame of faces in young adulthood and old age. *Memory and Cognition, 19,* 177–188

Brainerd, C.L., & Reyna, V.F. (1998). When things that were not experienced are easier to "remember" than things that were not experienced. *Psychological Science, 9,* 484–489.

Brainerd, C.L., Reyna, V.F., & Kneer, R. (1995). False-recognition reversal: When similarity is distinctive. *Journal of Memory and Language, 34,* 157–185.

Craik, F.I.M., Anderson, N.D., Kerr, S.A., & Li, K.Z.H. (1995). Memory changes in normal aging.

In A.D. Baddeley, B.A. Wilson, & F.N. Watts (Eds.), *Handbook of memory disorders* (pp. 211–241). New York: Wiley.

Deese, J. (1959). On the prediction of occurrence of particular verbal intrusions in immediate recall. *Journal of Experimental Psychology, 58,* 17–22.

Donaldson, W. (1993). The role of decision processes in remembering and knowing. *Memory and Cognition, 24,* 523–533.

Dywan, J., & Jacoby, L. (1990). Effects of aging on source monitoring: Differences in susceptibility to false fame. *Psychology and Aging, 5,* 379–387.

Glisky, E.L., Polster, M.R., & Routhieaux, B. (1995). Double dissociation between item and source memory. *Neuropsychology, 9,* 229–235.

Grady, C.L., McIntosh, A.R., Horwitz, B., Maisog, J.M., Ungerleider, L.G., Mentis, M.J., Pietrini, P., Shapiro, M.B., & Haxby, J.V. (1995). Age-related reductions in human recognition memory due to impaired encoding. *Science, 269,* 218–221.

Henkel, L.A., Johnson, M.K., & De Leonardis, D.M. (1998). Aging and source memory: Cognitive processes and neuropsychological correlates. *Journal of Experimental Psychology: General, 127,* 251–268.

Hintzman, D.L. (1988). Judgments of frequency and recognition memory in a multiple-trace memory model. *Psychological Review, 95,* 528–551.

Hintzman, D.L., & Curran, T. (1994). Retrieval dynamics of recognition and frequency judgments: Evidence for separate processes of familiarity and recall. *Journal of Memory and Language, 33,* 17–18.

Isingrini, M., Fontaine, R., Taconnat, L., & Duportal, A. (1995). Aging and encoding in memory: False alarms and decision criteria in a word-pair recognition task. *International Journal of Aging and Human Development, 41,* 79–88.

Jacoby, L.L. (this issue). Deceiving the elderly: effects of accessibility bias in cued-recall performance. *Cognitive Neuropsychology, 16,* 417–436.

Jacoby, L.L. (1999). Ironic effects of repetition: Measuring age- related differences in memory. *Journal of Experimental Psychology: Learning, Memory, and Cognition, 25,* 3–22.

Johnson, M.K., Foley, M.A., Suengas, A.G., & Raye, C.L. (1988). Phenomenal characteristics of memories for perceived and imagined autobiographical events. *Journal of Experimental Psychology: General, 117,* 371–376

Koutstaal, W., & Schacter, D.L. (1997). Gist-based false recognition of pictures in older and younger adults. *Journal of Memory and Language, 37,* 555–583.

Koutstaal, W., Schacter, D.L., & Galluccio, L., & Stofer, K. (in press). Reducing gist-based false recognition in older adults: Encoding and retrieval manipulations. *Psychology and Aging.*

Light, L.L. (1991). Memory and aging: Four hypotheses in search of data. *Annual Review of Psychology, 42,* 333–376.

Mather, M., Henkel, L.A., & Johnson, M.K. (1997). Evaluating characteristics of false memories: Remember/know judgments and memory characteristics questionnaire compared. *Memory Cognition, 25,* 826–837.

McClelland, J.L., & Chappell, M. (1998). Familiarity breeds differentiation: A subjective-likelihood approach to the effects of experience in recognition memory. *Psychological Review, 105,* 724–760.

McDermott, K.B. (1996). The persistence of false memories in list recall. *Journal of Memory and Language, 35,* 212–230.

McDermott, K.B. (1997). Priming on perceptual implicit memory tests can be achieved through presentation of associates. *Psychonomic Bulletin and Review, 4,* 582–586.

McIntyre, J.S., & Craik, F.I.M. (1987). Age differences in memory for item and source information. *Canadian Journal of Psychology, 41,* 175–192.

Moscovitch, M., & Winocur, G. (1992). The neuropsychology of memory and aging. In F.I.M. Craik & T.A. Salthouse (Eds.), *The handbook of aging and cognition* (pp. 315–372). Hillsdale, NJ: Lawrence Erlbaum Associates.

Multhaup, K.S. (1995). Aging, source, and decision criteria: When false fame errors do and do not occur. *Psychology and Aging, 10,* 492–497.

Norman, K.A., & Schacter, D.L. (1997). False recognition in younger and older adults: Exploring the characteristics of illusory memories. *Memory and Cognition, 25,* 838–848.

Payne, D.G., Elic, C.J., Blackwell, J.M., & Neuschatz, J.S. (1996). Memory, illusions: Recalling, recognizing and recollecting events that never occurred. *Journal of Memory and Language, 35,* 261–285.

Rabinowitz, J.C., Craik, F.I.M., & Ackerman, B.P. (1982). A processing resource account of age differences in recall. *Canadian Journal of Psychology, 36,* 325–344.

Rankin, J.S., & Kausler, D.H. (1979). Adult age differences in false recognition. *Journal of Gerontology, 34,* 58–65.

Reyna, V.F., & Brainerd, C.J. (1995). Fuzzy-trace theory: An interim synthesis. *Learning and Individual Differences, 7,* 1–75.

Roediger, H.L., & McDermott, K.B. (1995). Creating false memories: Remembering words not presented in lists. *Journal of Experimental Psychology: Learning, Memory and Cognition, 21,* 803–814.

Schacter, D.L. (1987). Memory, amnesia, and frontal lobe dysfunction. *Psychobiology, 15,* 21–36.

Schacter, D.L., Buckner, R.L., Koutstaal, W., Dale, A.M., & Rosen, B.R. (1997a). Late onset of anterior prefrontal activity during true and false recognition: An event-related fMRI study. *NeuroImage, 6,* 259–269.

Schacter, D.L., Israel, L., & Racine, C. (1999): Suppressing false recognition in younger and older adults: The distinctiveness heuristic. *Journal of Memory and Language, 40,* 1–24.

Schacter, D.L., Koutstaal, W., Johnson, M.K., Gross, M.S., & Angell, K.A. (1997b). False recollection induced via photographs: A comparison of older and younger adults. *Psychology and Aging, 12,* 203–215.

Schacter, D.L., Koutstaal, W., & Norman, K.A. (1997c). False memories and aging. *Trends in Cognitive Science, 1,* 229–236.

Schacter, D.L., Norman, K.A., & Koutstaal, W. (1998a). The cognitive neuroscience of constructive memory. *Annual Review of Psychology, 49,* 289–318.

Schacter, D.L., Osowiecki, D., Kaszniak, A.W., Kihlstrom, J.F. & Valdiserri, M. (1994). Source memory: Extending the boundaries of age-related deficits. *Psychology and Aging, 9,* 81–89.

Schacter, D.L., Savage, C.R., Alpert, N.M., Rauch, S.L., & Alpert, N.S. (1996a). The role of hippocampus and frontal cortex in age-related memory changes: A PET study. *NeuroReport, 7,* 1165–1169.

Schacter, D.L., Verfaellie, M., Anes, M.D., & Racine, C. (1998b). When true recognition suppresses false recognition: Evidence from amnesic patients. *Journal of Cognitive Neuroscience, 10,* 668–679.

Schacter, D.L., Verfaellie, M., & Pradere, D. (1996b). The neuropsychology of memory illusions: False recall and recognition in amnesic patients. *Journal of Memory and Language, 35,* 319–334.

Shiffrin, R.M., Huber, D.E., & Marinelli, K. (1995). Effects of category length and strength on familiarity in recognition. *Journal of Experimental Psychology: Learning, Memory and Cognition, 21,* 267–287.

Shimamura, A.P. (1995). Memory and frontal lobe function. In M.S. Gazzaniga (Ed.) *The cognitive neurosciences* (pp. 803–814). Cambridge, MA: MIT Press.

Smith, A.D. (1975). Partial learning and recognition memory in the aged. *International Journal of Aging and Human Development, 6,* 359–365.

Snodgrass, J.G., & Corwin, J. (1988). Pragmatics of measuring recognition memory: Applications to dementia and amnesia. *Journal of Experimental Psychology: General, 117,* 34–50.

Spencer, W.D., & Raz, N. (1995). Differential effects of aging on memory for content and context: A meta-analysis. *Psychology of Aging, 10,* 527–539.

Stadler, M.A., Roediger, H.L., & McDermott, K.B. (in press). Norms for word lists that create false memories. *Memory and Cognition.*

Tun, P.A., Wingfield, A., Rosen, M.J., & Blanchard, L. (1998). Older adults show greater susceptibility to false memory than young adults: Temporal characteristics of false recognition. *Psychology and Aging, 13,* 230–241.

COGNITIVE NEUROPSYCHOLOGY, 1999, 16 (3/4/5), 417–436

DECEIVING THE ELDERLY: EFFECTS OF ACCESSIBILITY BIAS IN CUED-RECALL PERFORMANCE

Larry L. Jacoby
New York University, USA

Two experiments examined age-related differences in a misinformation paradigm. Young and elderly participants studied a list of related word pairs (e.g. bed sheet) and were then given a cued-recall test ("bed s_ee_" presented as cues for recall of "sheet"). A "prime" stimulus was presented briefly before each test trial. On congruent trials the prime was the target word from study (sheet) whereas on incongruent trials the prime was a related word that was a plausible response but not the target (sleep). On baseline trials, the prime was a string of ampersands. When forced to respond (Expt. 1), both young and elderly participants demonstrated a bias to respond with the prime word, although the elderly showed a larger false memory effect as measured by higher false recalls on incongruent relative to baseline trials. When given the option to pass (Expt. 2), elderly participants continued to exhibit a large bias toward the prime word whereas young participants tended to pass when they were unable to recall the target. Results are interpreted in terms of an accessibility bias, which influences guessing and is a basis of responding independent of recollection. Discussion focuses on the importance of studying age-related changes in bias and recollection along with neural correlates of these changes.

INTRODUCTION

"I told you earlier that ..." My wife recently informed me that her mother was coming for a visit. When I expressed surprise, she responded that she had informed me earlier of the upcoming visit. However, I was unable to remember her having done so. One possibility is that, perhaps as a result of ageing, I am suffering a deficit in recollection. Another possibility, an unlikely one in this case, is that I was a victim of a "scam"—the earlier conversation may not have occurred but, rather, been invented as a convenience by my wife. A possibility of that sort is one for which elderly people need be alert. Any memory deficit suffered by the elderly might make them particularly vulnerable to untrue claims about past events. Much more than an unexpected visitor can be at stake.

The elderly are a favourite target for fraud, and some fraudulent practices rely on the victim accepting a false "I-told-you" claim. According to the Cleveland Better Business Bureau (http: / /www.cleveland.bbb.org / alerts / senior.html), in one such scam, con artists telephone seniors and chat with them, in the process collecting as much personal information as possible. In a subsequent callback, the con artists ask questions based on the personal information collected in the first phone

---

Requests for reprints should be addressed to Larry L. Jacoby, Department of Psychology, McMaster University, 1280 Main Street West, Hamilton, ON L8S 4K1, Canada (Phone: (905) 525-9140; Fax: (905) 529-6225; E-mail: jacoby@mcmaster.ca).

This research was supported by grants to Larry L. Jacoby from the National Institute on Aging (NIA) #AG 13845-02 and from the Natural Sciences and Engineering Research Council of Canada (NSERC) #OGP0000281.

The author would like to express thanks to Jim Debner and Ann Hollingshead for their assistance in this research.

call. If the senior fails to recollect the previous conversation, the con artists exploit the memory deficit by means of a false claim about an earlier event. As an example, the senior might be told: "We received your cheque for $1200, but it should only have been for $950. Send us another cheque for $950 and we'll simply return the first cheque to you." Actually, no cheque had been sent earlier, but victims of the scam respond by sending a cheque out of guilt or embarrassment.

Does an I-told-you claim create a false memory for the supposed earlier conversation? Other misinformation effects have been explained in that way. Loftus (1975; Loftus & Palmer, 1974) found that exposure to misleading questions about an experience resulted in an apparently permanent loss from memory of details of the original experience. Memory for the original experience was said to be replaced or "overwritten" by the misleading information. Similarly, the misinformation provided by a false I-told-you claim might be added to memory, and replace memory for what was actually said in a prior conversation. However, alternative accounts of misinformation effects have been offered (for a review, see Ayers & Reder, 1998). By a "blocking" account, exposure to incorrect information impairs access to memory for the correct information but does not replace it (e.g. Bekerian & Bowers, 1983; Chandler, 1991). A "source memory" account of misinformation effects also holds that memory for an original experience co-exists with memory for misleading information. However, rather than blocking retrieval of memory for the original experience, misinformation is said to be accepted because of confusion regarding its source (e.g. Ayers & Reder, 1998; Lindsay & Johnson, 1989).

It seems improbable that effects of a false I-told-you claim are fully reliant on memory alteration. In part, at least, I-told-you effects are likely because of an influence on bias or guessing. A false claim might be effective only if people are unable to remember the original experience, and then it may only serve as a source for guesses. The possibility of a particular prior experience having occurred is made more accessible by the I-told-you claim. However, acceptance of the claim might rely on a person's forgetting of the original experience and willingness to guess that the claim is a valid one. Similarly, McCloskey and Zaragoza (1985; Zaragoza, McCloskey, & Jamis, 1987) argued that apparent memory impairment found in misinformation effect studies might be due to task demands along with forgetting and influences on guessing rather than to real changes in memory.

Cohen and Faulkner (1989) found that elderly participants were more often misled by false information in an eyewitness testimony paradigm and were also more confident in their erroneous responses than were younger participants. The goal of the experiments reported here was to determine whether elderly participants are also more vulnerable to misinformation in a situation that is similar to the I-told-you example. The procedure of the experiments is outlined in Fig. 1. In Phase 1, people studied a list of related word pairs (e.g. bed sheet, eagle bird, knee bone) that they were told to remember for a later test. In Phase 2, memory was tested by presenting the first word (the cue word) along with a fragment of the second word (the target word) of each pair (e.g. knee b_n_) as cues for recall of the studied target word. Participants were informed that the target word was related semantically to the presented cue word and would complete the fragment. For "incongruent" tests, a "prime" word that would fulfill those requirements but was *not* the target word was presented immediately prior to the presentation of the test cue (e.g. sleep; bed s_ee_). In contrast, for baseline tests, no prime word was presented (e.g. &&&&&; eagle b__d). For a third type of test, a "congruent" test, the prime word was the same as the target word (e.g. bone; knee b_n_). Participants were warned that the prime word often would be misleading, and were instructed to recall the earlier-studied target word rather than being misled.

Presenting a prime that is plausible but invalid (incongruent test condition) is akin to a false I-told-you claim. Elderly participants, as compared to university students, were expected to show a larger misinformation effect by more often giving the invalid prime as a response. However, that difference simply might reflect elderly participants' poorer ability to remember the target words. Even for baseline tests, for which primes are not pre-

PHASE 1 STUDY	PHASE 2 TEST Prime	Cue Word Word Fragment	TEST CONDITIONS
bed		bed	Incongruent
sheet	sleep	s_ee_	(invalid prime)
:			
eagle		eagle	Baseline
bird	&&&&	b__d	(no prime)
:			
knee		knee	Congruent
bone	bone	b_n_	(valid prime)

Fig. 1. *The basic procedure used for all the experiments.*

sented, elderly participants are likely to recall fewer studied words. As an attempt to eliminate that baseline difference, a second group of young participants studied pairs under conditions of divided attention. We expected that for baseline tests, the performance of elderly participants would not differ from that of young participants whose attention was divided during study (e.g. Craik, 1982; Rabinowitz, Craik, & Ackerman, 1982) and that the performance of both groups would be poorer than that of young participants who studied under conditions of full attention.

Unlike other paradigms used to investigate misinformation effects (e.g. Loftus, 1975), the source of (mis)information provided by a prime was made obvious by presenting primes immediately prior to the memory tests. Otherwise, the arrangements for investigating effects of an invalid prime were the same as for investigating other misinformation effects. However, prior investigations of misinformation effects have not included a congruent test condition. Rather, investigators have relied on comparisons between a condition in which misinformation is presented (invalid prime) and a control condition in which misinformation is not presented to measure false memory. Following that convention, we use "false-memory effect" to refer to findings that participants were more likely to mistakenly claim to have earlier studied a word presented as an invalid prime than they would have been had the prime not been presented (baseline condition). Later, we describe advantages of using performance on congruent tests in combination with performance on incongruent tests to analyse the bases for false-memory effects.

After studying under conditions of full attention, the false-memory effect produced by invalid primes was expected to be larger for elderly than for young participants (cf. Cohen & Faulkner, 1989). Dividing young participants' attention during study was expected to produce performance on baseline tests that was the same as that found for elderly participants who devoted full attention to study, but result in a level of false memory that was intermediate to that found for young, full-attention and elderly participants. That is, even if dividing attention of young participants during study did equate performance on baseline tests, we still expected elderly participants to be more vulnerable to misinformation effects. A popular justification for a prediction of this sort is to claim that elderly participants suffer a deficit in their ability to inhibit (e.g. Hasher & Zacks, 1988) preponderant responses. Hasher and Zacks proposed a general theory of cognitive ageing that postulates age-linked deficits in inhibitory processes, and have since reported a great deal of evidence to support their theory. Zacks and Hasher (1997) briefly reviewed the supporting evidence and responded to critics (Burke, 1997; McDowd, 1997) of their approach. Although elderly participants do show greater interference effects (e.g. Winocur & Moscovitch, 1983), we did *not* base our predictions on differences in inhibitory processes.

By an inhibition-deficit account, elderly participants are unable to inhibit giving an invalid prime word as a response even though, had they been able to do so, they would have been able to recall the earlier-studied word correctly. As an example, they might fail to correctly recall "sheet" when given the cue "bed s_ee_" because they were unable to inhibit giving the invalid prime (sleep) as a response. However, against that account, the causative sequence might be in the opposite direction: Elderly participants might be more likely to produce the invalid prime as a response *because* they are less able to remember the study word. That is, false recall of an invalid prime might be a consequence, rather than the cause, of memory failure. Anderson and Bjork (1994) noted that a similar ambiguity exists for interpreting the tip-of-the-tongue (TOT) phenomenon. The TOT state is one in which a person is temporarily unable to produce a sought-after word although absolutely certain that they know the word. A common interpretation of the TOT phenomenon is that it arises because of failure to inhibit alternative responses and, in line with that interpretation, people do often report alternate, competing words that come to mind during a TOT. However, the alternative responses might come to mind *because* of failure to recall the sought-after word rather than being responsible for that failure. Problems in word finding are well documented as increasing with age and older adults suffer more TOTs. However, older adults are *less* likely to report alternate words than young adults during TOTs in either the laboratory or everyday life (Burke, MacKay, Worthley, & Wade, 1991; Cohen & Faulkner, 1986; Maylor, 1990). The report of fewer alternates is inconsistent with the claim that an age-linked deficit in ability to inhibit alternative responses causes the greater likelihood of a TOT state (Burke, 1997).

Performance on congruent test items in combination with that on incongruent test items can be used to show that people produce the prime as a response only when they are unable to remember the target. When people do not remember the earlier-studied target word, they might be more likely to produce the prime word as a guess because of its increased accessibility (relative to the baseline test where there is no prime). If people were forced to give a response for each test item, an accessibility bias of this sort would result in the probability of correct recall on congruent and incongruent tests being symmetrical around that on baseline tests. Relative to baseline, giving the prime word as a guess when recollection fails would increase the probability of correct recall for congruent tests but would produce a perfectly offsetting decrease in that probability for incongruent tests. The effect should be perfectly offsetting because materials were constructed such that there were only two acceptable responses for each test item—the target and its alternate. Consequently, if responding is forced, a decrease in correct recalls on an incongruent test must be accompanied by an increase in false recalls (i.e. a larger misinformation effect).

For all groups (young full-attention; young divided attention; and elderly), we expected symmetric effects of valid and invalid primes to show that priming effects do reflect accessibility bias. Given that result, differences in false memory could, at least, in part be explained as because of differences in recollection. Because of a deficit in ability to recollect, elderly participants more often guess and, so, show a larger effect of the prime. For the same reason, dividing attention of young participants during study should increase the likelihood of false memory. However, any difference in false memory between elderly and divided-attention young participants could not be explained as due to a difference in recollection, not if performance on baseline tests was equated.

Strategic avoidance of the prime as a response would allow one to counter accessibility bias when the target word could not be remembered, and differences in strategic avoidance would explain age-related differences in false memory that occur when recollection is equated. Avoidance of the prime as a response when unable to remember the target word is seen as being a strategy that is similar to reversing claims made by an untrusted salesperson so as to avoid being gullible. Reliance on such a strategy would be reasonable in our situation because participants were warned that the prime word often would be misleading. However, although avoiding the prime would avoid false memory, it would carry the cost of decreasing the probability of correct responding on congruent tests. Also, avoiding the prime requires that one be able to generate a suitable alternative response; in this case, a word other than the prime that completes the word fragment and is semantically related to the cue word. Doing so likely requires a good deal of cognitive effort along with vigilance to the possibility of being misled by the high accessibility of the prime word. We expected elderly adults to be more gullible—less likely to strategically avoid the prime when unable to remember the target word.

In sum, our experiments were designed to show that there are two means by which a misinformation effect can be avoided. First, presenting misinformation in the form of an invalid prime was only expected to have an effect when people were unable to remember the target and, so, ability to remember protects one from being misled. Symmetrical effects of valid and invalid primes would show that primes had their effect by means of accessibility bias, a basis for responding that comes into play only when memory fails. Second, when memory does fail, accessibility bias can be countered by strategically avoiding the prime so as to avoid false memory. Elderly participants were expected to be more vulnerable to misinformation both because of their poorer ability to remember and because of their being less likely to avoid the prime strategically when unable to remember. Yet a third means of avoiding a misinformation effect is simply not to respond when unable to remember. Experiment 2 examined age-related differences in willingness to respond. In contrast to Experiment 1, participants in Experiment 2 were allowed to say "pass" when unable to remember the target word rather than being forced to guess. The question was whether allowing participants not to respond would reduce age-related differences in false memory. In the General Discussion, we further emphasise the advantages of using congruent and incongruent tests to separate the contributions of different bases for responding rather than only examining false memory. Also, we speculate that the different means of avoiding being misled might have different anatomical bases.

EXPERIMENT 1

Method

Participants

Seventy-two young adults and 24 older adults participated in the experiment. The young adults were New York University undergraduates who received credit for an introductory psychology course. Forty-eight of the young adults were selected randomly and assigned to the full attention at study condition, while the remaining 24 were assigned to the divided attention at study condition[1]. The older adults were community-dwelling volunteers from the New York City area who were reimbursed for travel expenses. The older adults ranged in age from 64 to 89 years (mean = 73.6 years, SD 7.2), and had a mean of 16.9 years of education. All the older adults were tested in the full attention at study condition. Participants were tested individually.

Materials and design

A pool of 87 cue words, each paired with two associatively related responses (e.g. knee bend, knee bone), was selected mainly from the norms reported by Jacoby (1996). Some additional pairs were constructed based on the same criteria as used in Jacoby's norms. Both associatively related responses

[1] This experiment was run as two separate experiments. One experiment manipulated attention between groups (full vs. divided) with only young participants, and the other experiment looked at different age groups (young vs. elderly) under full-attention conditions. The experiments were identical in all other aspects so they were combined into one which resulted in there being twice as many participants in the young full-attention group than in the other two groups. No Mill Hill Vocabulary test scores were collected on these groups of participants.

contained the same number of letters and could be used to complete the same word fragment (e.g. knee b_n_; bone/bend). Three sets of 25 cue words along with their 2 associatively related responses were selected, and with each response word acting equally often as the target response word, this resulted in 6 sets. All sets had an equal distribution of word frequencies (as indexed by Thorndike & Lorge, 1944) for the cue words as well as the two response words, and equal probabilities of completing the word fragments when new (mean = 0.33 for both response words). The sets were balanced also on word length for the cue words (mean = 5.2 letters) and the response words (mean = 4.7 letters). With regard to the placement of the missing letters within each fragment, particular care was given to the first letter so that each set had an equal number of fragments missing the first letter (mean = 9.3 words). Each response set was rotated through each of three test conditions: congruent, incongruent, and baseline. This design resulted in 6 formats (2 response groups × 3 test conditions). To avoid primacy and recency effects, the remaining 12 items in the stimulus pool were used as buffer items with 6 items being presented at the beginning and at the end of the study list. The buffer items stayed constant across all formats.

This setup resulted in a study list of 87 pairs made up of 75 critical pairs and 12 buffer pairs. A test list of 75 items consisted of the 75 critical items from the study phase, with 25 items each presented as congruent, incongruent, and baseline trials. The 12 buffer items from the study phase were used in a separate practice test with 4 items each representing the 3 experimental test conditions. In all phases of the experiment, order of presentation was random with the restrictions that no more than three items representing the same combination of conditions could be presented in a row and all conditions were presented evenly throughout the list.

The listening task used in the divided-attention condition was one previously used by Craik (1982). In this task, participants monitored an auditory list of digits (1 to 9) to detect target sequences of three consecutive odd numbers (e.g. 9, 3, 7). The digits were random with the restriction that a minimum of one number and a maximum of three numbers occur between the end of one target sequence and the beginning of the next target sequence. Digits were recorded at a 1.5sec rate.

Procedure

Words were presented and responses were collected on an IBM-compatible computer with a VGA colour monitor, using Micro Experimental Laboratory (MEL) software (Schneider, 1990). Words were presented in lower-case white letters (approximately 3 × 5mm in size), on a black background in the centre of the computer screen.

In the study phase for both attention conditions, participants were told they would see a list of associatively related word pairs presented one pair at a time with one word placed immediately above the other in the middle of the screen. The pairs were presented for 2sec each with a 0.5sec intertrial interval during which the screen was blank. Participants in both conditions were instructed to pronounce the words out loud and to remember each pair for a later memory test. Participants in the divided-attention condition were told also that they would be required to do a listening task at the same time as doing the reading task. They were informed that it was very important not to miss a target sequence in the listening task. Participants responded by tapping the table whenever they detected a target sequence. Performance on the listening task was monitored by the experimenter. The number tape was presented alone for 15sec prior to the reading task to allow the participants to settle into one task before starting the other.

In the test phase, which followed immediately after the study phase, participants were told they would be required to alternate between two tasks. That is, they would have to study briefly presented single words (the prime words) for a later test as well as do a cued-recall test for the word pairs that they studied in the first part of the experiment. They were informed that we were interested in their ability to memorise the briefly presented single words without confusing those single words with the words they were trying to recall. It was mentioned that this would be a difficult task because sometimes the single word would be the same as the word they were trying to recall but other times it would be a different word. For the cued-recall test, the participants were told they would be presented with a cue word and a fragmented word, a word with some of the letters replaced with underscores. They were to use the word and fragment as cues to help them recall the word (the target word) that accompanied the cue word in the study phase of the experiment. They were instructed to try to recall but, if they couldn't recall, they were to guess but to keep in mind that their guess must be a word related to the cue word and also must fit the fragment. They were again warned not to be misled by the briefly presented single word when doing the recall task. Lastly, they were informed that on some trials no single word would be presented but rather just a string of symbols (&&&&&&&). For these trials, they were told there was no word to remember for later and that they should just do the recall task. It was explained that these trials allowed us to look at recall performance without the interference of the other task. A demonstration of the test procedure using the example cherry p__ (pie/pit) was presented prior to the practice test.

Each test trial started with a pair of plus signs (10 spaces apart), which were presented for 1sec. The plus signs marked the location on the screen where the single word (prime) appeared. The prime was presented for 500msec followed by an interstimulus interval of 500msec of blank screen. The cue word and word fragment were then presented with the word fragment presented in the same location as the prime while the cue word was on the line immediately above. The cue word and fragment stayed on the screen until the participant either gave a response or 20sec elapsed, at which time the screen cleared and the next trial was presented. The participants were to give their responses out loud. The experimenter keyed in the response and after an intertrial interval of 500msec, the next trial was presented. There was no test of memory for the prime words.

Results and Discussion

In the divided-attention condition, the probability of young adults failing to detect a target sequence for the listening task was .16 (SD = 11).

Although participants were instructed to respond to each test item, they did not always do so. Rather, they sometimes allowed the response interval to lapse without responding or, more rarely, produced a response that was not one of the two responses that we chose for the test item. Errors of this sort were more common for baseline tests than for congruent or incongruent tests (tests preceded by a valid or an invalid prime), and were less common for young participants who studied under conditions of full attention than for participants in the other two groups (Table 1), as indicated by a significant interaction of test condition and group [$F(4,186) = 4.05$, $MSe = 0.003$]. This pattern of results is consistent with the suggestion that presentation of a word as a prime increased its accessibility as a response. For baseline tests, participants' inability to think of the alternate as a possible response probably helped to protect against its false recall when they were unable to remember the target. Presenting the alternate as an invalid prime made it more accessible as a response and thereby made it less likely that participants would allow the response interval to lapse without responding.

Because of the rather high probability of failure to respond for baseline tests, it was necessary to examine both correct and false recalls when using those tests to evaluate memory performance. Recall performance was corrected for guessing by subtracting the probability of false recall from that of correct recall. Analysis of these corrected scores revealed that memory performance was higher for young participants who devoted full attention to study (.51) than for elderly participants (.24) or young participants who studied under conditions of divided attention (.22) [$F(2,91) = 26.55$,

Table 1. *Proportion of Trials on Which Participants Failed To Give Either the Target Response or the Alternate Response across Groups and Tests in Experiment 1*

	Type of Test		
Group	*Congruent*	*Baseline*	*Incongruent*
Young, full attention	.01	.10	.03
Young, divided attention	.02	.16	.03
Elderly	.02	.17	.02

*MS*e = 0.036] A posthoc Newman-Keuls analysis revealed that the difference in performance between the latter two conditions did not approach significance. That is, dividing attention of young participants during study was successful as a means of equating performance of young and elderly participants in their performance on baseline tests.

Examining probabilities of false recall on baseline and incongruent tests revealed that elderly participants showed a much larger false-memory effect than did young full-attention participants (Fig. 2b). For elderly participants, the probability of false recall was much higher on incongruent tests than on baseline tests, whereas this difference was smallest for young full-attention participants and intermediate for young divided-attention participants [$F(2,91) = 9.23$, *MS*e = 0.030]. In part, the differences in magnitude of the false-memory effect reflect differences in ability to recall the target item. Young participants who devoted full attention to study were better able to recall target words, as shown by their performance on baseline tests, and so were less likely to show false recall of the prime word for incongruent tests.

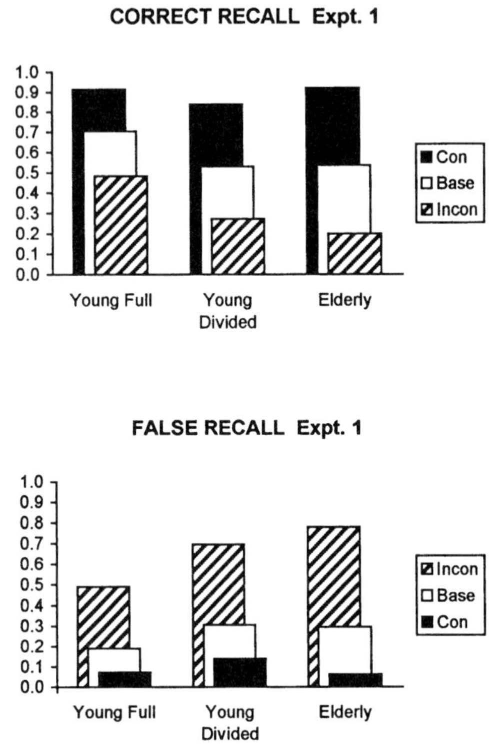

Fig. 2. *Probability of (a) correct recall and (b) false recall for each group for each test condition for Experiment 1.*

Accessibility Bias

Analysis of the probabilities of correct recall revealed a highly significant interaction between Test Condition and Groups [$F(4,186) = 13.13$, *MS*e = 0.013]. For each of the groups of participants, probabilities of correct recall on congruent and incongruent tests were almost perfectly symmetrical around performance on baseline tests (Fig. 2a). That is, presenting a valid prime (congruent test) increased the probability of correct recall by an amount that was nearly identical to the decrease in the probability of correct recall that resulted from presentation of an invalid prime (incongruent test). This is the pattern of results that would be expected if participants gave the prime word as a guess when they were unable to remember the earlier-studied target word.

Strategic Avoidance of the Prime

Comparisons of performance of young divided-attention participants with performance of elderly participants was of particular interest because performance of those two groups was equated on baseline tests. Although the two groups were equal in their ability to remember the earlier-studied target word, they did differ in effects of accessibility bias revealed by their performance on congruent and incongruent tests (Fig. 2a). Young divided attention participants were more likely, as compared to elderly participants, to respond correctly on incongruent tests but less likely to respond correctly on congruent test [$F(1,46) = 7.74$, *MS*e = 0.019 for the interaction of Type of Test and Group.

Analysis of the false recalls revealed convergent results. That is, young divided-attention participants, as compared to elderly participants, were less likely to be misled by an invalid prime word on incongruent tests (i.e. fewer false recalls) but more likely to avoid a valid prime word on congruent tests (i.e. more false recalls), [$F(1,46) = 7.62$, *MS*e = 0.020 for the interaction of Type of Test and

Group]. Indeed, for the congruent test (prior to which the alternate solution had never been shown), the divided-attention participants incorrectly responded with the alternate solution more than twice as often as did the elderly group (.14 and .06, respectively).

These results show that elderly participants were less likely to strategically avoid the effects of accessibility bias. Young participants who divided attention during study were aware of their poor ability to remember the target word and were more vigilant of the possibility of being misled by the prime than were elderly participants. To counter accessibility effects, they sometimes strategically avoided the prime word by generating the alternative completion as a guess when unable to remember the target word. Their doing so reduced the probability of being misled by the prime on incongruent tests but carried the cost of their being less likely to correctly recall the target word on congruent tests.

EXPERIMENT 2

Results of Experiment 1 showed that elderly participants were more vulnerable to an I-told-you effect than were younger participants. Presenting a potential response, as a valid or invalid prime, that fit the constraints of an immediate situation increased the likelihood that participants would give that primed response. Their doing so produced a misinformation effect when the prime was invalid—the incongruent test condition. However, the misinformation effect was because of guessing rather than because the invalid prime created a false memory or because of a failure to inhibit the prime. The decrease in correct recall produced by presenting an invalid prime was nearly identical to the increase in correct recall produced by presenting a valid prime. This pattern of results would be expected if presentation of the prime had its effect by an influence on guessing.

In part, elderly participants' greater vulnerability to false memory was a result of their poorer ability to remember the earlier-studied target word. Young participants who devoted full attention to study, as compared to elderly participants, were better able to remember the target word for baseline tests, and showed a smaller false-memory effect. An I-told-you effect can be avoided if one is able to remember the relevant earlier experience. However, equating memory performance on baseline tests did not equate the magnitude of the false-memory effect shown by young, as compared to elderly, participants. Young participants who studied under conditions of divided attention performed the same as elderly participants on baseline tests, but differed from elderly participants in their performance on congruent and incongruent tests. Young participants strategically avoided misleading effects of the prime by sometimes generating a completion word other than the prime to be given as a guess when they were unable to remember the target word. Their doing so reduced the magnitude of the false-memory effect but carried the cost of also reducing the probability of correctly responding when the prime was valid. Indeed, the probability of correct recall on congruent tests was lower for young divided-attention participants than for elderly participants.

Experiment 2 was designed to reduce the misinformation effect observed in Experiment 1. A study manipulation was meant to increase memory for the target word in Experiment 2; participants focused on the meaning of the members of word pairs by judging whether the words were related. Materials were the same as in Experiment 1 except that some pairs of unrelated words were added to the study list to legitimatise the participants' task of judging whether members of a pair were related. Memory for words in those unrelated pairs was not tested. As in Experiment 1, elderly participants and one group of young participants devoted full attention to words presented during the study phase whereas young participants in a second group divided their attention between judging the relatedness of words in pairs and engaging in a listening task. Dividing attention during the study phase was expected to equate performance on baseline tests of young participants with that of elderly participants.

Did participants experience their false recall of invalid primes as resulting from a guess or did they mistakenly experience those words as having been earlier studied? Perhaps the large false-memory effects observed in Experiment 1 were owed to participants being forced to respond to each test item. For the cued-recall tests in Experiment 2, participants were told to try hard to recall the earlier-studied word but were given the option of responding "pass" if they were unable to do so. Giving people the option not to guess was expected to reduce the false-memory effect produced by presenting invalid primes. Age differences in the effect of allowing a "pass" response were of particular interest. Some (e.g. Basowitz & Korchin, 1957; Botwinick, 1959; Botwinick, Brinley, & Robbin, 1958) have found that older, as compared to younger, adults are more conservative—more likely to withhold responding to avoid an error when allowed to do so. However, such differences are not reliably found (e.g. Ferris, Crook, Clark, McCarthy, & Rae, 1980; Harkins, Chapman, & Eisdorfer, 1979).

Method

Participants

Forty-eight young adults and 24 older adults participated in the experiment and were drawn from the same participant pool as in Experiment 1. Twenty-four young adults were assigned randomly to two between-participant conditions in which attention was manipulated during study (full attention and divided attention). The mean age for the full-attention group was 19.2 years (SD 1.2) and for the divided-attention group was 19.5 years (SD 2.0). On the Mill Hill Vocabulary test (Raven, 1965), average scores of 51% and 57% were obtained by the full-attention and divided-attention groups respectively. The older adults ranged in age from 57 to 89 years (mean = 72.6 years, SD 7.1), and had an average of 16.7 years of education. They scored an average of 77% on the Mill Hill Vocabulary test. An analysis of the vocabulary scores showed a main effect of Group [$F(2,69) = 30.965$, $MSe = 0.015$]. A posthoc Newman-Keuls analysis revealed that the elders' score was significantly greater than the two young groups, which did not differ from each other.

Design and procedure

The design and procedure of Experiment 2 were very similar to Experiment 1. The major differences were in the study manipulation and in the cued-recall test instructions. In the study phase, the participants judged the relatedness of the pairs of words. In order to facilitate this procedure 25 unrelated foils were added to the related critical pairs in the study list. The related pairs that formed the foils were selected based on the same criteria used for the critical items. Only one target response word for each cue word was chosen to be used and then the response words were shuffled to create unrelated pairs. The foils were distributed evenly throughout the study list. Four primacy and four recency buffers (seven related and one unrelated) were added to the main list. This setup resulted in a study list of 108 trials: 75 critical, 8 buffer, and 25 foil pairs. A separate practice of five related and three unrelated pairs was presented prior to the critical study list in order to give the participants some experience in responding within the allotted time. The foils, buffers, and practice items remained constant across all formats.

The young divided-attention group responded verbally whenever they heard a sequence of three odd digits in the distractor task so as not to interfere with their manual responding to the relatedness question. Also there was a change in the stimulus display on the monitor. The words in each pair were presented side by side instead of one above the other in both the study and test phases. In the test phase, the prime word was presented in the same location on the screen as the word fragment, but the cue word was presented immediately to the left of the word fragment in the recall task. Otherwise, the test procedure remained the same as in Experiment 1.

In the study phase, it was explained that we were interested in people's judgements about the relatedness of words. Participants were informed that the two words in each pair were related meaningfully to each other in some of the pairs and unrelated in other pairs. Examples were given to demonstrate the various aspects of relatedness (e.g. doctor nurse, cherry pie, scream yell) and unrelatedness (phone ankle). Each pair appeared for 2.5sec followed by 0.5sec of blank screen. The task was to decide if each pair was related and to press the "1" key on the numberpad to enter a "yes" (the pair is related) and the "2" key to enter a "no" (the pair is not related). Participants were instructed that since 2.5sec was a very short time for judging some of the pairs and since relatedness was not always a straightforward matter, that they should try to base their judgements on their first impression about the relatedness of the pair because it was important that they stay apace of the presentation rate. The young participants in the divided-attention condition were given the same instructions as the full-attention conditions along with the instructions used in Experiment 1 for the distractor task. The only change in these instructions was that they were to say "now" aloud whenever they heard a sequence of three consecutive odd numbers. The divided-attention condition had 15sec of practice with the number monitoring task prior to the start of the study phase.

The test instructions were identical to those of Experiment 1 with the added instruction in the cued-recall test that if participants were unable to recall the earlier presented study word, they should respond "pass." However, they were encouraged to try hard to remember rather than give up easily.

Results and Discussion

In the divided-attention condition, the probability of the young adults failing to detect a target sequence for the listening task was .19 (SD = 13). Consistent with the results of the Mill Hill Vocabulary score, the proportion of correct relatedness judgements within the 2.5sec deadline in Phase 1 was lower for the two groups of young participants (mean = .84 for divided and .90 for full attention) than for the elderly participants (mean = .95).

In Experiment 2, participants were allowed to "pass" if they could not recall the studied word. As in Experiment 1, we analysed the proportion of trials on which neither of the two chosen responses was given (i.e. passes, timeouts, and other responses). Analysis revealed a main effect of Test Condition [$F(2,138) = 74.13$, $MSe = 0.004$] and of Group [$F(2,69) = 13.22$, $MSe = 0.007$], with no interaction [$F < 1$]. As can be seen in Table 2, failure to respond with either the target or the alternate was highest for the baseline test (as in Experiment 1) compared to the other two types of test.

Table 2. *Proportion of Trials on Which Participants Failed To Give Either the Target Response or the Alternate Response across Groups and Tests in Experiment 2*

	Type of Test		
Group	*Congruent*	*Baseline*	*Incongruent*
Young, full attention	.02	.15	.06
Young, divided attention	.07	.21	.12
Elderly	.02	.14	.03

More interestingly young participants who studied under conditions of divided attention were more likely not to give the target or alternate as a response than were either young full-attention participants or elderly participants. The smaller number of failures to respond made by young full-attention participants is understandable if they were better able to remember the target word than were young divided-attention participants. However, we expected elderly participants not to differ from young divided-attention participants in their ability to remember and, perhaps, be more conservative. The higher probability of not responding for young divided-attention participants might reflect that they were more aware of their poor memory for target words than were elderly participants and therefore sought to avoid being misled. Even though given the option to pass, elderly participants responded in a way that risked producing a misinformation effect. That is, results were opposite to what would be expected if the elderly were more conservative than the young participants (e.g. Basowitz & Korchin, 1957).

As shown by performance on baseline tests, young participants in the full-attention condition were better able to remember target words than were participants in the other two groups. Recall performance was corrected for guessing by subtracting the probability of false recall from that of correct recall. Analysis of these corrected scores revealed that memory performance was higher for young participants who devoted full attention to study (.66) than for elderly participants (.46) or young participants (.44) who studied under conditions of divided attention [$F(2,67) = 11.38$, MSe = 0.031].

Examining probabilities of false recall on baseline and incongruent tests (Fig. 3b) revealed that elderly participants showed a false-memory effect that was twice as large as that shown by participants in the young full-attention condition whereas there was little difference between the two groups of young participants in the magnitude of the misinformation effect [$F(2,67) = 11.74$, $MSe = 0.036$].

Analysis of the probabilities of correct recall on congruent and incongruent tests revealed a highly significant interaction between Test Condition and Groups [$F(4,138) = 13.92$, $MSe = 0.013$]. For all participants, probabilities of correct recall on congruent and incongruent tests were symmetrical around performance on baseline tests (Fig. 3a). That is, for correct recall, the congruent test was higher than the baseline test by nearly the same amount that the incongruent test was lower than baseline. As in Experiment 1, this result supports the claim that guessing is biased by the prime word. That the symmetry for the elderly group was not as striking as that for the two young groups merely reflects a ceiling effect on the congruent test. Elderly participants produced such a large decrease in correct recalls on the incongruent test that it would have been impossible for them to increase by the same amount on the congruent test.

Comparing the young divided-attention participants and the elderly participants again revealed differences in strategic avoidance of the prime. Even though both groups were given the option to pass when they failed to recall, and even though the groups were equated on baseline tests, the elderly were much more likely to be swayed by the prime word (Fig. 3a). Examining the data for correct recalls, elderly participants, as compared to young divided-attention participants, were more likely to respond correctly on congruent tests but less likely to respond correctly on incongruent tests [$F(1,46) = 16.20$, $MSe = 0.026$ for the interaction of test and group]. Also, elderly, as compared to young divided-attention participants, made more false recalls on incongruent tests but fewer false recalls on the congruent tests [$F(1,46) = 20.43$, $MSe = 0.027$ for the interaction of type of Test and Group]. As in Experiment 1, divided-attention participants incorrectly responded with the alternate solution on congruent tests more often than did the elderly group (mean = .10 and .03, respectively).

Together with the first experiment, these results highlight age-related differences in the countering of accessibility bias. Young participants who divided attention during study were aware of their poor ability to remember the target word and took steps to avoid being misled by the prime. To counter accessibility effects, divided-attention participants sometimes avoided the prime word by generating the alternative completion as a guess when they were unable to remember the target word. They also responded less often than did the elderly participants on congruent and incongruent tests (Table 2). So, when faced with a situation in which they could not remember the target, young

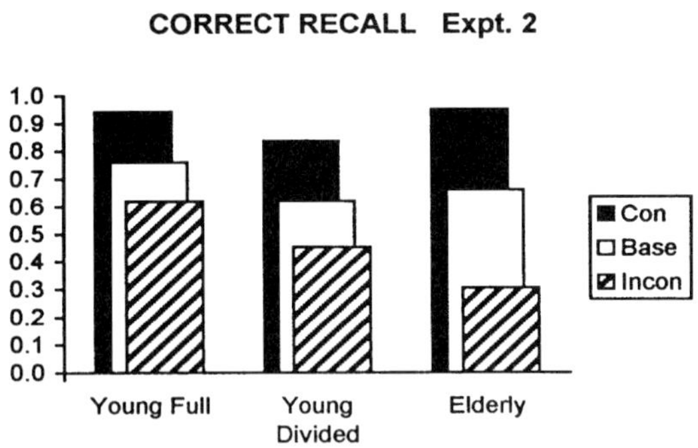

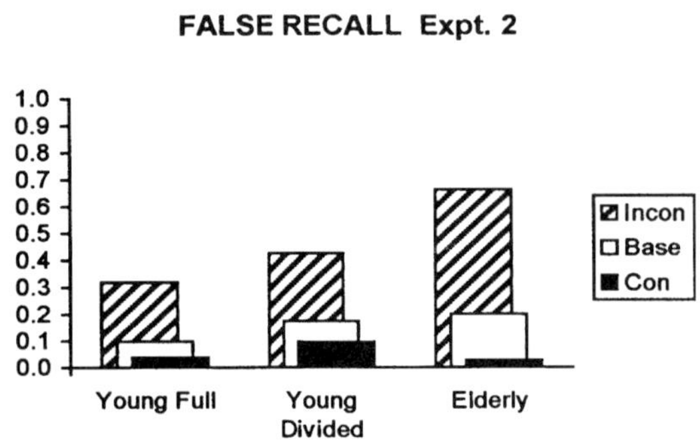

Fig. 3. *Probability of (a) correct recall and (b) false recall for each group for each test condition for Experiment 2.*

divided-attention participants were willing to withhold responding rather than risk being misled by the prime, and when they did respond, they sometimes did so by generating an alternative to the prime. Elderly participants faced with the same situation were inclined to go with the prime.

GENERAL DISCUSSION

Elderly, as compared to younger, adults are more vulnerable to deception in a situation similar to that of being faced with a false I-told-you claim. If we had used only incongruent and baseline tests, as has been done in other investigations of misinformation effects, this would be all that we could conclude. However, by using congruent tests as well as incongruent and baseline tests we were able to analyse the bases responsible for the larger effect shown by elderly participants. The strategy of combining performance from different types of tests to separate effects on accessibility bias from differences in memory is the same as the process-dissociation approach (e.g. Jacoby, 1991, 1998). In the discussion that follows, we consider results from the current experiments in the context of that approach.

Accessibility Bias Reflects a Basis of Responding That Is Independent of Recollection

By using results from congruent tests in combination with those from baseline and incongruent tests, we were able to show that the I-told-you effect arose from an influence of accessibility bias. The probability of a correct response after valid and invalid primes was symmetrical around performance on baseline tests, just as would be expected if presentation of the prime only influenced guessing. In part, the greater vulnerability of elderly participants to misinformation resulted from their poorer ability to remember a relevant earlier event, making it necessary for them to guess more often than did young participants.

As well as showing a larger misinformation effect, elderly participants show larger interference effects in a variety of tasks (e.g. Winocur & Moscovitch, 1983). Poorer ability to remember is sometimes responsible for those larger effects. Just as is found for congruent and incongruent primes, habit can also serve as a source of accessibility bias. The elderly, because of their poorer ability to recollect, are more vulnerable to misleading effects of habit. Recent studies have utilised the process-dissociation procedure to separate experimentally developed habits from recollection (Hay & Jacoby, 1996, in press). In those studies, habits were established during a training phase, where cue words were paired with a typical response on 75% of the occasions (e.g. knee bone) and an atypical response on 25% of the occasions (e.g. knee bend). A condition in which the two responses appeared equally often, 50%, served as a baseline. In a second phase, participants studied lists of word pairs that included some word pairs for which the cue word was paired with a typical response, some word pairs for which the cue word was paired with an atypical response, and some baseline items. After studying each list, memory was tested by presenting the cue word along with a fragment of the response word (e.g. knee b_n_). That is, the experiments were comparable to those reported in this article except congruent and incongruent tests were created by means of prior training rather than by presenting valid and invalid primes.

Correct recall of typical pairs could be based either on memory for the list (R) or on the habitual response (H). Assuming independence of recollection and habit, the probability of correct recall for typical pairs can be represented as: Prob (typical) = R + H(1-R). People sometimes respond incorrectly with the typical response after having studied an atypical pair. Such a "memory slip" or false memory indicates that habit, in the absence of recollection, determined their response. The probability of such errors after study of atypical pairs is represented by: Prob (typical) = H (1-R).

The different levels of habit for typical and atypical responses produced probabilities of correct responding that were symmetrical around baseline tests, just as has been found for valid and invalid primes (Fig. 4). Because responding was forced and participants were able to produce a response for all test items, probabilities of correct and false recall

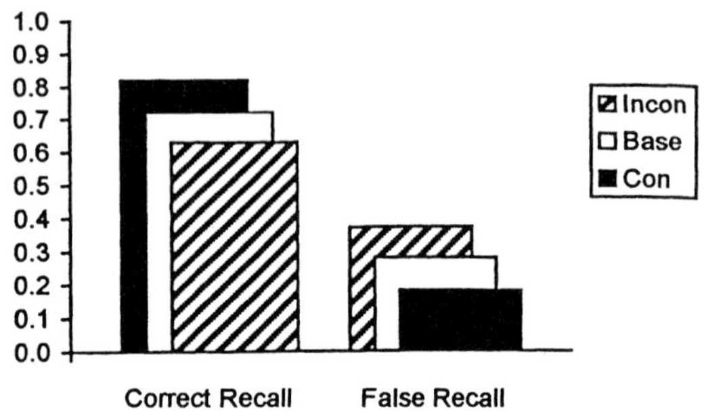

Fig. 4. *Probability of correct recall and false recall for Hay and Jacoby (1996), Experiment 1.*

summed to 1.0. Hay and Jacoby used the above equations to solve for estimates of the contributions of habit (H) and memory (R) to cued-recall performance. They found that manipulating the strength of the habit established in the training phase did not affect the estimates of R in later cued recall, but did affect the estimates of H. The estimates of habit matched the probabilities established in the training phase. Manipulations of the presentation rate of the study list and response deadline in cued recall affected the estimates of R, but did not affect the estimates of H. Hay and Jacoby (in press) showed that cued-recall performance of elderly and young participants differed only because elderly participants were less able to recollect, the contribution of habit was age invariant. These dissociations support the assumption that habit and memory make independent contributions to performance, and converge with results from experiments using other variants of the process-dissociation procedure (for a review, see Jacoby, Jennings, & Hay, 1996).

The finding that estimates of habit show probability matching suggests that habit is a form of implicit learning. Reber (e.g., 1989) has argued that probability matching reflects implicit learning of an event sequence that is acquired independently of a conscious effort to learn and without intentional strategies. Knowlton, Squire, and Gluck (1994) described probability learning as a task that relies primarily on the form of memory preserved by amnesics who have suffered damage to the hippocampus. They found that such amnesics show evidence of probability learning but perform more poorly than people with normally functioning memory. They suggested that the poorer probability learning of amnesics is a result of their inability to recollect (declarative memory), a type of memory used by people with normal memory to supplement the more automatic, unintentional form of memory (procedural memory) that is fully relied on by those with amnesia. Performance in probability learning tasks is unlikely to serve as a pure measure of more automatic bases of responding (e.g. implicit learning or habit) in cued-recall performance. The process-dissociation procedure offers the advantage of separating the contributions of different forms or uses of memory within a task, rather than identifying processes with different tasks.

Ratcliff and McKoon (1997) presented a "counter" model that describes effects of implicit memory as produced by bias. They noted that in experiments using indirect tests of memory, prior presentation of an item can increase both hits and false alarms, which is the signature of bias effects (e.g. Ratcliff & McKoon, 1995). We (e.g. Jacoby, Toth, & Yonelinas, 1993) agree that automatic influences of memory (implicit memory) can be expressed as bias. However, we see the term "bias" as synonymous with the claim that an automatic influence of memory, such as that produced by habit or a prime, can serve as an alternative to recollection as a basis for responding. Jacoby, McElree, and Trainham (in press) have shown that results reported by Ratcliff and McKoon (1997) as support for their counter model, when re-analysed, reveal striking dissociations that are the same as those found by Hay and Jacoby (1996).

Implicit memory from a single prior presentation of a word can serve as a source of accessibility bias. Smith and Tindell (1997) found that word fragments were not as likely to be correctly completed when an orthographically similar but incorrect completion word was earlier presented as compared to a baseline condition in which a dissimilar prime was presented. In contrast, prior presentation of the completion word itself facilitated correct completion of the fragment. These priming effects were largely symmetrical around the baseline condition, and occurred even when participants were warned about the effects and told not to try to remember the prime. This and other details of the effects support the authors' claim that they originated from implicit memory for the primes.

Repetition can have a strengthening effect and, thereby, increase the likelihood of later false memory. Jacoby (1999) required participants to read words one, two, or three times and then listen to a second list of words. For a later test of recognition memory, participants were instructed to respond "old" only if the test word was one that had earlier been *heard*. They were correctly informed that none of the words that they read were in the list of words that they heard. For elderly participants, repeatedly reading a word increased the probability of its later being falsely recognised as having been earlier heard. In contrast, repetition had an opposite effect for young adults—repeatedly reading a word made it *less* likely the word would later be falsely recognised as earlier heard. An experiment reported in the same article used the process-dissociation procedure to show that repeatedly reading a word increased its familiarity equally for elderly and young participants. However, elderly participants were less able to recollect earlier reading a word as a means of excluding the word as earlier heard. The opposite effects of repetition resulted from elderly participants mistakenly accepting earlier-read words because of their familiarity, whereas young participants were able to use recollection successfully to counter the increased familiarity produced by repetition. Similarly, Kensinger and Schacter (this issue) found that repetition of words that were all associated to a nonpresented target did not reduce false recognition of the nonpresented target for elderly adults but did so for young adults. Using similar procedures, Schacter, Verfaellie, Anes, and Racine (1998b) showed that, for Korsakoff amnesic patients, repeated presentation and testing of lists of semantic associates produced an *increase* in the probability of false recognition.

A Deficit in Recollection vs. an Age-linked Deficit in Inhibitory Processes

Results reported by Hay and Jacoby (1996, in press) show that interference does *not* differentially influence young and elderly participants' ability to recollect an earlier event. Rather, by using congruent along with incongruent test conditions, prior training was shown to only influence accessibility bias—the probability of recollection was invariant across the different forms (congruent, incongruent, and baseline) of prior training. Similarly, results of the experiments reported in this article suggest that presenting a valid versus an invalid prime did *not* influence participants' ability to recollect earlier-studied words. Rather, the symmetric effect of valid and invalid primes on the probability of correct recall, relative to baseline tests, suggests that effects were because of an influence on accessibility bias. Results are only suggestive because symmetry was not found for false recalls, presumably because participants were sometimes unable to think of the alternative response and, so, did not respond rather than falsely recalling the alternative. Invariance in recollection is most easily shown if participants respond with one of the two alternative words for each test item.

An experiment that was recently completed eliminated failures to respond by requiring participants to read each of the two possible responses to a context word and fragment (e.g. bed sheet; bed sleep) in a first phase of the experiment. Otherwise, the experiment was the same as those reported here. Results showed that prefamiliarisation of the alternatives eliminated failures to respond, allowing it to be demonstrated that presenting an invalid versus a valid prime does not influence recollection but, rather, influences only accessibility bias. Recollection for baseline tests was the same as for conditions in which valid and invalid primes were presented. Results are the same as found for manipulations of habit. These dissociations cannot be explained in terms of differential interference that results from an age-linked deficit in ability to inhibit *responses*. A deficit in inhibiting responses would not predict the invariances in recollection that are found across manipulations of prior training or priming (Hay & Jacoby, in press; Jacoby, 1999).

Recent interest in inhibitory processes has been inspired by findings from special populations, such as patients who have suffered frontal lobe damage (e.g. Shimamura, 1995) and by connectionist models that acknowledge the existence of inhibitory as well as excitatory connections between neural units and formally specify the role of both types of connections (e.g. McClelland & Rumelhart, 1981). However, more informal theorising about inhibitory processes has failed to specify the locus at which inhibitory processes operate. (As an example, see criticisms by Burke, 1997 and McDowd, 1997 of Hasher and Zacks' inhibition theory.) When not explicitly specified, the tone of arguments about inhibitory processes is often such as to imply that the inhibition in question operates only after a candidate response has already been computed and serves the function of allowing inappropriate responses to be withheld (e.g. Dempster, 1992). In contrast, within connectionist models, inhibitory links are intermixed with excitatory links at levels prior to the level at which a response is computed.

Our dissociations are consistent with connectionist models that postulate inhibitory connections at levels prior to the computation of a response. In particular, our results are consistent with the proposal by McClelland, McNaughton, and O'Reilly (1995) of complementary learning systems in the hippocampus and neocortex. The hippocampal system is described as fast learning and as having the characteristics that we have ascribed to recollection, whereas neocortical synapses are said to change slowly across repetitions of a pattern, in ways required for development of a habit. Both memory systems probably rely on inhibitory as well as excitatory connections. That is, it is likely to be the configuration of connections, rather than the presence or absence of inhibitory connections, that differentiates the two learning systems. The model that McClelland et al. (1995, p. 445) proposed for combining outputs from the learning systems to determine performance is based on an independence assumption and is expressed in equations that are essentially identical to those used by the process-dissociation procedure. O'Reilly, Norman, and McClelland (1997) provided a connectionist model of recollection, subserved by the hippocampus, in recognition memory. The goal of their model was to capture characteristics of recollection revealed by use of process-dissociation procedures (e.g. Yonelinas, 1994, 1997).

Almost certainly, recollection involves inhibitory as well as excitatory processes and the same might be true for strategically avoiding a prime. However, the two means of preventing false memory are likely to involve inhibition of different sorts. Jacoby, Kelley, and McElree (in press) distinguish between early selection and late correction means of gaining cognitive control of performance, and discuss the relation between memory monitoring and self-monitoring in social settings. They describe recollection as illustrating an early selection means of control. In contrast, strategic avoidance of a prime might rely on a late correction method of control by requiring the conscious assessment of a candidate response so as to measure its adequacy and make any necessary corrections prior to output. Regardless, the two means of cognitive control differ in that recollection relies on a form or use of memory that has been identified with the hippocampus, whereas strategic avoidance of a prime provides a means of countering attempts at deception when recollection fails. Strategic avoidance of a prime might most heavily rely on frontal lobe functions. Glisky, Polster, and Routhieaux (1995) reviewed evidence showing age-related decline in both hippocampal and frontal functions, and used a battery of neuropsychological tests to measure decline in the two types of function separately (also, see Henkel, Johnson, & De Leonardis, 1998).

Countering Deception: Generating Alternatives and Knowing When Not To Respond

Even when performance was matched on baseline tests, elderly adults were more vulnerable to deception in the form of a misinformation effect than were young adults. Young adults countered effects of accessibility bias by generating the alternative to the prime as a response, whereas elderly adults were more likely to give the prime as a guess when unable to remember the target word. Countering effects of accessibility did not confer any overall advantage to young over elderly participants in accuracy of responding. Avoiding the prime reduced the probability of being misled by invalid primes but also reduced the probability of responding correctly after valid primes. However, had the primes been invalid most of the time, as is the case in attempts to deceive, the young participants' countering of accessibility bias would have been advantageous. Elderly participants not countering effects of accessibility might reflect their inability to generate an alternative to the prime as a guess when they did not remember the target word.

Ability to counter deception by strategically avoiding a prime probably reflects frontal lobe function. Verbal fluency is required to generate an alternative to a prime so as to avoid deception. Reduction in verbal fluency, as measured by the FAS test, is treated as indicative of a deficit in frontal lobe function and is correlated with poor source memory shown by older adults (e.g. Craik, Morris, Morris, & Loewen, 1990). Also, as revealed by their performance on a cognitive estimation task, patients suffering a deficit in frontal lobe function are less able to make a sensible guess when an answer is unknown (Shallice & Evans, 1978). Instead, they seem to give an answer that is most accessible, without using general knowledge or constraints provided by a situation to restrict their guesses. Frontal lobe deficits also have been associated with findings of confabulation (Moscovitch, 1989; Schacter, Norman, & Koutstaal, 1998a) as well as interference effects (Shimamura, 1995). Showing a large misinformation effect could be described as "situation-assisted" confabulation. The prerequisites for confabulation are the same as for false memory: A failure to recollect in combination with a willingness to give any response that readily comes to mind, without questioning the reasons for its accessibility.

Another way to avoid being misled is to refuse to respond unless one is able to recollect. When given the choice to withhold responding if unsure, young participants whose attention was divided during study did respond less often so as to reduce the probability of being misled. In contrast, elderly participants did not reduce their probability of responding. Koriat and Goldsmith (1996) discuss the role of monitoring and control processes in the strategic regulation of memory accuracy. When given the freedom to withhold responding, increasing the accuracy of responding requires the ability to accurately monitor memory. Snodgrass and Corwin (1988) suggested that measures of bias, defined as willingness to respond, might identify members of special populations better than do measures of discriminability. For example, they found that participants with dementia associated with Alzheimer's and Parkinson's disease were more liberal in their responding compared to normal controls.

Neural bases for false memory is a research topic that has generated much interest (e.g. Schacter et al., 1998a). Further progress toward specifying brain-behaviour relations requires more analytic procedures to measure the contributions of different forms or uses of memory (Aggleton & Brown, in press). Most research on false memory has been done from the perspective of eyewitness testimony. In contrast, our research focuses on deceiving the elderly. Defrauding the elderly is a growth industry and it is important to identify those who are most at risk. Because of a deficit in recollection, older, as compared to younger, adults are more prone to errors that reflect inappropriate reliance on habit and other forms of accessibility bias such as that produced by an invalid I-told-you claim. It is important to devise means to measure such deficits in recollection for purposes of diagnosis and treatment (Hay & Jacoby, in press). Further, differences in ability to counter effects of accessibility bias by strategic means are as important as are differences in ability to recollect. Ability to generate an alternative to a response or an interpretation that is highly accessible but potentially misleading is the key to avoiding deception when recollection fails. The "send a cheque" scam described at the beginning of this article depends as much on an inability to generate alternatives as on a deficit in memory. To avoid being a victim of the scam, it would only be necessary to ask that the supposed, earlier-sent cheque be returned prior to sending a new one—a reasonable request in any case.

REFERENCES

Aggleton, J.P., & Brown, M.W. (in press). Episodic memory, amnesia, and hippocampal-anterior thalamic axis. *Behavioural and Brain Sciences.*

Anderson, M.C., & Bjork, R.A. (1994). Mechanisms of inhibition in long-term memory. A new taxonomy. In D. Dagenbach & T.H. Carr (Eds.), *Inhibitory processes in attention, memory and language* (pp. 265–326). San Diego, CA: Academic Press.

Ayers, M.S., & Reder, L.M. (1998). A theoretical review of the misinformation effect: Predictions from an activation-based memory model. *Psychonomic Bulletin and Review, 5*, 1–21.

Basowitz, H., & Korchin, S.J. (1957). Age differences in the perception of closure. *Journal of Abnormal Social Psychology, 54*, 93–97.

Bekerian, D.A., & Bowers, J.M. (1983). Eyewitness testimony: Were we misled? *Journal of Experimental Psychology: Learning, Memory and Cognition, 9*, 139–145.

Botwinick, J. (1959). Drives, expectancies, and emotion. In J.E. Birren (Ed.), *Handbook of aging and the individual* (pp. 639–768). Chicago IL: University of Chicago Press.

Botwinick, J., Brinley, J.F., & Robbin, J.S. (1958). The interaction effects of perceptual difficulty and stimulus exposure time on age differences in speed and accuracy of response. *Gerontologia, 2*, 1–10.

Burke, D.M. (1997). Language, aging, and inhibitory deficits: Evaluation of a theory. *Journal of Gerontology: Psychological Sciences, 52B*, P254–P264.

Burke, D.M., MacKay, D.G., Worthley, J.S., & Wade, E. (1991). On the tip of the tongue: What causes word finding failures in young and older adults? *Journal of Memory and Language, 30*, 542–579.

Chandler, C.C. (1991). How memory for an event is influenced by related events: Interference in modified recognition tests. *Journal of Experimental Psychology: Learning, Memory and Cognition, 17*, 115–125.

Cohen, G., & Faulkner, D. (1986). Memory for proper names. Age differences in retrieval. *British Journal of Developmental Psychology, 4*, 187–197.

Cohen, G., & Faulkner, D. (1989). Age differences in source forgetting: Effects on reality monitoring and eyewitness testimony. *Psychology and Aging, 4*, 10–17.

Craik, F.I.M. (1982). Selective changes in encoding as a function of reduced processing capacity. In F. Klix, J. Hoffman, & E. van der Meer (Eds.), *Cognitive research in psychology* (pp. 152–161). Berlin: Deutscher Verlag der Wissenschaffen.

Craik, F.I.M., Morris, L.W., Morris. R.G., & Loewen, E.R. (1990). Aging, source amnesia, and frontal lobe functioning. *Psychology and Aging, 5*, 148–151.

Dempster, F.N. (1992). The rise and fall of the inhibitory mechanism: Toward a unified theory of cognitive development and aging. *Developmental Review, 12*, 45–75.

Ferris, S.H., Crook, T., Clark, E., McCarthy, M., & Rae, D. (1980). Facial recognition memory deficits in normal aging and senile dementia. *Journal of Gerontology, 35*, 707–714.

Glisky, E.L., Polster, M.R., & Routhieaux, B.C. (1995). Double dissociation between item and source memory. *Neuropsychology, 9*, 229–235.

Harkins, S.W., Chapman, C.R., & Eisdorfer, C. (1979). Memory loss and response bias in senescence. *Journal of Gerontology, 34*, 66–72.

Hasher, L., & Zacks, R.T. (1988). Working memory, comprehension, and aging: A review of a new view. In G.H. Bower (Ed.), *The psychology of learning and motivation* (Vol. 22, pp. 193–225). New York: Academic Press.

Hay, J.F., & Jacoby, L.L. (1996). Separating habit and recollection: Memory slips, process dissociations and probability matching. *Journal of Experimental Psychology: Learning, Memory and Cognition, 22*, 1323–1335.

Hay, J.F., & Jacoby, L.L. (in press). Separating habit and recollection in young and elderly adults. Effects of elaborative processing and distinctiveness. *Psychology and Aging.*

Henkel, L.A., Johnson M.K., & De Leonardis, D.M. (1998). Aging and source monitoring: Cognitive processes and neuropsychological correlates. *Journal of Expermental Psychology: General, 127*, 251–268.

Jacoby, L.L. (1991). A process dissociation framework: Separating automatic from intentional uses of memory. *Journal of Memory and Language, 30*, 513–541.

Jacoby, L.L. (1996). Dissociating automatic and consciously-controlled effects of study/test compatability. *Journal of Memory and Language, 35*, 32–52.

Jacoby, L.L. (1998). Invariance in automatic influences of memory: Toward a user's guide for the process-dissociation procedure. *Journal of Experimental Psychology: Learning, Memory. and Cognition, 24.* 3–26.

Jacoby, L.L. (1999). Ironic effects of repetition: Measuring age-related differences in memory. *Journal of Experimental Psychology: Learning, Memory and Cognition, 25*, 3–22.

Jacoby, L.L., Jennings, J.M., & Hay, J.F. (1996). Dissociating automatic and consciously controlled processes: Implications for diagnosis and rehabilitation of memory deficits. In D.J. Herrmann, C.L. McEvoy, C. Hertzog, P. Hertel, & M.K. Johnson (Eds.), *Basic and applied memory research: Theory in context*, Vol.1 (pp. 161–193). Mahwah, NJ: Lawrence Erlbaum Associates Inc.

Jacoby, L.L., Kelley, C.M., & McElree, B. (in press). The role of cognitive control: Early selection vs. late correction. In S. Chaiken & Y. Trope (Eds.), *Dual process theories in social psychology*. New York: Guilford Press.

Jacoby, L.L., McElree, B., & Trainham, T.N. (in press). Automatic influences as accessibility bias in memory and Stroop-like tasks: Toward a formal model. In A. Koriat & D. Gopher (Eds.), *Attention and performance XVII*. Cambridge, MA: MIT Press.

Jacoby, L.L., Toth, L.P., & Yonelinas, A.P. (1993). Separating conscious and unconscious influences of memory: Measuring recollection. *Journal of Experimental Psychology: General, 122*, 139–154.

Kensinger, E.A., & Schacter, D.L. (this issue). When true memories suppress false memories: Effects of aging. *Cognitive Neuropsychology, 16*, 399–415.

Knowlton, B.J., Squire, L.R., & Gluck, M.A. (1994). Probabilistic classification learning in amnesia. *Learning and Memory, 1*, 106–120.

Koriat, A., & Goldsmith, M. (1996). Monitoring and control processes in the strategic regulation of memory accuracy. *Psychological Review, 103*, 490–517.

Lindsay, D.S., & Johnson, M.K. (1989). The eyewitness suggestibility effect and memory for source. *Memory and Cognition, 17*, 349–358.

Loftus, E.F. (1975). Leading questions and the eyewitness report. *Cognitive Psychology, 7*, 560–572.

Loftus, E.F., & Palmer, J.C. (1974). Reconstruction of automobile destruction: An example of the interaction between language and memory. *Journal of Verbal Learning and Verbal Behaviour, 13*, 585–589.

Maylor, E.A. (1990). Age, blocking and the tip of the tongue state. *British Journal of Psychology, 81*, 123–134.

McClelland, J.L., McNaughton, B.L., & O'Reilly, R.C. (1995). Why there are complementary learning systems in the hippocampus and neocortex: Insights from the successes and failures of connectionist models of learning and memory. *Psychological Review, 102*, 419–457.

McClelland, J.L., & Rumelhart, D.E. (1981). An interactive activation model of context effects in letter perception: Part I. An account of basic findings. *Psychological Review, 88*, 375–407.

McCloskey, M., & Zaragoza, M. (1985). Misleading post-event information and memory for events: Arguments and evidence against memory impairment hypotheses. *Journal of Experimental Psychology: General, 114*, 1–16.

McDowd, J.M. (1997). Inhibition in attention and aging. *Journal of Gerontology: Psychological Sciences, 52B*, P265–P273.

Moscovitch, M. (1989). Confabulation and the frontal systems: Strategic versus associative retrieval in neuropsychological theories of memory. In H.L. Roediger & F.I.M. Craik (Eds.), *Varieties of memory and consciousness: Essays in honour of Endel Tulving* (pp. 133–156). Hillsdale, NJ: Lawrence Erlbaum Associates Inc.

O'Reilly, R.C., Norman, K.A., & McClelland, J.L. (1997). A hippocampal model of recognition memory. In M.I. Jordan, J.J. Kearns, & S.A. Solla (Eds.), *Advances in neural information processing systems 10*. Cambridge, MA: MIT Press.

Rabinowitz, J.C., Craik, F.I.M., & Ackerman, B.P. (1982). A processing resource account of age differences in recall. *Canadian Journal of Psychology, 36*, 325–344.

Ratcliff, R., & McKoon, G. (1995) Bias in the priming of object decisions. *Journal of Experimental Psychology: Learning, Memory and Cognition, 21*, 754–767.

Ratcliff, R., & McKoon, G. (1997). A counter model for implicit priming in perceptual word identification. *Psychological Review, 104*, 319–343.

Raven, J.C. (1965). *Mill Hill Vocabulary Scale*. London: H. K. Lewis.

Reber, A.S. (1989). Implicit learning and tacit knowledge. *Journal of Experimental Psychology: General, 118*, 219–235.

Schacter, D.L., Norman, K.A., & Koustaal, W. (1998a). The cognitive neuroscience of constructive memory. *Annual Review of Psychology, 49*, 289–318.

Schacter, D.L., Verfaellie, M., Anes, M.D., & Racine, C. (1998b). When true recognition suppresses false recognition: Evidence from amnesic patients. *Journal of Cognitive Neuroscience, 10*, 668–679.

Schneider, W. (1990). *Micro experimental laboratory* [Computer program, Version 1.0]. Pittsburgh, PA: Psychology Software Tools.

Shallice, T., & Evans, M.E. (1978). The involvement of the frontal lobes in cognitive estimation. *Cortex, 14*, 294–303.

Shimamura, A.P. (1995). Memory and frontal lobe function. In M.S. Gazzaniga (Ed.). *The cognitive neurosciences* (pp. 803–813). Cambridge, MA: MIT Press.

Smith, S.M., & Tindell, D.R. (1997). Memory blocks in word fragment completion caused by involuntary retrieval of orthographically related pairs. *Journal of Experimental Psychology: Learning, Memory and Cognition, 23*, 355–370.

Snodgrass, J.G., & Corwin, J. (1988). Pragmatics of measuring recognition memory: Applications to dementia and amnesia. *Journal of Experimental Psychology: General, 117*, 34–50.

Thorndike, E.L., & Lorge, 1. (1944). *The teachers' handbook of 30,000 words*. New York: Columbia University.

Winocur, G., & Moscovitch, M. (1983). Paired-associate learning in institutionalized and non-institutionalized old people: An analysis of interference and context effects. *Journal of Gerontology, 38*, 455–464.

Yonelinas, A.P. (1994). Receiver-operating characteristics in recognition memory: Evidence for a dual-process model. *Journal of Experimental Psychology: Learning, Memory and Cognition, 20*, 1341–1354.

Yonelinas, A.P. (1997). Recognition memory ROCs for item and associative information: The contribution of recollection and familiarity. *Memory and Cognition, 25*, 747–763.

Zacks, R., & Hasher, L. (1997). Cognitive gerontology and attentional inhibition: A reply to Burke and McDowd. *Journal of Gerontology: Psychological Sciences, 52B*, P274–P283.

Zaragoza, M.S., McCloskey, M., & Jamis, M. (1987). Misleading postevent information and recall of the original event: Further evidence against the memory impairment hypothesis. *Journal of Experimental Psychology: Learning, Memory and Cognition, 13*, 36–44.

COGNITIVE NEUROPSYCHOLOGY, 1999, 16 (3/4/5), 437–458

STEREOTYPE RELIANCE IN SOURCE MONITORING: AGE DIFFERENCES AND NEUROPSYCHOLOGICAL TEST CORRELATES

Mara Mather, Marcia K. Johnson, and Doreen M. De Leonardis
Princeton University, USA

This study provides evidence that when source-specifying features are less available, people will rely more on their general knowledge to attribute memories to sources. Two factors (ageing and emotional self-focus) that, in general, are associated with poorer source identification performance both led to a greater reliance on stereotypes when participants attempted to remember who had said statements in a video they had watched earlier. In addition, correlations between older adults' ability to attribute statements correctly and their scores on a battery of neuropsychological tests suggests that both frontally based processes and medial temporally based processes affect accuracy of source identification, but do so to different degrees depending upon the nature of the source identification tasks.

INTRODUCTION

Our general knowledge about the world is invaluable in guiding us through our daily lives, helping us perceive, structure, and remember what we encounter. However, sometimes our knowledge can lead us astray. For example, when trying to remember which student in a seminar made a particularly interesting comment, you may misattribute the comment to the student who you know often says interesting things, rather than to the usually quiet student who actually made the remark. According to the Source Monitoring Framework (SMF) outlined by Johnson and her colleagues (e.g. Johnson, Hashtroudi, & Lindsay, 1993; Johnson & Raye, 1981, in press; Mitchell & Johnson, in press), general knowledge about how particular sources may relate to a remembered event is a critical part of attributing a source to the event.

The purpose of the present study was to investigate two factors that are likely to affect how much people rely on general knowledge (in this case, stereotypes) when making source judgements: (1) age; and (2) whether participants focus their attention inwardly or outwardly at encoding. In addition, this study investigates how two neuropsychological test batteries (comprised of tests often used to assess medial-temporal and frontal brain region functioning) correlate with the use of stereotypes in source monitoring.

Types of Information Used to Make Source Attributions

As outlined by the SMF, two main classes of information can be used to make source attributions for remembered information. The first consists of the

Requests for reprints should be addressed to Mara Mather, Psychology Dept., Princeton University, Princeton, NJ 08544-1010, USA (Tel: 609-258-4459; Fax: 609-258-1113; E-mail: tmmather@princeton.edu).

This research was supported by National Institute of Aging grant AG09253 and a Grant-In-Aid of Research from Sigma Xi. We wish to thank Sean Lane, Karen Mitchell, Carol Raye, and John Reeder for their helpful comments on previous drafts of this paper and Eli Massar, Maria Neimark, and Christine Voegeli for their help in testing participants.

qualitative characteristics of the information that come to mind, such as associated emotional reactions, associated cognitive operations, and semantic, perceptual, temporal, and spatial detail. The quality and quantity of particular types of characteristics can be used to distinguish one source from another. For example, because memories for perceived events tend to include more perceptual and contextual detail than memories for imagined events (e.g. Hashtroudi, Johnson, & Chrosniak, 1990; Henkel, Johnson, & De Leonardis, 1998; Johnson, Foley, Suengas, & Raye, 1988; Johnson, Raye, Foley, & Kim, 1982; Mather, Henkel, & Johnson, 1997; Norman & Schacter, 1997; Schooler, Gerhard, & Loftus, 1986; Suengas & Johnson, 1988), the amount of perceptual and contextual detail associated with a particular memory can help one determine whether the event was perceived or imagined. Even in situations in which imagined events seem indistinguishable from perceived events, inducing participants to focus on perceptual and contextual memorial characteristics can increase their source monitoring accuracy (Lane & Villa, 1997; Mather et al., 1997).

The second class of information that can be used to make memory source attributions includes beliefs, supporting memories, plausibility, schemas, stereotypes, and category information. We know from many different lines of research that our general knowledge and beliefs about the world can have a powerful effect on the way we perceive and remember the world, helping us to organise information (so that we do not have to remember all the details to retain the meaning), but sometimes leading to systematic errors (e.g. Bartlett, 1932, Bransford & Johnson, 1973; Devine, 1989; Fiske & Neuberg, 1990; Owens, Bower, & Black, 1979; Ross, 1989; Taylor & Crocker, 1981).

To date, most studies investigating source monitoring processes have focused on the use of more specific attributes such as perceptual detail and cognitive operations and not on the role of more general, abstract knowledge in determining the source of information. Conversely, most studies investigating the effects of stereotypes and schemas on memory have focused on the fact that schema-consistent errors occur, rather than on the source attribution processes that account for why the errors occur.

However, in daily life specific attributes and general knowledge often act in concert to help determine how we remember events. Both types of information are continuously activated, weighted, and used in ongoing source attributions that are integral parts of all remembering. For example, in trying to remember who gave you permission to do something, in which store you purchased a particular item, or when you last had a tetanus shot, both specific qualities of the memory and general knowledge guide attribution of information to sources (e.g. who, where, when, etc.). One question is how these two types of information interact. Do people change how much they weight one type of information depending upon how much access they have to the other type of information? The present study uses an explicit source identification task to explore the interplay between specific feature information and general knowledge in remembering.

Using Category or Stereotype Knowledge to Make Memory Attributions

Using our knowledge about typical members of a category to attribute information to a member of that category can be quite a useful strategy. For example, if one were trying to remember who was talking about a great new fitness centre, one might be more likely to attribute the information to an athletic friend than to a nonathletic friend. However, if it happened to be a nonathletic friend who made the remark, relying only on stereotype knowledge would lead to an incorrect attribution. Such misattributions could have a much more serious impact than just making it difficult to find the phone number of the new fitness centre. For example, an eyewitness might misattribute a crime to someone other than the actual perpetrator because it seems more consistent with their race or gender.

One type of study that has examined the effects of general categorical knowledge on source attributions has been concerned with distinguishing category-based and person-based memory (Brewer, Weber, & Carini, 1995; Taylor & Falcone, 1982; Taylor, Fiske, Etcoff, & Ruderman, 1978; see also

Stangor, Lynch, Duan, & Glass, 1992). In these studies, participants were presented with a video (or slides and tape-recording) of a group of people talking. The composition of the groups was varied, such that discussants could be split into groups based on some feature such as race, gender, or the colour of their sweatshirt. In general, when later asked to attribute the statements that had been made to their speaker, participants made more misattributions within a category (e.g. misattributing something one female said to another female) than between categories (e.g. misattributing something a female said to a male). This difference in error rates was interpreted as suggesting that participants relied on the categories to some extent when attributing the source of the statements. Similar findings have been used to argue that source information is not an all-or-none proposition—instead, memories represent different amounts of partial source information (Dodson, Holland, & Shimamura, 1998). We may remember that a female said a statement, but not know which female said it. These studies (e.g. Dodson et al., 1998; Taylor et al., 1978) provide evidence consistent with the idea that category knowledge can play a role in making source attributions. However, they do not distinguish between two factors—both assumed to be important within the SMF—attributions based on abstract category information and attributions based on partial item-specific information (e.g. remembering a voice was high-pitched, but not more discriminating perceptual information). In addition, the stereotypicality of the content of the information to be attributed was not manipulated in those studies.

Studies that have manipulated how well the content of items corresponds with stereotypes about target sources have found that content can play an important role in source attributions. For example, unfriendly behaviours were more likely to be misattributed to a skinhead than were friendly behaviours (Sherman & Bessenoff, in press). Another study (Stangor, 1988) had participants read about actors performing actions (e.g. "Pam met a friend for coffee") and then had them recognise which statements they had previously read. Participants were instructed to reject statements if the actors had been switched (e.g. "Don met a friend for coffee"). Participants were more likely to falsely recognise gender-consistent pairings of actors and behaviours than gender-inconsistent pairings. Gender stereotypes also played a role for participants presented with a recently read name and asked to decide whether or not it belonged to a famous person (Banaji & Greenwald, 1995). Participants were more likely to categorise the name incorrectly as being famous if it was a male name than if it was a female name. In a related vein, in a study of conversation memory (Holtgraves, Srull, & Socall, 1989), participants who believed the speaker was of higher status than his conversational partner were more likely to falsely recognise assertive paraphrases of the speaker's remarks than participants who believed the two speakers were of equal status (e.g. "Tell them to hurry things up" when what had actually been said was "You could ask them to hurry things up"). Knowledge about a particular source also affected source attributions in a study in which participants were more likely to say they had heard a particular speaker say a word (that had actually not been spoken) if they had heard that speaker say a list of words semantically related to the new word than if they had heard the other speaker say the related words (Mather et al., 1997). Thus, knowledge or beliefs about what sort of things are typically associated with a particular source can sometimes lead to false source attributions.

The present study investigated two factors (age and emotional focus) that should affect how much people rely on stereotypes when trying to identify the source of remembered information. Participants watched a videotape of two women making statements. Each woman said some statements that matched her stereotyped description in the instructions (speaker-consistent statements; e.g. "We need to invest in rehabilitating criminals, rather than just punishing them" said by a woman previously described as a Democrat) and some statements that did not match the speaker's established stereotype but rather matched the description of the other speaker (speaker-inconsistent statements; e.g. "Illegal immigrants shouldn't receive public services" also said by the Democrat). This comparison between performance on items in which the actual source and the probable source (based on knowledge about the speaker) are the same (speaker-consistent) and items for which the actual source and the probable source are different (speaker-inconsistent) allowed us to separate the influence of categorical knowledge from that of more specific qualitative characteristics.

Ageing and Reliance on Stereotypes

The majority of studies investigating how stereotypes may affect memory for social information have involved only college students. However, as we age, the way we process and remember information changes (e.g. Light, 1996; Salthouse, 1992; Schacter, Koutstaal, & Norman, 1997). Older adults often show a deficit in making source identifications, even when they are as good as younger adults at recognising that items were previously presented (e.g. Brown, Jones, & Davis, 1995; Ferguson, Hashtroudi, & Johnson, 1992; Henkel et al., 1998; McIntyre & Craik, 1987; Spencer & Raz, 1995).

Of particular interest for this study is the possibility that older adults rely more than younger adults do on abstract, stereotypical (i.e. categorical) cues in making attributions about the source of a remembered item. For example, in studies in which younger and older adults heard words spoken by either two similar sources (two females) or two dissimilar sources (male and female) (Ferguson et al., 1992; Johnson, De Leonardis, Hashtroudi, & Ferguson, 1995), older adults were worse than younger adults at identifying the source of a word when both speakers had been female. Yet when the speakers were male and female, older adults were just as good as younger adults at identifying the source of words. In a related study (Bayen & Murnane, 1996) in which the distinctiveness of both gender (two males vs. one male and one female) and temporal context (speakers' statements alternated vs. were blocked) were varied, older adults performed as well as younger adults only in the condition in which both the speaker's gender and temporal context of the statement could discriminate between the sources.

These experiments, however, do not necessarily indicate that older adults rely more on categorical information to make source attributions than younger adults. The categories in these studies (i.e. male and female, temporal context) were associated with different qualitative characteristics of the memory for the items (i.e. voice qualities suggesting gender, distinctiveness of the memory trace, or particular associations suggesting when it was presented). It may be that the older adults generally have fewer (or less vivid) perceptual/contextual qualitative characteristics available to make source judgements (e.g. Hashtroudi et al., 1990), but that when these qualitative characteristics are different enough, older adults can make quite accurate source judgements in spite of an overall lower level of qualitative information (e.g. Dodson et al., 1998). In contrast, in the present study, the categorical information (e.g. political affiliation) does not arise from any physical qualities of the speaker or from the context in which the statement was said, allowing us to examine the influence of categorical knowledge separately from the influence of source similarity of physical or contextual features.

Some previous studies do provide direct evidence of increased reliance on general knowledge during source monitoring in older adults. For example, older adults are more likely to identify an object incorrectly as having been present in a visual scene if the object typically belongs in that context than if it does not (e.g. a sink vs. a television in a kitchen scene), and the difference between their false recognition of new but thematically associated items and new unassociated items is greater than it is for the young (Hess & Slaughter, 1990). In other studies, age differences in memory decrease as the relevance and typicality of the target information increases (Hess, Donley, & Vandermaas, 1989) and also as test stimuli are more meaningfully organised (Waddell & Rogoff, 1981), suggesting that older adults are able to take advantage of general knowledge during remembering. Thus, in the current study, we expected older adults to show less of a memory disadvantage relative to younger adults when attributing speaker-consistent statements than when attributing speaker-inconsistent statements.

We further expected that the ability to attribute the source of speaker-inconsistent statements correctly would be particularly difficult for older participants with low performance on measures of reflective or executive functions usually associated with frontal brain regions—activities such as planning, problem solving, metamemory, and evaluation and retrieval of information in memory (e.g. Johnson & Raye, 1998; Moscovitch & Winocur, 1995; Nolde, Johnson, & Raye, 1998b; Raz, Gunning-Dixon, Head, Dupuis, & Acker, 1998; Shimamura,1995; Stuss & Benson, 1986; West, 1996). In general, source identification decisions require more frontally based reflective activity than do old/new recognition decisions (Johnson, Kounios, & Nolde, 1996a). However, we expect that not all source identification tasks rely on frontal brain regions to the same extent. The level of reliance should depend upon the level of reflective activity demanded by the task (Nolde et al., 1998b). In the present context, processes supported by frontal regions should be essential (at both acquisition and test) to help resolve the contradictions between the schematic content of the statement that implies one source and the specific attribute details that imply another source.

In contrast, determining the source of the schema-consistent items should depend less upon frontal functioning. Correct attribution of these schema-consistent items should depend both on the ability to encode the general schema about each person and on the initial binding and subsequent reactivation of item-specific attributes (e.g. associating the speaker's emotional expression with the content of the statement). These processes are more likely to be supported by the medial-temporal regions (e.g. N.J. Cohen & Eichenbaum, 1993; Johnson & Chalfonte, 1994; Squire, 1992; Squire & Knowlton, 1995). In addition, we expected accurate old/new recognition of both types of statements to be supported by medial-temporal regions (e.g. Squire, 1992).

Normal ageing is likely to be accompanied by neuropathology in frontal (e.g. Haug & Eggers, 1991; Raz et al., 1998; West, 1996) and medial-temporal regions (e.g. Golomb et al., 1994; Jernigan et al., 1991). Thus, in order to investigate the brain mechanisms underlying source monitoring processes, we examined the older participants' memory performance in relation to their performance on two batteries of neuropsychological tests that have been used to assess frontal and medial-temporal brain region functioning (Glisky, Polster, & Routhieaux, 1995; Henkel et al., 1998). The frontal and medial-temporal test batteries are each composed of several tests for which performance has often been shown to be impaired in patients with lesions in frontal and medial-temporal brain regions, respectively. Any particular test may not specifically and uniquely assess functioning of frontal or medial-temporal brain regions (e.g. Reitan & Wolfson, 1994; Salthouse, Fristoe, & Rhee, 1996). Nonetheless, the frontal tasks generally tap more complex reflective or executive processes than the medial-temporal tasks, and thus differences in patterns of correlations between these batteries and other performance measures provide clues about processes and underlying brain regions.

Emotional Focus and Reliance on Stereotypes

Often when interacting with other people, we evaluate what was said by considering how we feel about it or how it relates to ourselves. Focusing on one's own emotional reactions to an event can result in a memorial trade-off. Because focusing on one's own feelings may distract one from the event itself, contextual and perceptual details are less likely to be bound to that event, making it more difficult later to identify the context in which the event was experienced. Instead, the external event may become linked with personal associations, possibly making it easier to recall or recognise the event itself later (but not its source). In general, distracted participants are more likely to base impressions on group knowledge than on individuating characteristics (Bargh & Thein, 1985; Kruglanski & Freund, 1983; Macrae, Hewstone, & Griffiths, 1993; Pratto & Bargh, 1991; Rothbart, Fulero, Jensen, Howard, & Birrell, 1978), suggesting that an emotional self-focus may have similar effects.

The simultaneous positive and negative memorial effects of self-focus were reflected in a study in which participants hearing statements thought about either how they felt or how the speakers felt about what was being said (Johnson, Nolde, & De Leonardis, 1996b). Participants who thought about their own feelings later recognised the content of the statements better than did participants who thought about the speakers' feelings. However, self-focus resulted in poorer identification of the source of the statement than did other-focus. In addition, in a subsequent study, older adults were affected by the direction of focus in the same way as younger adults (De Leonardis, Nolde, & Johnson, 1996). Emotional self-focus also increases the number of elaborations that later embellish an account of an event (Hashtroudi, Johnson, Vnek, & Ferguson, 1994). Interestingly, self-focus when reviewing an event can lead to a particular pattern of memory distortion, in which events are remembered as being more internally consistent (and thus more schematic) than they actually were (Mather & Johnson, 1998).

Therefore we manipulated the direction of emotional focus in this study. We predicted that participants in the present study who focused on how they felt about the statements they heard would be better at recognising the statements but worse at identifying the source of the statements than participants who focused on how the speakers felt about the statements. Of particular interest was the form of the source identification deficit in the self-focus condition. One possibility is that self-focus participants will show a uniform source memory deficit for both consistent and inconsistent items. However, the tendency for emotional self-focus to lead to more schematic recall in Mather and Johnson (1998) and previous studies, which found that distracted participants were more likely to form impressions based on stereotypes or general knowledge about a group, suggest that self-focus may lead to a greater reliance on stereotypes in source identification. If so, emotional self-focus would lead to a source memory deficit that is greatest for the inconsistent items.

There is some evidence that older adults may focus more on affective information when experiencing events. For example, they report greater memory for thoughts and feelings experienced at the time of a remembered event than do younger adults (Hashtroudi et al., 1990). Focusing on thoughts and feelings when thinking about an event can reduce the salience of the event's contextual and sensory characteristics (Suengas & Johnson, 1988). Thus, age differences in remembering information may sometimes be related to the type of focus preferred by each age group. In addition, even when both older and younger adults engage in an emotional focus, it can have more of an effect (relative to a more factual focus) on older adults' performance (Hashtroudi et al., 1994). Consequently, we were interested in whether the direction of emotional focus may affect one's reliance upon stereotypes any differently for older adults than for younger adults.

Another question addressed is how the direction of focus affects the forming of a stereotype on-line. In this study, participants were given a stereotype label for each speaker before watching the videotape; thus they did not have to form an impression on-line in order to be able to tell that certain statements were consistent or inconsistent with the speaker's label. To see how the direction of focus may affect the use of stereotypes when the stereotype must be formed as the video is watched, we also had each speaker say a set of statements that were from a second, unrelated schema set (secondary-schema statements). These statements were irrelevant to the speaker's dominant schema, but were internally consistent for each speaker. Thus if a speaker was described as a Republican, she might also make some statements consistent with being athletic. We were also interested in whether age (in particular, medial-temporal functioning) might be related to the likelihood of forming stereotypes on-line.

Experiment Overview

In summary, in this study we investigated how age and emotional self-focus affect participants' reliance on stereotypes when making source judgements from memory. For this purpose, we gave participants a source identification test that included both old and new statements that fit particular stereotypes. Some statements had been said by a speaker with a stereotype label consistent with the content of the statement and some had actually been said by the other speaker. By contrasting participants' ability to attribute the source of the speaker-consistent statements with their ability to attribute speaker-inconsistent statements, we derived a measure of stereotype reliance that could be compared across conditions. In addition, we included secondary-schema items (all of which were consistent with their speaker), for which the stereotype could be learned only by listening to the statements throughout the video, in order to compare how the different conditions affected the likelihood of acquiring and applying a schema on-line. For the older adults, we also administered batteries of neuropsychological tests associated with frontal and medial-temporal brain region functioning. We correlated source identification and recognition performance with scores on these test batteries to investigate neuropsychological correlates of stereotype reliance in this situation.

METHOD

Participants

Forty-eight older adults (ages 62–85 years; mean = 72) and 48 undergraduates (ages 17–21 years; mean = 19) participated. All of the older adults and some of the younger adults received financial compensation for their participation. The rest of the younger adults received credit toward a course requirement. Three additional older adults participated, but their data were discarded because they indicated that they had difficulty hearing 12 or more of the statements on the video. One other older adult participated but was replaced because she took notes while watching the video.

Materials

Two pairs of schemas were used. One pair included a Republican and a Democrat schema and the other pair included a writer and an athlete schema. One-paragraph descriptions (see Appendix A) and 24 related items corresponding to each schema were created (see Table 1 for some example statements from each schema).

The related items were designed such that they were associated with their corresponding schema, but could be said by someone not associated with that schema without undermining that other speaker's schema (e.g. although being a Democrat is more associated with being pro-choice for abortion, a Republican might happen to be pro-choice). In addition, there were four filler items for each schema that were unambiguously associated with the schema (e.g. "Writing is my passion in life" for the writer schema; "My parents were also

Table 1. *Examples of Statements Associated with Schemas*

Athlete
I work out almost every day.
It's hard to find good athletic clothing.
I enjoy competing in athletic events.
I think many of the Olympic athletes are such amazing role models.
A coach I once had told me not to worry about winning or losing, but just to have a great time doing it.

Writer
I was the editor of the paper in high school.
I can type faster than I write.
I don't have enough bookcases to hold my books.
In the evenings, I usually curl up on the couch with a good book.
My mother always said I shouldn't read in dim light.

Republican
Most college professors are liberal, so students get a distorted view of reality.
I think welfare creates a cycle of dependency.
Divorce laws should be tougher so that people take marriage seriously.
We need stricter measures to prevent illegal immigration.
Affirmative action discriminates against white males.

Democrat
I'm pro-choice.
I seriously considered serving in the Peace Corps.
There are many gross inequities in our society today.
The death penalty is a cruel and unusual punishment.
The federal government must do more to protect our environment.

Democrats" for the Democrat schema). For counterbalancing purposes, eight acquisition videotapes were created in which two middle-aged women randomly alternated reading statements (with the constraint that neither speaker said more than two statements in a row). After each statement, there was a 15-second pause, followed by a beep and the next statement. In each videotape, each of the women had a dominant schema that was explicitly described in the instructions (e.g. Democrat). Half (12) of the statements she read corresponded to that schema. Another six of the statements each woman read corresponded to the dominant schema of the other woman in the videotape (e.g. Republican). Each woman also had a secondary schema (e.g. athlete), and the six other statements she read were from that schema. This schema was not described for the subjects and there were no statements inconsistent with it. Thus, it could develop on-line as the video advanced. In addition to these 24 target items each woman also read the 4 filler items corresponding to her dominant schema (2 at the beginning of the videotape and 2 at the end). The materials were counterbalanced such that: (1) The dominant schemas were equally as often Republican/Democrat as they were writer/athlete; (2) there was every possible pairing of dominant schemas with secondary schemas (such that there were both Republican-athlete and Republican-writer characters); (3) the actors who read the statements played an athlete, a writer, a Republican and a Democrat equally often; and (4) each statement was presented as a consistent, inconsistent, and secondary schema item as often as was every other statement.

For the memory test, each participant read 72 statements, randomly ordered. All 48 critical statements that had been heard in the video were on the list (the filler items were not included). There were also 24 new statements. Six of these corresponded to each of the two speaker's secondary schemas and six corresponded to each speaker's dominant schema[1].

Procedure

Before participating in the experiment, participants were asked if they felt comfortable using a computer mouse. If they did not, they were given a computer-run tutorial to familiarise them with pointing and clicking the mouse. Subsequently, participants viewed the video either alone or in pairs. If there were two participants in the same session, one was randomly assigned to the self-focus condition and the other to the other-focus condition. The focus conditions and the video counterbalancing conditions were crossed such that three self-focus and three other-focus participants viewed each of the eight videotapes in each of the age groups.

Participants were given written instructions and a pen to fill out a rating form corresponding to their condition. In the self-focus condition, the first line of the instructions was "We are interested in how much people agree in the strength of their feelings to various types of statements." In the other-focus condition, the first line was "We are interested in people's ability to perceive other people's emotions." Then both instructions continued as follows:

> We have videotaped a number of people saying statements about different sorts of things and had them rate the strength of their feelings about what they said. In the videotape you will see, you will hear Sandy and Patricia saying statements. Before recording the videotape, they were asked to write down a number of statements that were opinions they hold or facts about themselves. During the videotape, they were cued by the experimenter to read the statements they had written.

Subsequently, self-focus participants were instructed to think about how strongly they felt about what was said after they heard each statement, and then rate how strongly they felt about it on the rating sheet provided. Other-focus participants were instructed to think about how strongly they thought the speaker felt about what she had said, and then to rate how strongly they thought the speaker felt on their rating sheet. Participants were given an example of how to rate a sentence. Then

[1] Note that new items were always consistent with one of the two speaker's schemas, either the dominant or secondary one.

participants were instructed that if they had difficulty understanding what was said for any particular statement they should draw a line through that item on their sheet, and not to discuss anything with the other participant if there was someone else watching the video at the same time.

Participants then turned the page and read descriptions of the two speakers. The descriptions they read corresponded with the dominant schema of each speaker in that counterbalancing condition (see Appendix A for descriptions). Participants were shown photographs of each speaker with their name so they would know which description corresponded with which speaker on the video. As they watched the video, participants rated each statement on a 5-point scale with the endpoints of either *the speaker does not feel strongly/the speaker feels strongly or I do not feel strongly/I do feel strongly.*

After watching the video, participants moved to another room, where they were seated at a computer (if there were two participants, they were seated with their backs to each other so they could not see what the other person was doing). They were given a computer-presented recognition test, with the photos and names of the women available to look at, in case they forgot which name corresponded with which speaker. Each statement in the test was displayed at the top of the screen. Participants first clicked on a button displayed on the screen to indicate that either "yes," the statement had been said in the video, or "no," the statement had not been said in the video. Then they rated each old/new judgement on a scale from 1 for not at all confident to 5 for very confident. If they said that the item was not said in the video, they were presented with the next statement. If, however, they had said the item was in the video, they were asked to make a source judgement by choosing either Sandy or Patricia as the speaker of the statement and then to make a confidence rating (using the same scale as for the old/new judgement) for the source judgement. They were then presented with the next statement.

When participants had completed the memory test, they were debriefed and paid or given course credit. Forty of the 48 (20 self-focus and 20 other-focus) older participants returned for a separate session to complete the neuropsychological tests (Glisky et al., 1995). Frontal lobe measures were: the modified Wisconsin Card Sorting Test (Hart, Kwentus, Wade, & Taylor, 1988), the Controlled Oral Word Association Test (Benton & Hamsher, 1976), the Mental Arithmetic Test from the Weschler Adult Intelligence Scale-Revised (Weschler, 1981), and the Mental Control Test and Backward Digit Span Test from the Weschler Memory Scale-Revised (Weschler, 1987). Medial-temporal lobe measures were: Logical Memory 1, Verbal Paired Associates 1, and Visual Paired Associates II (all from the Weschler Memory Scale-Revised), and the Long-Delay Cued Recall measure from the California Verbal Learning Test (Delis, Kramer, Kaplan, & Ober, 1987).

RESULTS

An alpha level of .05 was assumed for all of the following statistical tests. If a participant had marked that he or she had difficulty hearing or understanding a statement during the video, that item was excluded from the analysis of their memory test results (proportions reported included only the items they did hear).

Correct Recognition of Old Items

A 2 (Age: old, young) × 2 (Focus: self, other) × 3 (Item Type: consistent, inconsistent, secondary) ANOVA for old items that were correctly recognised as old (see Table 2) revealed main effects of Age [$F(1,92) = 29.29$, $MSe = 0.02$], and Focus [$F(1,92) = 13.38$, $MSe = 0.02$]. Younger adults were more likely to say correctly that a statement from the video had been in the video (mean = .94) than were older adults (mean = .85), and participants who had focused on their own feelings while watching the video were more accurate (mean = .93) than those who had focused on the speakers' feelings (mean = .86). There were no effects of item type and no interactions, indicating that whether the statement was consistent or

Table 2. *Correct Recognition and Source Identification for Younger and Older Participants*

	Younger		*Older*	
Item Type	*Self-focus*	*Other-focus*	*Self-focus*	*Other-focus*
Recognition of old items				
Consistent	.95	.91	.90	.80
Inconsistent	.97	.91	.89	.79
Secondary-schema	.97	.95	.89	.82
Source identification				
Consistent	.91	.93	.86	.90
Inconsistent	.75	.88	.40	.62
Secondary-schema	.84	.94	.78	.91

inconsistent with the speaker or whether it was from the speaker's primary or secondary schema did not affect whether it would be recognised later.

Source Identification

If participants relied solely on the stereotypes to make their source attributions, they should correctly attribute nearly all of the speaker-consistent statements and virtually none of the speaker-inconsistent statements. In contrast, if participants were not affected by the stereotypes at all in making their source attributions, they should have approximately the same proportion of correct attributions for the consistent and the inconsistent statements. Thus, the difference between each participant's proportion of correctly identified speaker-consistent statements and their proportion of correctly identified speaker-inconsistent statements (both shown in the bottom of Table 2) indicates the extent to which they relied on the stereotypes to make their attributions. We submitted these difference scores to a 2 (Age: younger, older) × 2 (Focus: self, other) ANOVA, which revealed main effects of both Age [$F(1,92) = 31.96$ $MSe = 0.05$] and Focus [$F(1,92) = 8.85$, $MSe = 0.05$] (see Fig. 1). Older adults were more likely than younger adults were to rely on the stereotypes (means = .37 and .11, respectively), and self-focus participants were more likely than other-focus participants to rely on the stereotypes (means = .31 and .17, respectively). There was no interaction of Age and Focus.

In addition, because we were interested in performance on each type of item, we conducted separate Age × Focus ANOVAs for correct source identification for each Item Type (consistent, inconsistent, and secondary; see Table 2 for means). For consistent items, there were no significant effects. Older adults and younger adults showed no difference in the probability they would identify the source of consistent old items and the focus at encoding also did not affect participants' ability to identify the source. For secondary items, there was a main effect of Focus [$F(1,92) = 12.55$, $MSe = 0.03$], with other-focus leading to better source accuracy (mean = .92) than self-focus (mean = .81). Thus, for both types of consistent items (secondary schema items were all consistent with their speaker), there were no age differences in source attributions. For inconsistent items, however, there was a main effect of Age, [$F(1,92) = 49.93$, $MSe = 0.05$], as predicted. When asked to identify the source of an item that was inconsistent with its speaker's dominant schema, older adults were much less accurate (mean = .51) than younger adults (mean = .81). There was also a main effect of Focus [$F(1,92) = 15.82$, $MSe = 0.05$], with self-focused participants less accurate (mean = .57) at attributing inconsistent statements than other-focused participants (mean = .75).

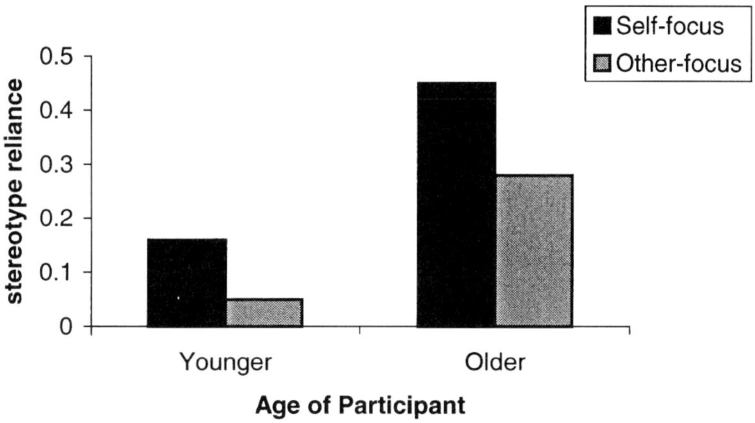

Fig. 1. *Reliance on stereotypes to make source attributions (reliance = proportion of speaker-consistent items correctly attributed – proportion of speaker-inconsistent items correctly attributed).*

False Alarms to New Items

Every new item was consistent with one of the two speakers, whether it was consistent with a speaker's primary (described in advance) or secondary (potentially picked up through watching the video) schema. Thus, every false alarm to a new item was attributed to a source that was either consistent or inconsistent with the content of the statement (see Table 3).

A 2 (Age: old, young) × 2 (Focus: self, other) × 2 (Schema Associated with Statement: primary, secondary) × 2 (False Alarm Attribution: consistent, inconsistent) ANOVA revealed a main effect of Age [$F(1,92) = 8.73$, $MSe = 0.004$]. Older adults were more likely to recognise new items falsely than were younger adults. In addition, participants were more likely to recognise a statement falsely from a speaker's primary schema than one from their secondary schema [$F(1,92) = 16.80$, $MSe = 0.002$]. A main effect of Type of False Alarm [$F(1,92) = 13.05$, $MSe = 0.003$], indicated that participants were more likely to attribute new items to the speaker with which the new items were consistent than to the other speaker. There were also several interactions[2] that were qualified by a four-way interaction of all the factors [$F(1,92) = 4.74$, $MSe = 0.003$]. This interaction was the result of the fact that, as can be seen in Table 3, older adults. were by far more likely to attribute primary schema new items to their consistent speaker than to make any other type of false alarm, a tendency which was even more likely when they had been self-focused (mean = .11) than when they had been other-focused (mean = .07). Thus, older adults were less likely than younger adults to screen out new items consistent with the primary schema of a speaker, especially if they had focused on their own feelings when hearing the statements.

Confidence Ratings

Recognition. We analysed confidence in correct and incorrect responses in a 2 (Age: younger, older) × 2 (Focus: self, other) × 2 (Response: correct, incorrect) ANOVA for each type of item[3]. There were main effects of Response for

[2] These other significant interactions were: Age by Focus, Age by Associated Schema, Age by False Alarm Attribution, Associated Schema by False Alarm Attribution, and a three-way interaction of Age, Associated Schema, and False Alarm Attribution.

[3] We analysed each type of item separately to minimise the impact of missing data points (some participants did not have any incorrect responses for a particular type of item and thus could not be included in the analysis for that type of item).

Table 3. *Proportion of False Alarms (FAs) to New Items for Younger and Older Participants*

	Self-focus		*Other-focus*	
	Cons. Attr.	*Incons. Attr.*	*Cons. Attr.*	*Incons. Attr.*
Younger participants				
Primary schema FAs	.02	.01	.05	.02
Secondary schema FAs	.01	.01	.01	.03
Older participants				
Primary schema FAs	.11	.01	.07	.01
Secondary schema FAs	.02	.03	.02	.01

Cons. Attr. = consistent attribution (e.g. Republican item attributed to a Republican speaker); Incons. Attr. = inconsistent attribution. The proportion of consistent and inconsistent attributions in each category (e.g. younger participants primary-schema self-focus condition), should be added (not averaged) to obtain the total proportion of false alarms in that condition for that type of item.

consistent [$F(1,73) = 190.99$, $MSe = 0.41$], inconsistent [$F(1,57) = 42.58$, $MSe = 0.67$], secondary [$F(1,48) = 66.44$, $MSe = 0.77$], and new items [$F(1,52) = 61.25$, $MSe = 0.44$], all indicating that participants were more confident in their correct responses than in their incorrect responses (see Table 4 for means). In addition, there were interactions of Age and Response for consistent [$F(1,73) = 4.64$, $MSe = 0.41$], secondary [$F(1,48) = 8.41$, $MSe = 0.77$], and new items [$F(1,52) = 5.36$, $MSe = 0.44$], such that older participants exhibited less difference between their confidence in their correct and incorrect responses than did younger adults. There were no other significant effects in the ANOVA analyses.

One possible explanation of the age deficit in confidence discriminability is that older adults used less of the scale when making their confidence ratings. However, in a t-test, there was not a significant difference between the standard deviations of older (mean = .88) and younger (mean = .93) adults' recognition confidence ratings. Thus, older adults use about as much of the scale as younger adults, but their ratings are less associated with their accuracy than those of younger adults.

Source Identification. As we did for recognition of old items, we analysed the average difference between confidence in correct and incorrect source attribution in a 2 (Age: younger, older) × 2 (Focus: self, other) × 2 (Response: correct, incorrect) ANOVA for consistent, inconsistent, and secondary items (it was not possible to make a correct attribution for new items). As found for recognition confidence, participants were more confident in their correct responses than in their incorrect responses for consistent [$F(1,64) = 76.69$, $MSe = 0.56$], inconsistent [$F(1,80) = 30.66$, $MSe = 0.46$], and secondary items [$F(1,49) = 25.42$, $MSe = 0.45$] (see Table 4 for means). In addition, older adults' confidence was less discriminating than younger adults' confidence, as indicated by the interactions of Age and Response for consistent [$F(1,64) = 6.61$, $MSe = 0.56$] and secondary items [$F(1,49) = 9.26$, $MSe = 0.45$][4]. For the source confidence ratings of the new items that were incorrectly recognised we conducted a 2 (Age: younger, older) × 2 (Focus: self, other) ANOVA. There was a main effect of Age [$F(1,52) = 6.70$, $MSe = 1.18$], indicating that older adults were more confident about their incorrectly attributed new items

[4] For both recognition and source identification, the interaction between Age and Response was not significant for inconsistent items, although it was in the same direction as for the other items.

Table 4. *Confidence Ratings for Younger and Older Participants for Correct and Incorrect Items*

	Correct	*Incorrect*
Old/New Recognition		
Younger Adults		
Consistent	4.77	3.09
Inconsistent	4.74	3.39
Secondary-schema	4.89	2.87
New	4.35	3.02
Older Adults		
Consistent	4.60	3.38
Inconsistent	4.56	3.71
Secondary-schema	4.55	3.59
New	4.35	3.63
Source Identification		
Younger Adults		
Consistent	4.47	3.01
Inconsistent	4.37	3.61
Secondary-schema	4.24	3.11
New		2.97
Older Adults		
Consistent	4.17	3.37
Inconsistent	4.07	3.66
Secondary-schema	4.06	3.78
New		3.76

For each type of item, the means are based on those subjects who made both correct and incorrect responses, corresponding with our analyses.

(mean = 3.76) than were younger adults (mean = 2.97).

As we did for the recognition confidence, we tested whether older adults were using a restricted range. Again, there was no significant difference between the average standard deviation of older (mean = .82) and younger (mean = .73) adults' confidence ratings.

Thus, across multiple types of confidence judgements, older adults' confidence ratings were less discriminating between correct and incorrect responses than younger adults' confidence ratings, although they selected just as large a variety of confidence scores as younger adults did. This difference was apparent even under circumstances in which older adults' memory responses were nearly as accurate as those of younger adults (source attributions of schema-consistent items).

Performance in Relation to Neuropsychological Test Scores

Scores on each test were converted to standardised z scores for each of the 40 older participants who completed the neuropsychological test batteries. For each participant, z scores were averaged across the five tests associated with a frontal factor and across the four tests associated with a medial-temporal factor (Glisky et al., 1995; Henkel et al., 1998). This yielded a frontal score and a medial-temporal score for each participant. Each participant was designated as a high frontal scorer if they scored above the mean and a low frontal scorer if they scored below the mean. The same was done for the medial-temporal scores. The distribution of high and low scorers across the two conditions was fairly evenly distributed (frequencies of high and low frontal and medial-temporal scores for the self-focus condition: HH = 4; HL = 6; LH = 4; LL = 6; for the other-focus condition: HH = 6; HL = 4; LH = 4; LL = 6), and the mean frontal and medial-temporal scores did not differ in the two conditions. Within the group of older participants, the oldest participants tended to have lower frontal ($r = -.27$) and medial-temporal scores ($r = -.22$), though neither correlation was significant.

Of particular interest is whether age-related neuropathology in medial-temporal and frontal brain regions may underlie the age deficits found in this study. Thus, to avoid confounding our analyses with other age-related factors, we used partial correlations to remove variance due to age for all of the following correlations. We correlated the frontal and medial-temporal scores with each participant's corrected recognition score (false alarms to new items subtracted from correct hits to old items) and correct source identification scores (we correlated the source identification scores for each type of item separately because we expected frontal processes to be more important for identifying the source of speaker-inconsistent than speaker-consistent items). In addition, we were interested in whether the age-related deficit in the difference in confidence scores between correct and incorrect responses (confidence discriminability) might be correlated with the neuropsychological test scores. Thus, we also correlated each participant's average difference in confidence for their correct and incorrect responses (for both recognition and source identification) with the neuropsychological scores. All of the correlations were done separately for the self-focus and other-focus conditions (see Table 5).

As might be expected from studies linking content memory and medial-temporal regions, medial-temporal test performance was positively correlated with recognition accuracy in both the self-focus condition ($r = .40$, $P < .1$) and other-focus ($r = .65$, $P < .005$) conditions (although the correlation was only marginally significant in the self-focus condition). In the other-focus condition, medial-temporal functioning seemed to affect not only memory performance, but also ability to evaluate the accuracy of one's responses, as indicated by the correlation between the confidence discriminability for recognition responses and medial-temporal scores ($r = .50$, $P < .05$).

Medial-temporal performance was also related to source monitoring performance. Participants with higher medial-temporal scores correctly attributed more secondary-schema items[5] than those with low scores ($r = .48$, $P < .05$; $r = .49$, $P < .05$ for self- and other-focus conditions, respectively) and, in the other-focus condition, correctly attributed more consistent items than those with low scores ($r = .47$, $P < .05$). As with recognition, medial-temporal functioning seemed to be related to participants' metamemory ability as well as to their actual performance: Medial-temporal scores were correlated with confidence discriminability for source judgements for both self-focus ($r = .57$, $P < .01$) and other-focus conditions ($r = .52$, $P < .05$). Thus, accurate metamemory judgements seem to depend on the ability to encode specific memorial qualitative characteristics.

Table 5. *Partial Correlations (Partialling Out Age) between Frontal and Medial-temporal Battery and Older Adults' Recognition Performance, Source Identification, and Confidence Ratings*

	Frontal Battery	*Medial-temporal Battery*
Self-focus Condition		
Corrected recognition	.05	.40
Source identification		
Stereotype reliance (C – I)	.30	–.28
Consistent	.15	–.05
Inconsistent	–.30	.34
Secondary-schema	.31	.48*
Confidence discriminability		
Recognition judgement	.10	.20
Source judgement	.03	.57*
Other-focus Condition		
Corrected recognition	.21	.65*
Source identification		
Stereotype reliance (C – I)	–.59*	–.16
Consistent	.02	.47*
Inconsistent	.62*	.38
Secondary-schema	.40	.49*
Confidence discriminability		
Recognition judgement	.34	.50*
Source judgement	.32	.52*

Stereotype reliance = consistent source identification – inconsistent source identification; confidence discriminability = average confidence for correct responses – average confidence for incorrect responses.
* $P < .05$.

Participants' stereotype reliance (consistent–inconsistent source identification) was negatively correlated with their frontal scores in the other-focus condition ($r = .59$, $P < .01$); participants with high frontal scores were less likely to rely on the stereotypes when making source identifica-

[5] Note that the secondary-schema items were all consistent with the speaker's secondary schema, and as such can be considered to be a type of speaker-consistent statements.

[6] As can be seen in Table 5, in the self-focus condition the correlation between stereotype reliance and frontal scores was actually in the opposite direction, with a positive value (although nonsignificant). This suggests that high frontal scorers may use different strategies depending upon the type of information available to them. Participants in the self-focus condition presumably had little source-specific information available, such that even if they attempted to retrieve specific memorial details about the item, those details would not have helped identify the source of the item. Thus, in the self-focus condition, high frontal scorers may have resorted to the best available strategy to complete the source identification task without the assistance of source-specific memorial information—using the schemas to identify who said which item.

tions than were participants with low frontal scores. This correlation was not significant in the self-focus condition[6]. Looking at the two components of stereotype reliance in the other-focus condition, there was a correlation between frontal scores and the ability to correctly attribute speaker-inconsistent items ($r = .62$, $P < .005$), but not between frontal scores and the ability to attribute speaker-consistent items.

The overall pattern of correlations suggests that not all source identification tasks require the same cognitive processes for optimal performance. These data suggest that when general knowledge and item-specific information are contradictory, performance on that task will rely upon frontal region functioning. The fact that the frontal correlation with stereotype reliance appeared in the other-focus condition but not the self-focus condition, whereas the correlations found with medial-temporal performance were generally consistent in the two conditions, suggests that the nature of the relationship between frontal functioning and performance is more dependent upon the type of focus than is the relationship between medial-temporal functioning and performance. Strategic frontal processes may be more flexible and likely to shift according to task demands than medial-temporal binding processes.

DISCUSSION

The results of this study demonstrate both the utility and the pitfalls of using general knowledge to help remember information. When the actual speaker and the probable speaker for a given statement were the same, neither emotional focus nor age affected participants' ability to attribute the statement to the correct speaker. Thus, under some circumstances, factors that generally make source monitoring less accurate can be counteracted with the use of general knowledge. This type of cognitive strategy can be very useful. Quite often, our memories do not have qualitative characteristics that are distinctive enough to determine the source of the remembered information. As long as potential sources act in a consistent manner, educated inferences about who said what will lead to correct source attributions. However, as also demonstrated by this experiment, relying on general knowledge can lead to problems when specific qualitative information and the knowledge about the source do not match. Emotional self-focus and ageing, factors associated with decrements in source identification (both presumably due in part to poor feature information), both led to a greater reliance on stereotypes for making source attributions for statements that had been heard.

A great deal of research has focused on when expectancy-congruent information is remembered better than expectancy-incongruent information, and vice versa (for a review, see Stangor & McMillan, 1992). One reason this question is interesting is that what is remembered can help determine when stereotypes will be maintained and when they will not. Our study suggests that source misattributions may be a mechanism through which stereotypes about particular individuals or groups may be maintained even when memory for the content of the consistent and the inconsistent information is equivalent. In particular, older adults and people in situations that encourage focusing more on oneself than on the source of information may be more likely to maintain their stereotypes through false (but stereotype-consistent) memories about the behaviour of particular individuals or groups. In general, increasing cognitive load through distraction or stress should have similar effects.

Also potentially leading to the maintenance of stereotypes is the fact that general knowledge affected the rates of false recognition to new statements. Items corresponding to the primary schema were more likely to be falsely recognised than items from the secondary schema. Participants were significantly more likely to attribute the new statements they falsely recognised to the speaker they were consistent with than to the other speaker (see Mather et al., 1997, for similar findings). It is possible that being able to associate a new statement with a particular speaker increased participants' confidence that they had actually heard the statement. Because we did not have any new items that were not associated with one of the two speakers, we cannot address this possibility with this study, but it would be an interesting question to pursue.

Neuropsychological Test Scores and Stereotype Reliance

The fact that older adults were more likely than younger adults to rely on schematic knowledge when making source attributions integrates two lines of research. First, in comparison to younger adults, older adults often show deficits in source identification tasks (e.g. Brown et al., 1995; G. Cohen & Faulkner, 1989; Ferguson et al., 1992; Henkel et al., 1998; McIntyre & Craik, 1987; Spencer & Raz, 1995), and second, older adults tend to rely more on schematic knowledge when trying to recall or recognise information (e.g. Hess et al., 1989; Hess & Slaughter, 1990; Hess & Tate, 1992). Thus, giving greater weight to schematic knowledge is one mechanism through which older adults can compensate for their decreased access to other types of source-specifying information (although we have also seen how schematic knowledge can lead them astray).

For older adults, source monitoring performance for different types of items was associated with scores on different neuropsychological test batteries. In the other-focus condition, correctly attributing statements that were not consistent with their speaker's schema (e.g. a Democratic statement spoken by a Republican) was correlated with performance on the frontal component of a neuropsychological test battery (Glisky et al., 1995). Frontal regions may contribute to this task through processes monitoring inconsistencies between a statement and the speaker at encoding or through systematic retrieval and evaluation processes engaged during the test. Because of the conflict at test between specific memorial information associated with who actually said the statement and the schematic knowledge about that person, it may be necessary to retrieve more information and evaluate it more closely. In contrast, correctly attributing speaker-consistent statements requires less reflection at encoding and a less complex retrieval/decision process (all one has to remember is the schema that was associated with that person). Indeed, speaker-consistent statements (and secondary-schema statements, which were also consistent with their speaker's schema) were not correlated with frontal scores, but instead with scores on the medial-temporal test battery. This finding suggests that the ability to remember the content of the schema and possibly to bind specific qualitative characteristics to the statement are important (whereas there is less of a need for strategic processes) in order to attribute the source of this type of item.

These findings help shed light on prior discrepancies in the literature regarding brain region functioning and performance. A number of researchers have suggested that memory for the content and the source of an event may be functionally dissociable (e.g. Craik, Morris, Morris, & Loewen, 1990; Glisky et al., 1995, Johnson & Raye, 1981; Schacter, Harbluk, & McLachlan, 1984) and neuropsychologically dissociable, with memory for content relying on medial-temporal lobe areas of the brain and memory for source relying on frontal areas of the brain (e.g. Glisky et al., 1995; Janowsky, Shimamura, & Squire, 1989; Schacter, 1987; Schacter et al., 1984; Shimamura, Janowsky, & Squire, 1990; Shimamura & Squire, 1987). For example, in one experiment, elderly participants' ability to remember sentences they had heard was correlated with their performance on a battery of tests often used clinically to measure medial-temporal lobe function but not with their performance on a battery used to measure frontal lobe function, whereas the reverse was true for their ability to remember the voice in which the sentence had been spoken (Glisky et al., 1995). However, although source memory is sometimes correlated with measures of frontal functioning in older adults, a reliable relationship is not always evident (e.g. Degl'Innocenti & Bäckman, 1996; Dywan, Segalowitz, & Williamson, 1994; Johnson et al., 1995; Schacter, Kaszniak, Kihlstrom, & Valdiserri, 1991; Spencer & Raz, 1995). In addition, source memory tasks are not necessarily exclusively associated with measures of frontal functioning. For example, determining whether an object was seen or imagined was found to be associated with measures of both frontal and medial-temporal region functioning in older adults (Henkel et al., 1998).

According to the SMF, accurate source monitoring requires both initial binding of multiple features of an event and later retrieval and evaluation of these features. Different types of source monitoring tasks depend to different degrees on these different processes. In particular, because frontal regions are critical for reflective activities such as strategic retrieval and evaluation (e.g., Burgess & Shallice, 1996; Gershberg & Shimamura, 1995; Johnson et al., 1993; Johnson & Raye, 1998, in press; Mangels, Gershberg, Shimamura, & Knight, 1996; Moscovitch, 1994; Schacter, Norman, & Koutstaal, 1998), the more reflective processing that is necessary to retrieve and evaluate the source of an event correctly, the more likely that source task is to be correlated with measures of frontal functioning. Democratic statements that were spoken by a Republican speaker require more systematic evaluation than speaker-consistent statements in order to be attributed correctly, and indeed, the likelihood of attributing speaker-inconsistent statements correctly was correlated with measures of frontal functioning, whereas speaker-consistent attributions were not. This differential relation to measures of frontal brain region functioning is consistent with recent brain-imaging studies suggesting that prefrontal region activity reflects the amount of reflective activity required at test (e.g. Johnson et al., 1996a; Nolde, Johnson, & D'Esposito, 1998a; Schacter, Alpert, Savage, Rauch & Albert, 1996). In addition, the fact that source identification for speaker-consistent statements was not correlated with frontal battery performance suggests that the degree to which a particular source task will rely on processes associated with medial-temporal or frontal brain regions will depend upon the demands of the particular task (Nolde et al., 1998b).

The finding of greater stereotype reliance among participants with low performance on the frontal test battery is also consistent with the argument that stereotypes are used as a means of simplifying complex judgement tasks (e.g. Bodenhausen & Lichtenstein, 1987; Fiske & Neuberg, 1990; Macrae, Milne, & Bodenhausen, 1994; Tajfel, 1981). Older participants whose low frontal battery scores suggest they have frontal brain region deterioration presumably have more difficulty engaging in reflectively demanding tasks and thus rely more on simpler, heuristic processes such as matching the statement to the speaker on the basis of the speaker's stereotype label.

Less Differentiated Confidence Ratings for Older Adults

Confidence ratings in this study indicate that, in general, participants had some information about the accuracy of their memory judgements. They tended to be less confident when they incorrectly recognised or attributed a statement than when they correctly remembered it. However, older adults' confidence ratings differentiated less well between correct and incorrect responses than did those of younger adults (see also Henkel et al., 1998). This was the case even when their accuracy was nearly as good as that of the younger adults (i.e. when attributing speaker-consistent statements). In addition, the average difference between older adults' confidence ratings for correct and incorrect items was correlated with their medial-temporal test performance, suggesting that the ability to make confidence judgements that reflect actual accuracy is aided by processes supported by medial-temporal brain regions. Presumably, these processes are critical for binding one qualitative characteristic (e.g. perceptual detail) to another (e.g. semantic detail) in memory.

Self-focus and Later Use of Stereotypes

Both older and younger participants who thought about how they felt about the statements (self-focus) rather than thinking about how the speakers felt (other-focus) were more likely to misattribute statements to the speaker for whom the statement would be more consistent. The higher reliance on schematic knowledge by self-focus participants was not due to poorer memory in general. Self-focus participants were actually more likely to recognise statements correctly from the video than were other-focus participants.

Instead, their schematic misattribution errors seem to be due to a lack of source-specifying memorial information, a result of their focus at encoding (Johnson et al., 1996b).

An interesting finding from this study is that self-focus increased the older adults' false recognition of new items but not that of the younger adults. Thinking about how strongly they felt about the statements led older adults to be particularly likely to say that they had heard new items that were consistent with a speaker's primary schema. These false alarms were almost always attributed to the speaker whose stereotype label was consistent with the content of the statement. This pattern suggests that after focusing on their own feelings when experiencing an event (and thus not encoding many source-specifying details for events) older adults may weight schema information more heavily when attributing related events to sources. Thus, older adults sometimes pay a greater cost for self-focus than do younger adults (e.g. Hashtroudi et al., 1994).

Conclusions

In summary, we found that the degree to which a person relies on stereotypes to determine the source of information depends both on the way they focused on the information when they first encountered it and also on age-related changes in processing. Thinking about our own feelings when listening to people talk might help us remember the content of the statements, but because it reduces the likelihood of binding source-specifying information to statements, it can also foster a greater reliance upon general knowledge when trying to remember who said the statement. In addition, the pattern of results with older adults was consistent with the hypothesis that frontal brain regions support the type of processes necessary to deal with possible contradictions between specific information and schematic knowledge.

Although we have investigated speaker as one type of source information, this general pattern of results would be expected to hold for conflicts between general knowledge and any type of source-specifying information (e.g. place, temporal information, colour, etc.). Similarly, although we used an explicit source identification task, the general pattern of findings are relevant to understanding performance in tasks that do not require explicit source identification but that require source monitoring nonetheless (exclusion tasks, e.g. Jacoby, Woloshyn, & Kelley, 1989; cryptomnesia paradigms, e.g. Marsh, Landau, & Hicks, 1997; free recall of stories, e.g. Mather & Johnson, 1998). In general, increased reliance on general knowledge as a result of a lack of source-specifying memorial qualitative characteristics can be dangerous. Assuming that the source that seems most consistent with an event was actually associated with the event can lead to errors that are difficult to detect because they seem so plausible.

REFERENCES

Banaji, M.R., & Greenwald, A.G. (1995). Implicit gender stereotyping in judgments of fame. *Journal of Personality and Social Psychology, 68*, 181–198.

Bargh, J.A., & Thein, R.D. (1985). Individual construct accessibility, person memory, and the recall-judgment link: The case of information overload. *Journal of Personality and Social Psychology, 49*, 1129–1146.

Bartlett, F.C. (1932). *Remembering: A study in experimental and social psychology.* Cambridge: Cambridge University Press.

Bayen, U.J., & Murnane, K. (1996). Aging and the use of perceptual and temporal information in source memory tasks. *Psychology and Aging, 11*, 293–303.

Benton, K.L., & Hamsher, K. (1976). *Multilingual Aphasia Examination manual.* Iowa City: University of Iowa.

Bodenhausen, G.V., & Lichtenstein, M. (1987). Social stereotypes and information-processing strategies: The impact of task complexity. *Journal of Personality and Social Psychology, 52*, 871–880.

Bransford, J.D., & Johnson, M.K. (1973). Considerations of some problems of comprehension. In W. Chase (Ed.), *Visual information processing* (pp. 383–438). New York: Academic Press.

Brewer, M.B., Weber, J. G., & Carini, B. (1995). Person memory in intergroup contexts: Categorization vs. Individuation. *Journal of Personality and Social Psychology*, *69*, 29–40.

Brown, A.S., Jones, E.M., & Davis, T. L. (1995). Age differences in conversational source monitoring. *Psychology and Aging*, *10*, 111–122.

Burgess, P.W., & Shallice, T. (1996). Bizarre responses, rule detection and frontal lobe lesions. *Cortex*, *32*, 241–259.

Cohen, G., & Faulkner, D. (1989). Age differences in source forgetting: Effects on reality monitoring and on eyewitness testimony. *Psychology and Aging*, *4*, 10–17.

Cohen, N.J., & Eichenbaum, H. (1993). *Memory, amnesia, and the hippocampal system*. Cambridge, MA: MIT Press.

Craik, F.I.M., Morris, L.W., Morris, R.G., & Loewen, E.R. (1990). Relations between source amnesia and frontal lobe functioning in older adults. *Psychology and Aging*, *5*, 148–151.

Degl'Innocenti, A., & Bäckman, L. (1996). Aging and source memory: Influences of intention to remember and associations with frontal lobe tests. *Aging, Neuropsychology, and Cognition*, *3*, 307–319.

De Leonardis, D.M., Nolde, S.F., & Johnson, M.K. (1996). *Direction of emotional focus and source memory in older and younger adults*. Paper presented at the eighth annual APS convention, June, San Francisco, CA.

Delis, D.C., Kramer, J., Kaplan, E., & Ober, B.A. (1987). *The California Verbal Learning Test*. San Antonio, TX: Psychological Corporation.

Devine, P.G. (1989). Stereotypes and prejudice: Their automatic and controlled components. *Journal of Personality and Social Psychology*, *56*, 5–18.

Dodson, C.S., Holland, P.W., & Shimamura, A.P. (1998). On the recollection of specific and partial source information. *Journal of Experimental Psychology: Learning, Memory, and Cognition*, *24*, 1121–1136

Dywan, J., Segalowitz, S.J., & Williamson, L. (1994). Source monitoring during name recognition in older adults: Psychometric and electrophysiological correlates. *Psychology and Aging*, *9*, 568–577.

Ferguson, S., Hashtroudi, S., & Johnson, M.K. (1992). Age differences in using source-relevant cues. *Psychology and Aging*, *7*, 443–452.

Fiske, S.T., & Neuberg, S.L. (1990). A continuum of impression formation, from category-based to individuating processes: Influences of information and motivation on attention and interpretation. *Advances in Experimental Social Psychology*, *23*, 1–73.

Gershberg, F.B., & Shimamura, A.P. (1995). The role of the frontal lobes in the use of organizational strategies in free recall. *Neuropsychologia*, *13*, 1305–1333.

Glisky, E.L., Polster, M.R., & Routhieaux, B.C. (1995). Double dissociation between item and source memory. *Neuropsychology*, *9*, 229–235.

Golomb, J., Kluger, A., de Leon, M.J., Ferris, S.H., Convit, A., Mittelman, M., Cohen, J., Rusinek, H., De Santi, S., & George, A.E. (1994). Hippocampal formation size in normal human aging: A correlate of delayed secondary memory performance. *Learning and Memory*, *1*, 45–54.

Hart, R.P., Kwentus, J.A., Wade, J.B., & Taylor, J.R. (1988). Modified Wisconsin Card Sorting Test in elderly normal, depressed and demented patients. *Clinical Neuropsychologist*, *2*, 49–56.

Hashtroudi, S., Johnson, M.K., & Chrosniak, L. D. (1990). Aging and qualitative characteristics of memories for perceived and imagined complex events. *Psychology and Aging*, *5*, 119–126.

Hashtroudi, S., Johnson, M.K., Vnek, N., & Ferguson, S.A. (1994). Aging and the effects of affective and factual focus on source monitoring and recall. *Psychology and Aging*, *9*, 160–170.

Haug, H., & Eggers, R. (1991). Morphometry of the human cortex cerebri and corpus striatum. *Neurobiology of Aging*, *12*, 336–338.

Henkel, L.A., Johnson, M.K., & De Leonardis, D.M. (1998). Aging and source monitoring: Cognitive processes and neuropsychological correlates. *Journal of Experimental Psychology: General*, *127*, 251–268.

Hess, T.M., Donley, J., & Vandermaas, M.O. (1989). Aging-related changes in the processing and retention of script information. *Experimental Aging Research*, *15*, 89–96.

Hess, T.M., & Slaughter, S.J. (1990). Schematic knowledge influences on memory for scene information in young and older adults. *Developmental Psychology*, *26*, 855–865.

Hess, T.M., & Tate, C.S. (1992). Direct and indirect assessments of memory for script-based narratives in young and older adults. *Cognitive Development*, *7*, 467–484.

Holtgraves, T., Srull, T.K., & Socall, D. (1989). Conversation memory: The effects of speaker status on memory for the assertiveness of conversation remarks. *Journal of Personality and Social Psychology*, *56*, 149–160.

Jacoby, L.L., Woloshyn, V., & Kelley, C. (1989). Becoming famous without being recognized:

Unconscious influences of memory produced by dividing attention. *Journal of Experimental Psychology: General, 118*, 115–125.

Janowsky, J.S., Shimamura, A.P., & Squire, L.R. (1989). Source memory impairment in patients with frontal lobe lesions. *Neuropsychologia, 27*, 1043–1056.

Jernigan, T.L., Archibald, S.L., Berhow, M.T., Sowell, E.R., Foster, D.S., & Hesselink, J.R. (1991). Cerebral structure on MRI, Part 1: Localization of age-related changes. *Biological Psychiatry, 29*, 55–67.

Johnson, M.K., & Chalfonte, B. L. (1994). Binding complex memories: The role of reactivation and the hippocampus. In D.L. Schacter & E. Tulving (Eds.), *Memory systems 1994* (pp. 311–350). Cambridge, MA: MIT Press.

Johnson, M.K., De Leonardis, D.M., Hashtroudi, S., & Ferguson, S.A. (1995). Aging and single versus multiple cues in source monitoring. *Psychology and Aging, 10*, 507–517.

Johnson, M.K., Foley, M.A., Suengas, A.G., & Raye, C.L. (1988). Phenomenal characteristics of memories for perceived and imagined autobiographical events. *Journal of Experimental Psychology: General, 117*, 371–376.

Johnson, M.K., Hashtroudi, S., & Lindsay, D.S. (1993). Source monitoring. *Psychological Bulletin, 114*, 3–28.

Johnson, M.K., Kounios, J., & Nolde, S.F. (1996a). Electrophysiological brain activity and memory source monitoring. *NeuroReport, 7*, 2929–2932.

Johnson, M.K., Nolde, S.F., & De Leonardis, D.M. (1996b). Emotional focus and source monitoring. *Journal of Memory and Language, 35*, 135–156.

Johnson, M.K., & Raye, C.L. (1981). Reality monitoring. *Psychological Review, 88*, 67–85.

Johnson, M.K., & Raye, C.L. (1998). False memories and confabulation. *Trends in Cognitive Science, 2*, 137 145.

Johnson, M.K., & Raye, C.L. (in press). Cognitive and brain mechanisms of false memories and beliefs. In D.L. Schacter & E. Scarry (Eds.), *Memory, brain, and belief.* Cambridge, MA: Harvard University Press.

Johnson, M.K., Raye, C.L., Foley, M.A., & Kim, J.K. (1982). Pictures and images: Spatial and temporal information compared. *Bulletin of the Psychonomic Society, 19*, 23–26.

Kruglanski, A.W., & Freund, T. (1983). The freezing and unfreezing of lay-inferences: Effects on impressional primacy, ethnic stereotyping, and numerical anchoring. *Journal of Experimental Social Psychology, 19*, 448–468.

Lane, S.M., & Villa, D. (1997). *Focusing on the characteristics of accurate memories reduces false memories.* Paper presented at the annual meeting of the Psychonomics Society, Philadelphia, PA.

Light, L.L. (1996). Memory and aging. In E.L. Bjork & R.A. Bjork (Eds.), *Memory* (pp. 443–490). San Diego, CA: Academic Press.

Macrae, C.N., Hewstone, M., & Griffiths, R.J. (1993). Processing load and memory for stereotype-based information. *European Journal of Social Psychology, 23*, 77–87.

Macrae, C.N., Milne, A.B., & Bodenhausen, G.V. (1994). Stereotypes as energy-saving devices: A peek inside the cognitive toolbox. *Journal of Personality and Social Psychology, 66*, 37–47.

Mangels, J.A., Gershberg, F.B., Shimamura, A.P., & Knight, R.T. (1996). Impaired retrieval from remote memory in patients with frontal lobe damage. *Neuropsychology, 10*, 32–41.

Marsh, R.L., Landau, J.D., & Hicks, J.L. (1997). Contributions of inadequate source monitoring to unconscious plagiarism during idea generation. *Journal of Experimental Psychology: Learning, Memory, and Cognition, 23*, 886–897.

Mather, M., Henkel, L.A., & Johnson, M.K. (1997). Evaluating characteristics of false memories: Remember/know judgments and memory characteristics questionnaire compared. *Memory and Cognition, 25*, 826–837.

Mather, M., & Johnson, M.K. (1998). *Emotional review and memory distortion.* Manuscript under review.

McIntyre, J.S., & Craik, F.I.M. (1987). Age differences in memory for item and source information. *Canadian Journal of Psychology, 41*, 175–192.

Mitchell, K.J., & Johnson, M.K. (in press). Source monitoring: Attributing (and misattributing) memories to sources. In E. Tulving & F.I.M. Craik (Eds.), *Oxford handbook of memory*. New York: Oxford University Press.

Moscovitch, M. (1994). Cognitive resources and dual-task interference effects at retrieval in normal people: The role of the frontal lobes and medial-temporal cortex. *Neuropsychology, 8*, 523–534.

Moscovitch, M., & Winocur, G. (1995). Frontal lobes, memory, and aging. *Annals of the New York Academy of Sciences, 769*, 119–150.

Nolde, S.F., Johnson, M.K., & D'Esposito, M. (1998a). Prefrontal activation during episodic remembering: An event-related MRI study. *NeuroReport, 9*, 3509–3514.

Nolde, S.F., Johnson, M.K., & Raye, C.L. (1998b). The role of the prefrontal cortex during tests of episodic memory. *Trends in Cognitive Sciences*, *2*, 399–406.

Norman, K.A., & Schacter, D.L. (1997). False recognition in younger and older adults: Exploring the characteristics of illusory memories. *Memory and Cognition*, *25*, 838–848.

Owens, J., Bower, G.H., & Black, J.B. (1979). The soap opera effect in story recall. *Memory and Cognition*, *7*, 185–191.

Pratto, F., & Bargh, J.A. (1991). Stereotyping based on apparently individuating information: Trait and global components of sex stereotypes under attention overload. *Journal of Experimental Social Psychology*, *27*, 26–47.

Raz, N., Gunning-Dixon, F.M., Head, D., Dupuis, J.H., & Acker, J.D. (1998). Neuroanatomical correlates of cognitive aging: Evidence from structural magnetic resonance imaging. *Neuropsychology*, *12*, 95–114.

Reitan, R.M., & Wolfson, D. (1994). A selective and critical review of neuropsychological deficits and the frontal lobes. *Neuropsychology Review*, *4*, 161–198.

Ross, M. (1989). Relation of implicit theories to the construction of personal histories. *Psychological Review*, *96*, 341–357.

Rothbart, M., Fulero, S., Jensen, C, Howard, J., & Birrell, P. (1978). Recall for confirming events: Memory processing and the maintenance of social stereotypes. *Journal of Experimental Social Psychology*, *14*, 237–255.

Salthouse, T.A. (1992). Why do adult age differences increase with task complexity? *Developmental Psychology*, *28*, 905–918.

Salthouse, T.A., Fristoe, N., & Rhee, S.H. (1996). How localized are age-related effects on neuropsychological measures? *Neuropsychology*, *10*, 272–285.

Schacter, D.L. (1987). Memory, amnesia, and frontal lobe dysfunction. *Psychobiology*, *15*, 21–36.

Schacter, D.L., Alpert, N.M., Savage, C.R., Rauch, S.L., & Albert, M.S. (1996). Conscious recollection and the human hippocampal formation: Evidence from positron emission tomography. *Proceedings of the National Academy of Sciences of the United States of America*, *93*, 321–325.

Schacter, D.L., Harbluk, J.L., & McLachlan, D.R. (1984). Retrieval without recollection: An experimental analysis of source amnesia. *Journal of Verbal Learning and Verbal Behavior*, *23*, 593–611.

Schacter, D.L., Kaszniak, A.W., Kihlstrom, J.F., & Valdiserri, M. (1991). The relation between source memory and aging. *Psychology and Aging*, *6*, 559–568.

Schacter, D.L., Koutstaal, W., & Norman, K.A. (1997). False memories and aging. *Trends in Cognitive Sciences*, *1*, 229–236.

Schacter, D.L., Norman, K.A., & Koutstaal, W. (1998). The cognitive neuroscience of constructive memory. *Annual Review of Psychology*, *49*, 289–318.

Schooler, J.W., Gerhard, D., & Loftus, E.F. (1986). Qualities of the unreal. *Journal of Experimental Psychology: Learning, Memory, and Cognition*, *12*, 171–181.

Sherman, J.W., & Bessenoff, G.R. (in press). Stereotypes as source monitoring cues: On the interaction between episodic and semantic memory. *Psychological Science*.

Shimamura, A.P. (1995). Memory and frontal lobe function. In M.S. Gazzaniga (Ed.), *The cognitive neurosciences* (pp. 803–813). Cambridge, MA: MIT Press.

Shimamura, A.P., Janowsky, J.S., & Squire, L.R. (1990). Memory for the temporal order of events in patients with frontal lobe lesions and amnesic patients. *Neuropsychologia*, *28*, 803–813.

Shimamura, A.R., & Squire, L.R. (1987). A neuropsychological study of fact memory and source amnesia. *Journal of Experimental Psychology: Learning, Memory, and Cognition*, *13*, 464–473.

Spencer, W.D., & Raz, N. (1995). Differential effects of aging on memory for content and context: A meta-analysis. *Psychology and Aging*, *10*, 527–539.

Squire, L.R. (1992). Memory and the hippocampus: A synthesis from findings with rats, monkeys, and humans. *Psychological Review*, *99*, 195–231.

Squire, L.R., & Knowlton, B.J. (1995). Memory, hippocampus, and brain systems. In M.S. Gazzaniga (Ed.), *The cognitive neurosciences* (pp. 825–837). Cambridge, MA: MIT Press.

Stangor, C. (1988). Stereotype accessibility and information processing. *Personality and Social Psychology Bulletin*, *14*, 694–708.

Stangor, C., Lynch, L., Duan, C., & Glass, B. (1992). Categorization of individuals on the basis on multiple social features. *Journal of Personality and Social Psychology*, *62*, 207–218.

Stangor, C., & McMillan, D. (1992). Memory for expectancy-congruent and expectancy-incongruent information: A review of the social and social developmental literatures. *Psychological Bulletin*, *111*, 42–61.

Stuss, D.T., & Benson, D.F. (1986). *The frontal lobes.* New York: Raven Press.

Suengas, A.G., & Johnson, M.K. (1988). Qualitative effects of rehearsal on memories for perceived and imagined complex events. *Journal of Experimental Psychology: General, 117*, 377–389.

Tajfel, H. (1981). *Human groups and social categories: Studies in social psychology.* New York: Cambridge University Press.

Taylor, S.E., & Crocker, J. (1981). Schematic bases of social information processing. In D.L. Hamilton (Ed.), *Cognitive processes in stereotyping and intergroup behaviour* (pp. 88–114). Hillsdale, NJ: Lawrence Erlbaum Associates Inc.

Taylor, S.E., & Falcone, H. (1982). Cognitive bases of stereotyping: The relationship between categorization and prejudice. *Personality and Social Psychology Bulletin, 8*, 426–432.

Taylor, S.E., Fiske, S.T., Etcoff, N.L., & Ruderman, A.J. (1978). Categorical and contextual bases of person memory and stereotyping. *Journal of Personality and Social Psychology, 36*, 778–793.

Waddell, K.J., & Rogoff, B. (1981). Effect of contextual organization on spatial memory of middle-aged and older women. *Developmental Psychology, 17*, 878–885.

Weschler, D. (1981). *Manual for the Weschler Adult Intelligence Scale-Revised.* New York: Psychological Corporation.

Weschler, D. (1987). *Weschler Memory Scale—Revised Manual.* New York: Psychological Corporation.

West, R.L. (1996). An application of prefrontal cortex function theory to cognitive aging. *Psychological Bulletin, 120*, 272–292.

APPENDIX A

Descriptions of Speakers

Athlete–Writer Pair

As a teenager, Sandy began running as a way to have some quiet time to herself at the beginning or end of each day. She used the time when she was running as a way to organise her thoughts. It soon became clear she had great talent as a runner. She competed in races while a student in college. For a while after she graduated, she stopped running. But she really missed the feeling of being in good shape, so she joined a running club and has been running and competing in local races ever since. It is difficult for her to run in the winter because of the early darkness and the ice on the roads, but she tries to stay in shape in other ways.

Patricia has always been interested in writing. An aunt gave her a journal for her thirteenth birthday. In addition to using the journal as a log of her daily activities, Patricia began to write short stories. Her high-school English teacher recognised her gift for writing and encouraged Patricia to submit her stories to local writing competitions. Patricia also began writing for her high school paper. She continued writing for the school paper at college, and her first job after college was for a local newspaper as a reporter.

Republican–Democrat Pair

Patricia was born in Arlington, Virginia. Her father was an officer in the military and her mother was a full-time housewife. She attended a private school for girls, where she developed a strong appreciation for religion. She still attends mass every Sunday. After Patricia graduated from college, she began working for RJ Reynolds, a tobacco company. She also became involved in local politics, campaigning for Republican candidates. She is still an active member of the Republican party and has been an important part of many local Republican campaigns. She enjoys being a part of the political process and feels that it is an important thing to do.

Sandy grew up in Newark, New Jersey. Her parents couldn't afford private schooling so Sandy attended the local public schools. Her sixth grade teacher introduced Sandy to a programme which involved reading to visually impaired children. Sandy continued to be active in this programme, throughout high school and also began volunteering in a local soup kitchen. In college, she realised that government action was a critical part of improving the lives of the poor, and so after she graduated she moved to Washington, DC and worked for several years with the Democratic party. She is an active member of the Democratic party—she attended the Democratic National Convention last year, and has frequently helped raise money for Democrat candidates. She enjoys discussing politics and feels that it is possible to make a difference as an individual citizen.

COGNITIVE NEUROPSYCHOLOGY, 1999, 16 (3/4/5), 459–488

MEMORY CONJUNCTION ERRORS IN YOUNGER AND OLDER ADULTS: EVENT-RELATED POTENTIAL AND NEUROPSYCHOLOGICAL DATA

Susan R. Rubin, Cyma Van Petten, Elizabeth L. Glisky, and Wendy M. Newberg
University of Arizona, Tucson, USA

In a study/recognition paradigm, new words at test were recombinations of studied syllables (e.g. BARLEY from BARTER and VALLEY), shared one syllable with studied words, or were completely new. False alarm rates followed the gradient of similarity with studied items. Event-related potentials to the three classes of false alarms were indistinguishable. False alarms elicited different brain activity than did hits, arguing against the idea that conjunction errors occur during encoding and are later retrieved liked genuine memories. In Experiment 2, with healthy older adults, neuropsychological tests sensitive to frontal lobe function predicted false alarm rate, but not hit rate. Performance on standardised memory scales sensitive to medial temporal/diencephalic function influenced the pattern of false alarm rates across the three classes of new words. The experiments suggest that false alarms to conjunction lures are not similar to true recollections, but are products of faulty monitoring at retrieval.

INTRODUCTION

Illusions of memory have provided a perennial source of fascination for psychologists. From Bartlett's famous 1932 *War of the Ghosts* study, through the groundbreaking work on eyewitness testimony done by Loftus and colleagues in the 1970s (e.g. Loftus, Miller, & Burns, 1978), and continuing today in the renewed interest in the converging associates paradigm (Deese, 1959), psychologists never cease to be amazed at how often, and with what confidence, people will claim to remember events that never occurred (Roediger & McDermott, 1995). It has been proposed that at least some false memories are caused by binding failures, namely that components of presented information are inappropriately recombined into episodes that never occurred, producing *memory conjunction errors* (Kroll, Knight, Metcalfe, Wolf, & Tulving, 1996; Reinitz, Verfaellie, & Milberg, 1996). For instance, after meeting several new colleagues, including a Mr. Waters and a Mr. Hanson, a person might later recognise "Watson" incorrectly. A laboratory paradigm for investigating such errors was introduced by Underwood and Zimmerman (1973). In this paradigm, people study two-syllable words that are recombined at test into words that are new as wholes but whose individual features (in this case syllables) have been studied. A person who studied SPANIEL and VARNISH might incorrectly judge the conjunction lure SPANISH to be an old word during

Requests for reprints should be addressed to Susan Rubin, Department of Psychology, University of Arizona, Tucson, AZ 85721, USA (Fax: (520) 621-9306; E-mail: rubin@u.arizona.edu).

The experiments were the Master's thesis of the first author. Financial support was provided by the National Institute of Aging (AG14792), National Institute of Neural Disorders and Stroke (NS30825), and the Flinn Foundation. We are grateful to Ava Senkfor, Roh Ohst, and Mark Bakarich for technical support, and to Cynthia P. May, Timothy Curran, and Mark Reinitz for comments on the paper.

recognition. Such conjunction errors have been found using diverse stimuli, including compound and noncompound words, nonsense words, word pairs, sentences, pictures, and faces, indicating that the phenomenon is not purely verbal (Dorfmann, 1994; Jha, Kroll, Baynes, & Gazzaniga, 1997; Kroll et al., 1996; Reinitz, Lammers, & Cochran, 1992; Reinitz et al., 1996; Underwood, Kapelak, & Malmi, 1976; Underwood & Zimmerman, 1973).

Storing the relations among diverse aspects of a single event is a core memory function. It has been suggested that a large proportion of the distortions observed in both normal and pathological memory result from incorrect amalgams of elements drawn from external events, inferences, and other mental events (Johnson & Raye, in press). The conjunction error paradigm offers a relatively direct window into the processes underlying miscombinations of features. Experiment 1 is designed to evaluate whether such miscombinations arise primarily from faulty encoding or faulty retrieval, using a combination of behavioural and brain activity measures. Experiment 2 investigates the neuropsychological correlates of memory conjunction errors in healthy older adults.

One interpretation of conjunction errors is that they reflect a binding failure during encoding, which may consist of a complete failure to encode relational information, weak or inefficient binding such that appropriate elements are not strongly linked, or excessive binding so that fragments that belong to separate events are indiscriminately linked (Kroll et al., 1996). Another interpretation is that these errors arise from separate encoding and storage of global structure and stimulus features, which may lead to conjunction errors at retrieval, when the parts must be recombined properly (Reinitz et al., 1996).

Encoding manipulations can be used to evaluate the idea that conjunction errors are due to faulty initial learning, but the evidence to date has been mixed. Reinitz and colleagues varied the task performed during the study phase, but found equivalent false alarm rates after semantic and orthographic study tasks (Reinitz et al., 1996). Dividing attention during encoding increases false alarms to conjunctions, but also increases other sorts of errors, and so may not indicate a specific role for encoding in the binding failure (Reinitz, Morrissey, & Demb, 1994; Reinitz et al., 1996).

The effects of dividing attention during retrieval have not been examined, but other evidence indicates that conjunction errors are sensitive to testing conditions. To date, the data on memory conjunction errors in free recall is mixed. Reinitz et al. (1992) reported finding memory conjunction errors in a recall task, using stimuli of the form "The X saw the Y". However Roder, Faneuf, Burch, and Connors (1996) found no such effect using noun pairs as stimuli. It is unclear if the ambiguity of these results is due to different types of stimuli, small numbers of trials, or other methodological issues. If additional experiments support the absence of conjunction errors in explicit recall, it will argue against the idea that a false memory is formed during study and later retrieved like a real memory.

Conjunction errors have been observed in some implicit memory tests but not others. Word fragments corresponding to conjunctions of studied items were solved more successfully than fragments with unstudied completions, but conjunction words fared no better than totally new words when they had to be identified in visual noise (Reinitz & Demb, 1994). It is something of a puzzle that conjunction errors have been found in recognition, but not consistently in either implicit or recall tasks. The data concerning the testing conditions that foster or prevent conjunction errors are still sparse, and present an intriguing area for future research.

One means of evaluating the hypothesis that conjunction errors arise from faulty binding at encoding is to measure the presence or absence of an elevated false alarm rate for test items sharing only one syllable with studied words (e.g. GARMENT when only BASEMENT was studied). An account based only on faulty binding would be likely to predict no difference between such *syllable lures* and new words because neither can be generated by miscombining studied syllables. The evidence to date has been inconclusive. Two studies report no significant difference for normal subjects (Kroll et al., 1996;

Reinitz et al., 1994), a third reports significantly more false alarms to feature lures using faces as stimuli (Reinitz et al., 1994), and a fourth includes no statistical comparison although the raw numbers indicate more false alarms to syllable lures than to completely new words (Reinitz et al., 1996). One likely reason for this murky picture is low statistical power; these studies included only four to six items per condition so that differences in false alarm rates may have been difficult to detect.

The question of when false conjunctions are formed thus remains open. A likely retrieval-based explanation involves *processing fluency*, in which familiarity at retrieval is responsible for automatic "yes" responses (Jacoby, 1991). Subjects may mistake the ease in processing studied syllables with familiarity of the whole word. If they have no strong recollection to oppose this impression, they may call the recombined word "old". In contrast to the pure binding hypothesis, the processing fluency account predicts an elevated false alarm rate for syllable lures relative to wholly new words because at least one part of the word is familiar.

Event-related potentials (ERPs) are particularly well-suited to discriminating between encoding and retrieval explanations of memory conjunction errors because brain activity can be recorded during both study and test phases. ERPs are summed synaptic potentials recorded from electrodes on the scalp; the activity elicited by a particular class of stimuli are separated from the background electroencephalogram by averaging responses timelocked to the stimuli of interest (Regan, 1989).

Previous research has shown that a late positive component (LPC) of the ERP is sensitive to mnemonic processes, but only to a subset of those processes that may influence behaviour. Studied words that elicit accurate recognition or cued-recall judgements also elicit larger LPCs than new items or unrecognised old items (Allan & Rugg, 1997; Neville, Kutas, Chesney, & Schmidt, 1986; Senkfor & Van Petten, 1998). Late positivities are also triggered by studied line-drawings, novel geometric shapes, and environmental sounds in recognition tasks, and by incidentally repeated words presented during other tasks that do not call for explicit memory judgements (Bentin & Peled, 1990; Berman, Friedman, & Cramer, 1991; Besson, Kutas, & Van Petten, 1992; Chao, Nielsen-Bohlman, & Knight, 1995; Swick & Knight, 1997; Van Petten & Senkfor, 1996). This old/new effect is enhanced by the same manipulations that improve accuracy in explicit memory tasks, such as "deep" or semantic study as compared to "shallow" or orthographic study tasks (Paller & Kutas, 1992). In studies using "remember/know" judgements, the LPC is largest for "remember" items as compared to "know" items or new words (Duzel, Yonelinas, Mangun, Heinze, & Tulving, 1997; Smith, 1993). In contrast, perceptual manipulations that increase or decrease priming effects in implicit memory tasks have no influence on the LPC (Paller & Gross, 1998; Paller, Kutas, & McIsaac, 1998; Rugg & Doyle, 1994). The available evidence supports the view that the memory-related LPC indexes conscious recollection rather than nondeclarative memory processes. Experiments using difficult-to-remember stimuli like scrambled faces or geometric shapes have thus yielded faster reaction times for repeated items in the absence of any LPC repetition effect, presumably because perceptual processes influenced by familiarity can drive behavioural output in the absence of conscious recollection (Bentin & McCarthy, 1994; Van Petten & Senkfor, 1996).

We have also observed that LPCs recorded during explicit recognition tasks distinguish correct old items (hits) from incorrect new items (false alarms), although both attract the same "yes" judgement (Van Petten & Senkfor, 1996). Our prior study evaluated only the garden-variety false alarms that occur in all recognition tests, rather than false alarms that are specially motivated by events occurring during the study phase. If conjunction errors are formed by inappropriate stimulus combinations during encoding, or during a post-encoding consolidation period, then these unstudied items may be distinct from garden-variety false alarms, and instead be retrieved much like genuine memories. The hypothesis of an initial binding failure thus predicts that ERPs to conjunction lure false alarms will look much like hits. In contrast, the processing fluency (retrieval) explanation predicts the standard result, in which hits look different from all other conditions that do not involve veridical memory traces for the whole words. Previous work suggests that mere familiarity or increased processing fluency leaves no LPC record, so that conjunction words may not differ from other new words in terms of the LPC if fluency alone is the relevant factor. Alternatively, if explicit recognition of individual syllables drives "yes" responses, we may observe a graded effect of similarity to studied items in the LPC in the following pattern: hits might have the largest LPC, followed by conjunction false alarms, then syllable lure false alarms, and finally false alarms to completely new items.

An additional factor investigated in both of the present experiments is recognition confidence for false alarms as compared to hits. As a general rule, incorrect responses (both false alarms and misses) are made with lower confidence than correct responses in recognition tests (Busey, Tunnicliff, Loftus, & Loftus, 1998; Clark, 1997; Gardiner & Java, 1990; Murdock & Dufty, 1972). In experiments designed to elicit false alarms, new items that are related to studied words yield higher confidence "yes" responses than unrelated new items, but these confidence ratings are still lower than those associated with correct "yes" responses (Roediger & McDermott, 1995). Decision confidence is almost certain to have some correlate in brain activity during recognition tests. Prior ERP studies have investigated decision confidence in non-memory tasks requiring difficult perceptual discriminations. As compared to low-confidence trials, high confidence decisions elicited larger P300s, a late positive potential in much the same latency range as the memory-sensitive late positive component (Hillyard, Squires, Bauer, & Lindsay, 1971; Paul & Sutton, 1972). This result suggests that it is critical to distinguish brain activity related to accurate memory performance from that related to confidence per se.

Two prior ERP studies have offered participants an opportunity to indicate that they were uncertain about a recognition judgement. Rugg and Doyle (1992) requested a second button-press response, which could either confirm a participant's old/new judgement or indicate that it was a guess. Wilding and Rugg (1996) offered three response alternatives of "old," "new," or "don't know." In both studies, the ERPs revealed a fairly standard old/new effect when the disconfirmed or "don't know" trials were excluded from the analyses. These studies suggest that the typical old/new difference observed in recognition ERPs may not be a reflection of differential confidence for correct old (hit) and correct new (correct rejection) judgements. However, neither study included enough trials to examine the ERPs elicited by trials with low confidence ratings, or to evaluate the impact of confidence during an erroneous recognition judgement. In Experiment 1 here, participants are offered a graded confidence scale for both "old" and "new" responses so that the interactions between confidence and accuracy can be examined.

EXPERIMENT 1

Method

Participants

Participants were 27 fluent English speakers with no history of neurological disorder, who gave informed consent (15 men, 12 women, age range 21–39 years). Three participants were excluded from the study because of unacceptably high artefact rejection rates. Of the remaining 24 participants, 21 were right-handed, 2 were left-handed, and 1 was ambidextrous. Eleven of the right-handers reported having a left-handed parent or sibling.

Materials

Materials included 440 triads of 2-syllable words. Each triad was structured so that the first syllable of the first word and the second syllable of the second word could be combined to make the third or conjunction word (e.g. BARTER/VALLEY/BARLEY). The syllables in the conjunction words were both spelled and pronounced the same as in the first two words of the triad, although we allowed variation in the stress pattern across words. As shown in Table 1, the recognition tests for each

Table 1. *Sample Stimuli in Study and Recognition Phases*

	Study		*Test*	
Words 1 and 2 (N = 220/110)	barter	valley	barley	*conjunction lure*
Word 2 (N = 110)	(spaniel)	varnish	spanish	*syllable lure*
Word 3 (N = 110)	(lobby gangster)	lobster	lobster	*old*
No study (N = 110)	(vulgar creature)	(vulture)	vulture	*new*
Single syllable studied (N = 140)	plaid		plaid	*old single*
Single syllable unstudied (P = 20)	(catch)		catch	*new single*

Parentheses denote words not presented during the study phase. A total of 580 words were presented for study, 600 for test (both split among 4 study/test cycles).

participant included all 440 conjunction words, but equal numbers of these served as *old* (studied) items, *new* (unstudied) items, *conjunction lures* (first two words of the triad studied), and *syllable lures* (second word of the triad studied)[1]. Assignment of conjunction words to one of the four conditions was rotated across participants, so that each word appeared equally often in each test condition.

This design maximises the number of trials in the critical conditions, but also results in only 25% of the critical items being truly old at recognition. Unequal probabilities of old and new items are undesirable, as they may encourage indiscriminate "yes" responses at test, or introduce probability effects in the ERP measures. Single syllable filler words were thus included to provide better balance between the proportions of old and new items; 140 were presented during the study and test phases (old items at test), and 20 only during the recognition phase (new items)[2].

The stimuli were split among four study-test cycles. Each study list thus included 110 two-syllable words, equally split between conjunction words, first and second members of a triad (presented in canonical order), and second members of a triad, together with 35 single-syllable filler words. Mean frequency of usage for all words was 45 (SD = 6; summed frequency of all regularly inflected forms, Francis & Kuçera, 1982); word length averaged 6 (SD = 0.1) letters. Care was taken to avoid inadvertent syllable overlap in either the study or test phases. For instance, if GARTER and SUDDEN appeared on a given study list (to suggest the conjunction GARDEN), that list would not include DENIM, nor would the syllable –DEN– appear in the other list presented in the same session, thereby avoiding ambiguity as to when it may have been acquired.

Procedure

The experiment was conducted in two sessions scheduled about a week apart, each consisting of a short practice list and two study-test cycles. Words were presented in the middle of the screen for 200 msec, at a rate of one every 3.2 sec at study and every 5 sec at test. Participants were informed of the upcoming memory test, but also assigned a study task of classifying each word as noun, verb, or modifier. At recognition, participants used three response keys with one hand to indicate Definite/Probable/Maybe Old, and three keys with the other hand for Definite/Probable/Maybe New.

[1] Experiment 2 indicated little difference in the recognition of unstudied words sharing the first versus second syllable of a studied word.

[2] None of the syllables in the single-syllable words were shared with the two-syllable words.

Left and right hands were counterbalanced across the two sessions.

The electroencephalogram (EEG) was recorded with tin electrodes mounted in a commercially available elastic cap. Midline central (Cz) and parietal (Pz) recording sites were used, along with lateral pairs of electrodes over the prefrontal (Fp 1, Fp2) and occipital (O1, O2) scalp as defined by the 10–20 system (Jasper, 1958). Three additional pairs of lateral electrodes were used: (1) a frontal pair placed midway between F7–8 and T3–4 (approximately over Broca's area and its right homologue, Bl and Br); (2) a temporoparietal pair placed 30% of the interaural distance lateral and 12.5% of the inion–nasion distance posterior to Cz (approximately over Wernicke's area and its right hemisphere homologue, Wl and Wr); and (3) a temporal pair 33% lateral to Cz (Tl and Tr). Each scalp site was referred to an off-line average of the left and right mastoids (see Van Petten & Kutas, 1988). Vertical eye movements and blinks were monitored via an electrode placed below the right eye referred to the left mastoid. Horizontal eye movements were monitored via a right to left bipolar montage at the external canthi.

The EEG was amplified by a Grass Model 12 polygraph with half-amplitude cutoffs of 0.01 and 100 Hz, digitised at an on-line sampling rate of 170 Hz. Trials with horizontal eye movement, excessive muscle activity, or amplifier saturation effects were rejected prior to averaging the single EEG trials into ERPs. Trials with blink artefacts were corrected using an algorithm developed by A. Dale.

Results

Behavioural Performance

The proportion of words called "old" in the four stimulus classes are shown in Fig. 1. Single-syllable filler words are not included in any of the figures or analyses as they were not of interest in this experiment. Conjunction lures elicited the highest false alarm rate, followed by syllable lures, and then new words. The false alarm rate for unrelated words was 21%, close to that of a previous study using study lists of similar length, but recognition lists in which all of the new words were unrelated to studied

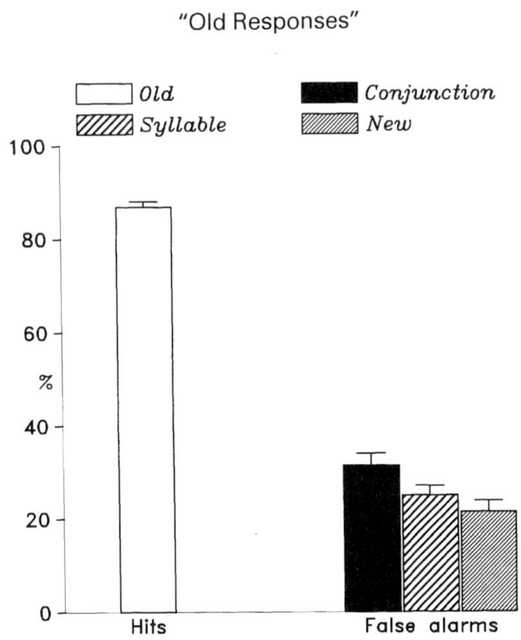

Fig. 1. *Mean percentage of items judged "old" during the recognition test (maximum = 100% in each category) of Experiment 1. Error bars show standard error of the mean. Single-syllable items are not included.*

words (Van Petten & Senkfor, 1996). Syllable lures elicited a 6% higher false alarm rate than new words, and conjunction lures elicited a 6% higher false alarm rate than syllable lures (standard error of these differences was 2%, with a 95% confidence interval of 2–10%). Conjunction lures elicited 12% more false alarms than unrelated new words (standard error of this difference was 2%, with a 95% confidence interval of 9–15%). Pairwise comparisons confirmed that each of the false alarm rates was significantly different from the others: conjunction lure vs. syllable lure, $F(1,23) = 19.2$, $P < .005$; syllable lure vs. new, $F(1,23) = 11.3$, $P < .005$.

Confidence levels were higher for hits (mean = 2.73, where "definite" = 3.0) than false alarms (mean = 2.05), correct rejections (mean = 2.31), and misses (mean = 2.06), all $Fs(1,23) > 49.15$, all $Ps < .0001$. Confidence levels for the two broad error categories—false alarms and misses—were equivalent ($F < 1$). Closer examination of the false alarms revealed no confidence differences among the three categories of conjunction lures, syllable lures, and new words (Fs < 2.61).

Reaction times are shown in Table 2, and were analysed by an initial 2 x 2 ANOVA with factors of accuracy and response type ("old" vs. "new"). One subject had no misses and was excluded from the above analysis. Accurate responses (hits and correct rejections) were faster than inaccurate (misses and false alarms), $F(1,22) = 9.96$, $P < .005$. "Old" responses were faster than "new", $F(1,22) = 18.2$, $P < .0001$, and there was a significant interaction of accuracy by "old/new", $F(1,22) = 5.03$, $P < .05$, reflecting the reaction time pattern of hits faster than correct rejections faster than false alarms that were equivalent to misses. A separate analysis revealed no reaction time differences among the three false alarm types. Not surprisingly, reaction times were correlated with confidence level. Collapsed across accuracy, reaction times ranged from a mean of 1354 msec for "definite" responses to 1772 msec for "probable" responses, to 2014 msec for "maybe" responses, $F(2,44) = 50.0$, $P < .0001$.

Event-related Potentials

Old versus New Items. Figure 2 shows that correctly recognised words (hits) elicited a substantially more positive ERP than correctly rejected new words, beginning at about 350 msec post-stimulus onset. Figure 3 shows a similar difference between hits and false alarms (all types collapsed) that was of somewhat longer duration. ERPs elicited at test were analysed in an early time window (300–600 m after stimulus onset) and a late time window (600–900 msec after stimulus onset), using 100msec of pre-stimulus activity as a baseline.[3] In the early time window, the mean amplitude of ERPs elicited by hits was significantly more positive than that of all correct rejections together, $F(1,23) = 42.2$, $P < .0001$, but there was no difference in the late time window. Hits were more positive than false alarms in both the early and late time windows, $F(1,23) = 24.4$ and 17.6, Ps < .0001 and .0005.

Figure 4 shows that the ERPs elicited by false alarms to conjunction lures, syllable lures, and new words were indistinguishable from one another at any latency. The ERPs elicited by correct rejections were also unaffected by word type, Fs$(2,46) < 2$, as shown in Fig. 5.

Because confidence was shown to vary systematically with accuracy and response type, we restricted our analyses from this point on to thc "definite" items to ensure that the observed effects were not due to this potentially confounding factor. This restriction decreased the trial numbers in each category since some individuals made very few high confidence errors. Subjects with less than 10 artefact-free trials in each category of interest were excluded from the analyses in order to preserve an adequate signal-to-noise ratio in the individual subject averages, which form the basis for all statistical comparisons. A minimum of 16 subjects were included in each analysis of high confidence responses.

After controlling for confidence, most of the ERP effects remained the same. "Definite" hits were still more positive than "definite" correct rejections in the early time window, $F(1,23) = 17.6$, $P < .001$. Hits were also more positive than "definite" false alarms in the late time window, $F(1,19) = 14.25$, $P < .001$, but the previously observed difference in the early time window faded into marginal significance, $F(1,19) = 3.94$, $P < .06$.

Table 2. *Means and standard errors of reaction times at test*

	All	*"Definites" only*
	Mean (SE)	*Mean (SE)*
Hits	1502 (67)	1053 (43)
Correct rejections	1687 (75)	1393 (57)
False alarms	1758 (81)	1262 (81)
Misses	1760 (106)	—

Not all subjects made misses with high confidence, so the mean for "definite" misses was not calculated.

[3] Electrode site was used as a factor (13 levels) in this and all subsequent ANOVAs. We report only main effects and interactions involving the condition factors in the text, as these serve as the most conservative tests of the experimental effects. As evident in Figs. 2 and 3, the ERP memory effects were widespread across the scalp and not confined to restricted scalp regions.

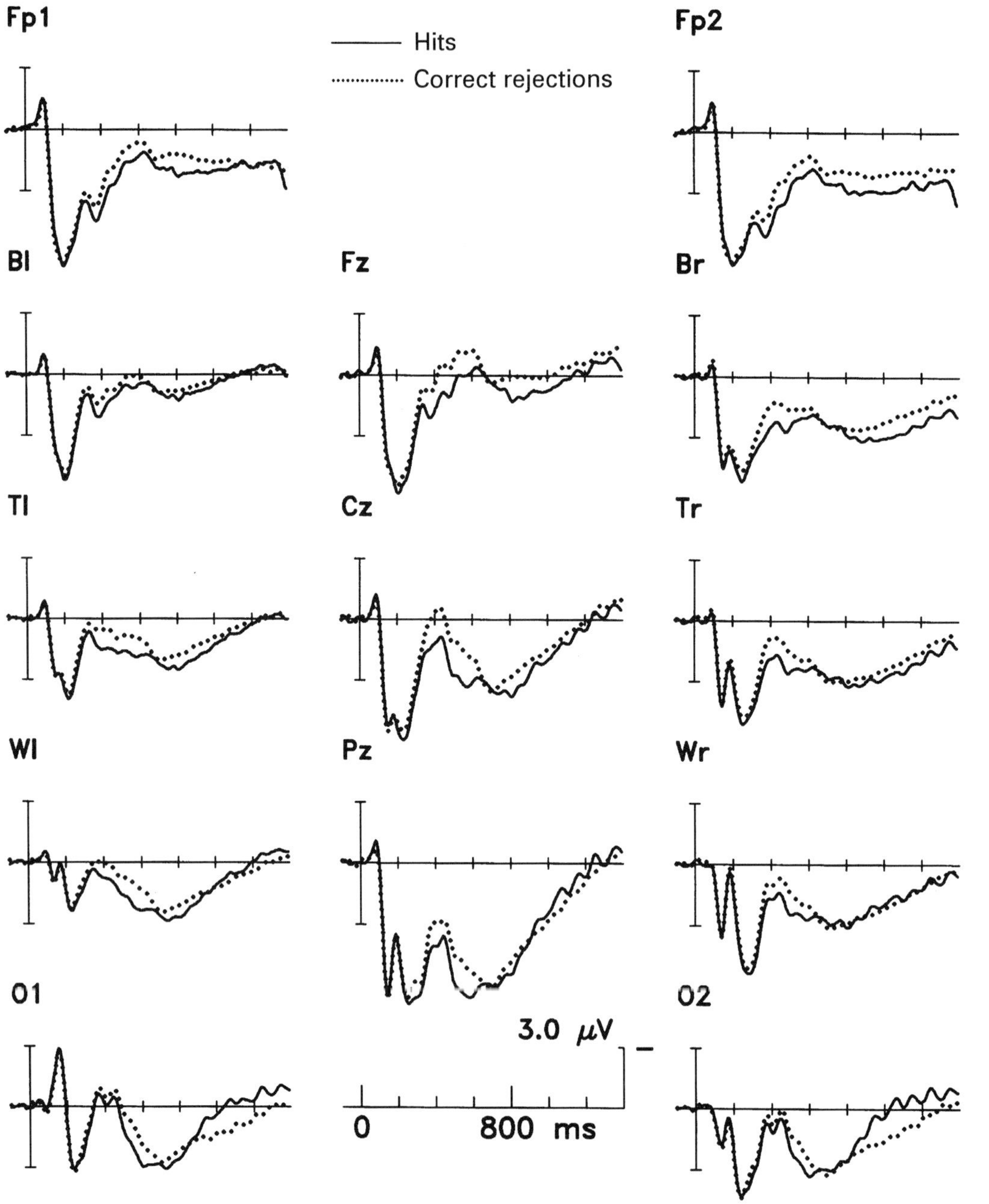

Fig. 2. *Grand average ERPs elicited by words correctly recognised (hits) and correctly rejected (correct rejections) at test. Single-syllable items are not included. Negative voltage is plotted up. Electrode sites over the left scalp are displayed in the left column, midline sites in the centre column, and sites over the right scalp in the right column. The most anterior scalp sites appear at the top and the most posterior sites at the bottom of the figure.*

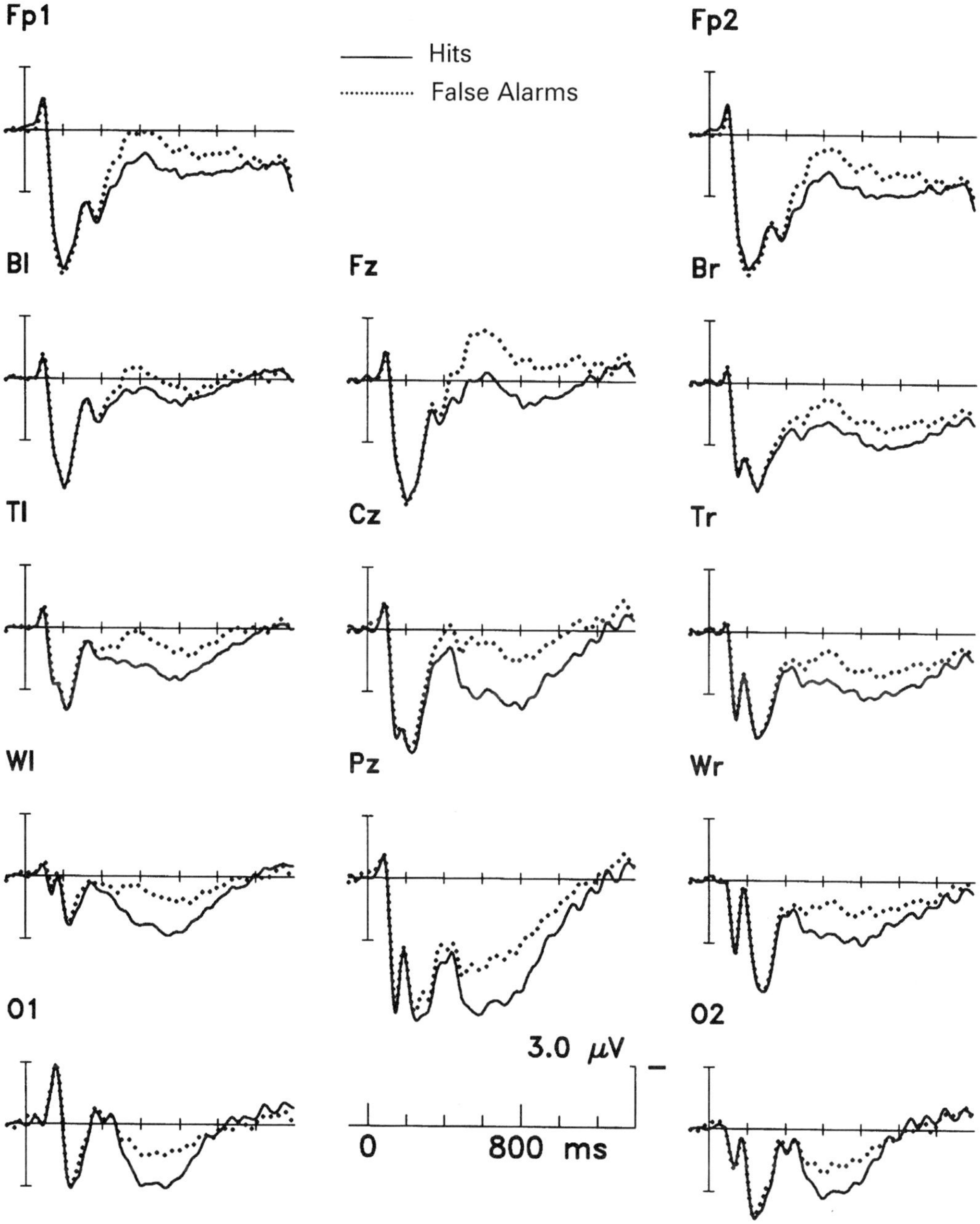

Fig. 3. *Grand average ERPs elicited by words correctly and incorrectly categorised as "old" (hits and false alarms) at test. Single-syllable items are not included.*

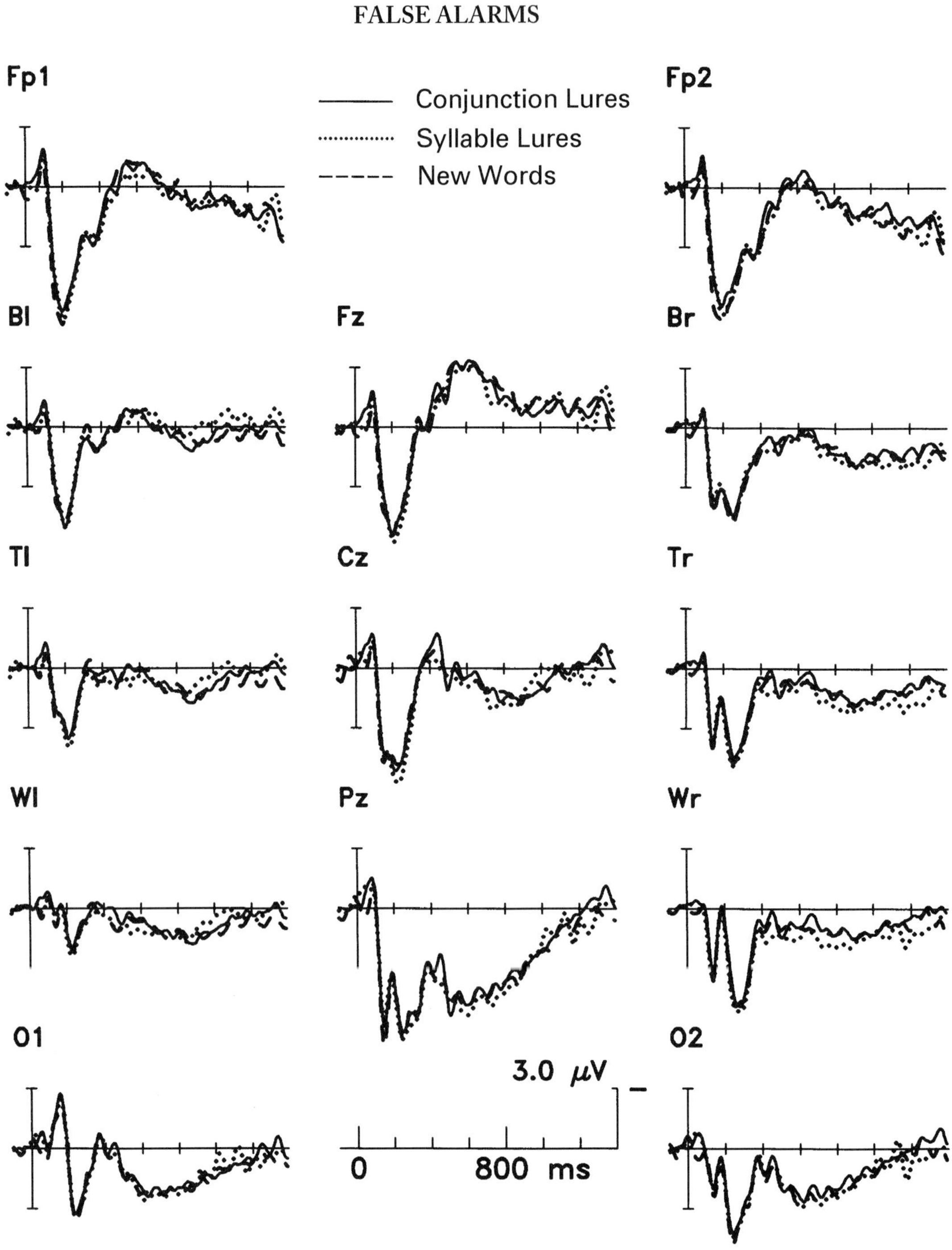

Fig. 4. *Grand average ERPs elicited by conjunction lures, syllable lures, and new words falsely categorised as "old" at test. Single-syllable items are not included.*

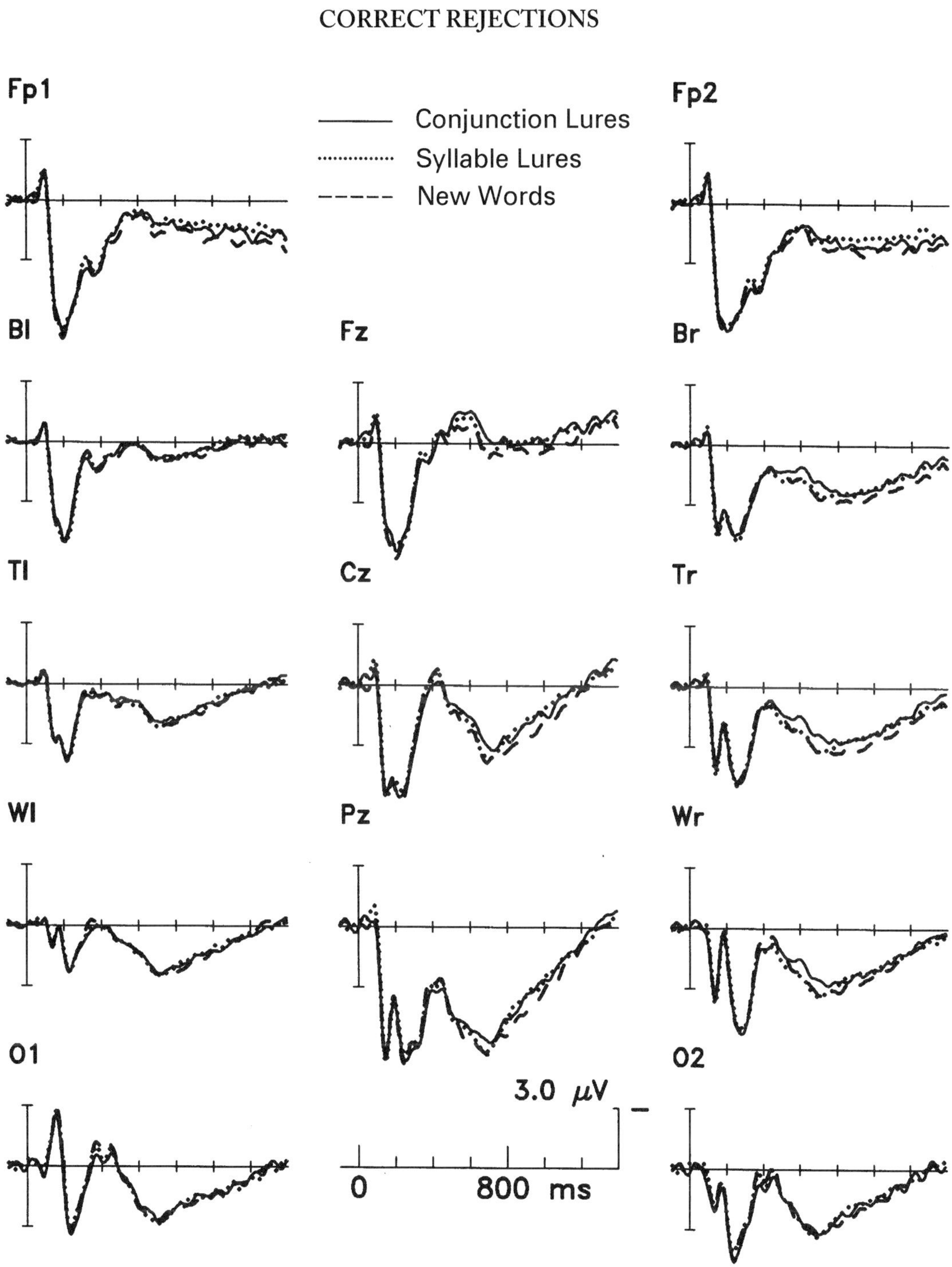

Fig. 5. *Grand average ERPS elicited by conjunction lures syllable lures, and new words correctly rejected as "new" at test. Single-syllable items are not included.*

Perhaps the most central comparison of the experiment is shown in Fig. 6, which contrasts the ERPs elicited by old words and conjunction lures when both were accompanied by "definite old" responses. The ERPs elicited by veridical recognition were significantly more positive than conjunction lure false alarms in the late time window, $F(1,15) = 7.72$, $P < .01$, and marginally more positive in the early time window, $F(1,15) = 4.20$, $P < .06$.

ERPs elicited during the study phase were examined for signs of differential encoding leading to correct or incorrect recognition judgements in the subsequent test. Too few studied words were missed at test to form reliable ERP averages for these words when they were initially studied. Three other categories of study-phase items were evaluated: (1) words subsequently presented, and recognised at test (*hits at test*) (2) words whose individual syllables were presented as parts of other words at test (i.e., the studied counterparts of the conjunction and syllable lures), and those test lure words were correctly rejected (*correct rejections at test*), and (3) words whose individual syllables were presented as parts of other words at test, and those test words were falsely categorised as old (*false alarms at test*). Figure 7 shows that there were no differences among these three categories, all Fs < 1.

Confidence Effects. The preceding analyses confirmed that the ERP differences between hits and new words (both correct rejections and false alarms) could not be attributed to differential confidence, because the differences were still evident when the analyses were restricted to "definite" responses. However, the relationship between decision confidence and accuracy, as well as the impact of confidence per se on the ERPs are also of interest. A priori, we can imagine two very different scenarios about the role of confidence in recognition ERPs. One possibility is that confidence exerts an independent influence on ERPs in all decision tasks, including recognition tests, so that this influence is additive with the old/new memory effects. This account predicts equivalent confidence effects (differences between high and low confidence responses) for hits, correct rejections, false alarms, and misses. An alternate possibility is that the influence of decision confidence on the ERPs elicited in a memory task is largely mediated by accurate retrieval; strong memory traces result in both high ratings of confidence, and a larger LPC in the ERP waveform. This latter account predicts a confidence effect for hits, and no confidence effect for misses or false alarms. The prediction of this account for correct rejections is less clear. If participants consult their memories for studied items in order to rule out these new items, correct rejections may also be subject to a confidence effect; but if making a correct rejection does not involve explicit retrieval, this process may leave no record in the memory-sensitive LPC.

We examined the relationship between decision confidence and accurate retrieval by comparing the ERPs elicited by hits, false alarms, and correct rejections at different confidence levels. There were too few misses to form ERP averages with an adequate signal-to-noise ratio. Similarly, very few correct responses (hits or correct rejections) were accompanied by "maybe" responses, so that it was not possible to form separate ERP averages for this lowest confidence ranking. Instead, "probable" and "maybe" responses were summed for comparison to "definite" responses. For the six categories of interest—hits, correct rejections, and all varieties of false alarm accompanied by "definite" and "probable/maybe" ratings—15 of the 24 subjects had at least 10 artefact free trials per category and the analyses here are based on those subjects.

Figure 8 shows that confident and correct judgements about old words elicited more positive ERPs than hits accompanied by lower confidence, beginning about 500msec post-stimulus onset. Confidence had a smaller impact in correct judgements about new words, and essentially no effect on incorrect judgements about new words. Analyses of mean amplitudes in the 600–900msec epoch thus yielded a significant confidence effect for hits [$F(1,14) = 8.78$, $P < .02$], a nonsignificant trend for correct rejections [$F(1,14) = 3.24$, $P < 10$], and no difference for false alarms [$F(1,14) = 1.40$]. Comparisons between hits and both categories of new items confirmed that the confidence effect was largest for correct old items

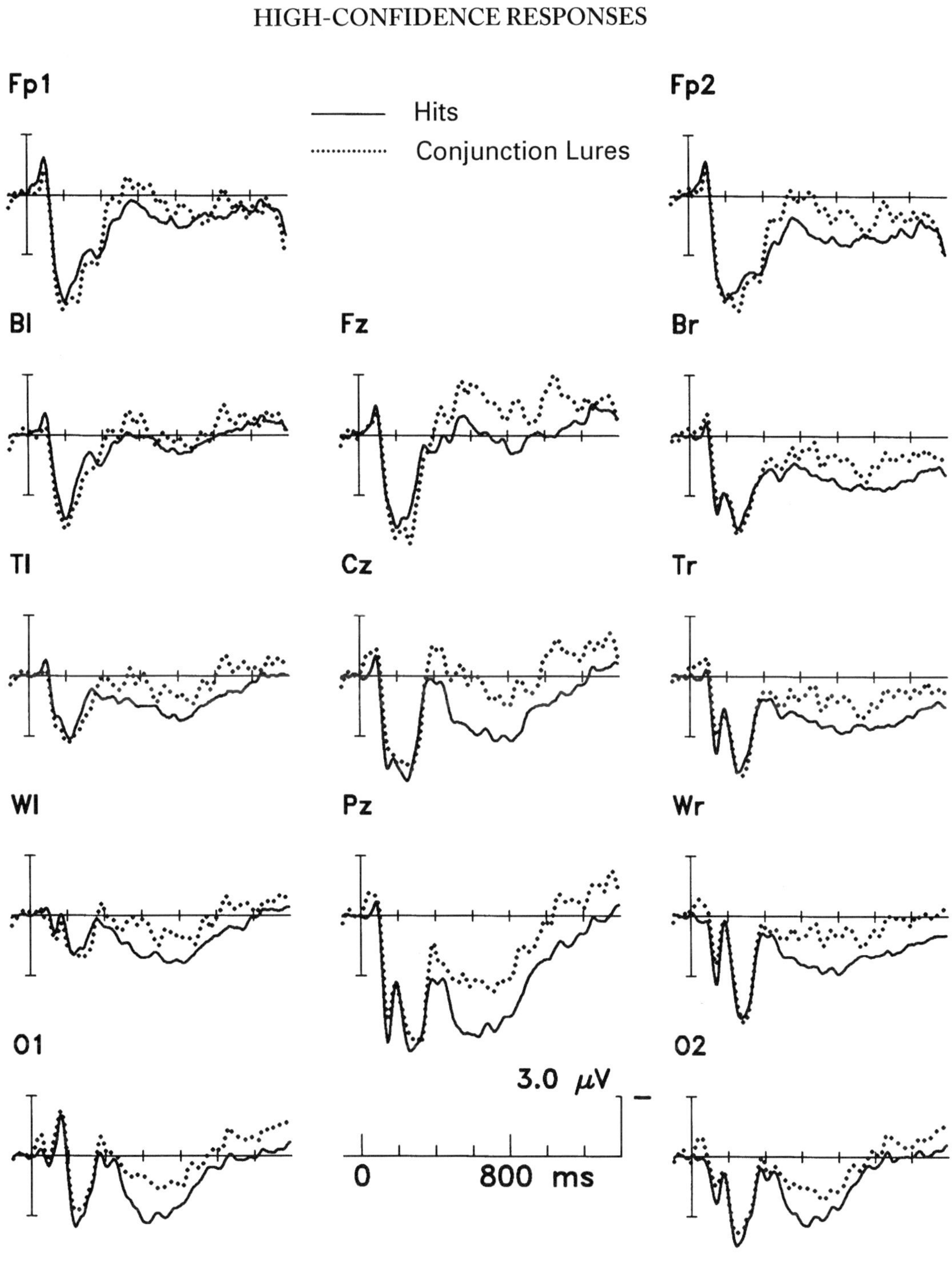

Fig. 6. *Grand average ERPs elicited by truly old words and conjunction lures caterorised as "definitely old" at test. Single-syllable items are not included.*

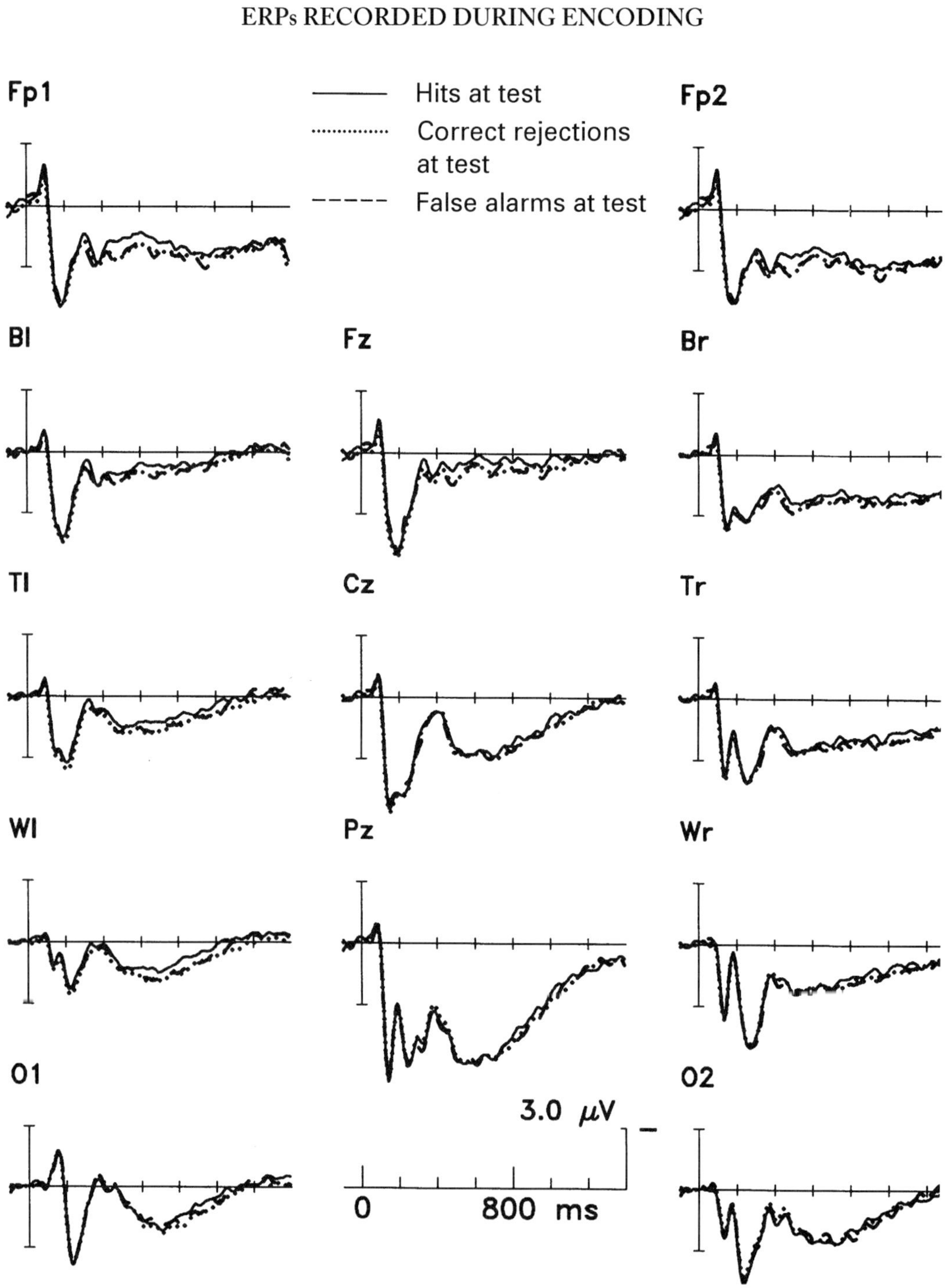

Fig. 7. *Grand average ERPs elicited during study by words later correctly categorised as "old" (hits) correctly categorised as "new" (correct rejections), and incorrectly categorised as "old" (false alarms) at test. Single-syllable items are not included.*

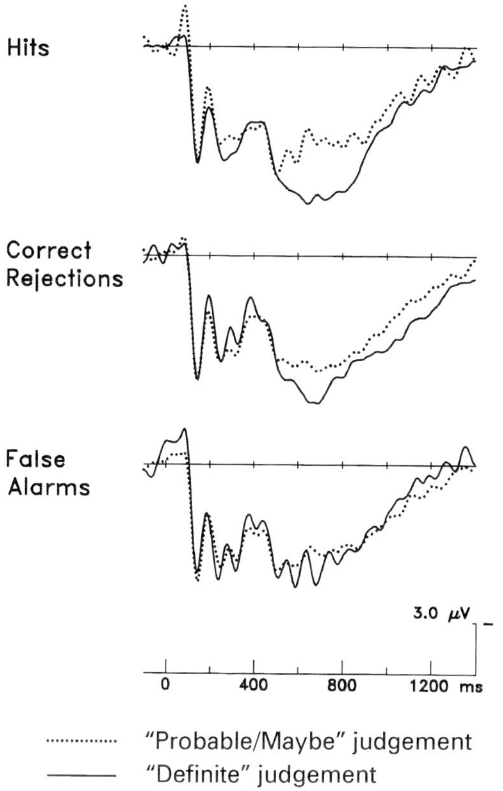

Fig. 8. *Effect of confidence on grand average ERPs elicited by different-response types (hits, correct rejections, and false alarms) at electrode site Pz. Single-syllable items are not included.*

[interaction of Old/New by Confidence: hits vs. correct rejections, $F(1,14) = 4.59$, $P < .05$; hits vs. false alarms, $F(1,14) = 8.43$, $P < .02$]. There were no significant confidence effects in analyses of the 300-600msec epoch.

The outcome of these confidence analyses is most compatible with the second hypothesis outlined earlier. Although it will be important to examine recognition misses in some future experiment that includes more highly confident misses, the present results suggest that the amplitude of the LPC is primarily driven by successful retrieval so that a clear recollection of a studied item will yield both high decision confidence and larger late positivities.

Discussion

Encoding versus Retrieval

Our results are most compatible with a processing fluency explanation of false alarms to conjunction lures. The critical piece of behavioural evidence is that subjects had consistently higher false alarm rates to syllable lures than to new words. If the binding hypothesis were correct, we would have expected no difference between these two word types. False alarms to syllable lures follow presentation of only one of the relevant syllables during encoding, so this type of error is unlikely to be attributable to inappropriate binding during the study phase. Two previous studies have reported no differences between syllable lures and new words, but these suffered from low statistical power due to small numbers of trials, which is not the case in the current study (Kroll et al., 1996; Reinitz & Demb, 1994). The graded pattern of false alarms (conjunction lures < syllable lures < new words) observed here is predicted by a processing fluency account since conjunction lures have two familiar components, syllable lures have one, and new words have none.

An even stronger argument against the binding hypothesis comes from the ERP data, which indicates that conjunction errors are formed at retrieval rather than encoding. The key finding here was that ERPs elicited by false alarms to conjunction lures, syllable lures, and new words at test were indistinguishable from one another, but all were significantly different from the ERPs elicited by hits. The largest LPC, previously thought to be sensitive to conscious recollection, was observed for hits. Moreover, high confidence hits elicited larger LPCs than low-confidence hits, providing further support for the idea that this component reflects the recollective experience of previously studied items. No differences were observed among the three types of false alarms, suggesting that these responses were not based on explicit recollection of words created by mis-binding during the study phase, or even of individual syllables viewed earlier, but on a feeling of familiarity, which led to a "yes" response. However, it is still unclear what this feeling of familiarity is based on. It could plausibly be due to orthographic, phonological, or visual similarity, and the current study cannot distinguish between these possibilities.

Although the ERPs elicited by false recognition of new items were clearly distinct from those elicited by accurate retrieval of old items, judgements of "old" and "new" for new items did not lead to identical ERPs. Comparison of Fig. 2 and 3 (as well as the statistical analyses) indicates that the difference between hits and false alarms is of longer duration than the analogous difference between hits and correct rejections. We have suggested that both false alarms and correct rejections differ from hits because they share one core feature: the absence of a clear recollective experience. But false alarms and correct rejections differ along other dimensions, some of which may be general to tasks that involve an element of target detection—accepting or rejecting an item as "old" in the case of a recognition task. Reaction times for high-confidence false alarm judgements were shorter than for correct rejections, although slower than for hits, which may reflect the absence of a clear conscious recollective experience on false alarm trials. There was also a large difference in the variability of reaction times across the three trial types: Table 2 shows that the standard error of the mean of the reaction time was substantially higher for false alarms than for either hits or correct rejections. This table shows the variability across subjects; examination of reaction times for individual subjects revealed a more striking difference. Even for high-confidence responses, the average within subject standard errors for hits and correct rejections were 31 and 40 msec respectively, whereas the average standard error for false alarms was 104 msec. Variability in the timing of cognitive processes also influences the appearance of ERP waveforms. Increased latency jitter across the individual trials contributing to an averaged ERP produces broader, flatter waveforms than averages with a narrower range of latency variability. The degree of latency variability within and between conditions can thus determine the duration of the difference between two ERP waveforms. The reaction times for hits and correct rejections showed relatively small and equivalent variability; Fig. 2 correspondingly shows a relatively short-duration difference between the ERPs in these two conditions. In contrast, the false alarm category showed substantially greater reaction time variability than the hit category; Fig. 3 correspondingly shows a long duration ERP difference between these two conditions.

In contrast to the robust difference between old and new words observed during the recognition tests, the ERPs recorded during the study phase did not reveal any encoding differences among items. In previous research, the typical analysis of study-phase ERPs has compared items that are subsequently recognised (hits at test) to those subsequently unrecognised (misses at test). A convenient term for this conventional analysis is Dm (difference according to memory). Under some study conditions, particularly those that include a "yes/no" study task (e.g. living vs. nonliving judgements), the Dm comparison reveals a larger late positivity for successfully encoded items (Fabiani & Donchin, 1995; Paller, Kutas, & Mayes, 1987; Van Petten & Senkfor, 1996). The present experiment did not allow this typical analysis because of the relatively small number of studied words that were unrecognised at test. Instead, we conducted a related analysis of study-phase words whose individual syllables were presented at test; in this analysis "good encoding" might lead to correct rejection of recognition lures containing only one studied syllable, whereas "poor encoding" might lead to incorrect acceptance of these lures. However, this prediction was not verified; no difference was observed between study-phase items whose related lures were rejected or accepted at test (Fig. 7). The null result of our study-phase analysis lends no support to the hypothesis that false alarms at test are due to a specific defect in prior encoding processes. However, the null result should also be interpreted with some caution for two reasons. First, the present analysis is a novel one, so that there are no prior studies in which "good encoding" is associated with both a correct rejection at test, and some demonstrable ERP effect during the study phase. Second, although the more conventional Dm analysis has yielded a distinction between good versus poor encoding in some dozen studies, two recent studies have also suggested that the presence or absence of a typical Dm effect is contingent on the exact form of the study-phase task (Senkfor & Van Petten, 1998; Van Petten & Senkfor, 1996). Because the non-binary "noun/verb/modifier" study task used in the present experiment is also novel, we do not yet know if it is well suited to detecting encoding differences.

Relationship to Prior Studies of Brain Activity and False Recognition

As noted in the Introduction, previous ERP studies have compared correct and incorrect "old" responses during recognition tests in which the new items bear no special relationship to studied items. These studies yielded the same results as those observed here: false alarms are accompanied by much smaller late positive ERP components than hits (Neville et al., 1986; Sanquist, Rohrbaugh, Syndulko, & Lindsley, 1980; Van Petten & Senlefor, 1996). We are aware of four recent studies examining brain activity when new items are closely related to studied items and thus elicit higher than typical false alarm rates. Each of these used the converging semantic associate paradigm in which the critical lures are semantically associated with studied words; all report great similarity between hits and false alarms (Duzel et al., 1997; Johnson et al., 1997; Schacter, Buckner, Koutstaal, Dale, & Rosen, 1997; Schacter, Reiman, et al., 1996).

Johnson and colleagues (1997) observed essentially identical ERPs for hits and false alarms to related lures, when these related lures were randomly intermixed with old words and unrelated new words. However, Johnson et al., observed larger late positivities for hits than false alarms in a separate experiment which presented old, new, and related new words in distinct blocks. Johnson and colleagues interpret the different pattern of results in the blocked and random versions as reflective of different response criteria. Although the contrast between hits and correct rejections was not analysed in this study, it appears that this basic old/new effect also differed between the participants in the two experiments, so that careful examination of response criteria, confidence levels, and/or individual differences in the converging semantic associates paradigm will be important avenues of future investigation.

Using a randomised design very similar to Johnson et al. (1997), Duzel and colleagues (1997) observed no late positive difference between hits and false alarms to related lures, but instead a larger N400 component for hits. A direct relationship between the N400 component and episodic memory has not been established, but N400 amplitude is exquisitely sensitive to semantic context (see Kutas & Van Petten, 1994, for review). The N400 result may reflect differential semantic context effects for old items and related lures in the specific implementation of the converging semantic associate paradigm used by Duzel and other investigators. Related lures are, by definition, related to a large number of studied items, some of which re-occur during the recognition test. Old items are subject to less semantic context at both study and test, because these words are selected for their semantic relationships to the critical related lures, but not for their relationships to each other (e.g. TOOTH is associated with the critical lure SWEET, but is not as strongly related to HONEY, SOUR, CANDY, etc). At test, old words may thus provide semantic context for the lures, but not for each other. Similarly, the semantic associations between old words and lures may not be directionally symmetric (e.g. SWEET may elicit TOOTH in a production norm, but TOOTH may not elicit SWEET). At test, the truly old items may thus serve as semantic context for the related lures, but the reverse is less likely to occur. Differential semantic context effects during recognition may account for the N400 difference between hits and false alarms observed by Duzel et al. (1997); the strength of this factor across studies using the converging semantic associate paradigm will depend on the exact composition and ordering of recognition word lists.

With positron emission tomographic (PET) measures, Schacter and colleagues (Schacter, Reiman et al., 1996) observed greater blood flow in left temporoparietal cortex during blocks of old words than blocks of related lures. Prefrontal cortex showed a statistical trend for greater blood flow during blocks of related lures. Relative to a fixation baseline, other brain regions such as the medial temporal lobe showed similar increases in blood flow for old words and related lures. The left temporoparietal result was attributed to the retrieval of auditory/phonological information for old words heard during the study phase, information that would be absent in the case of related lures. However, the proximity of this region to those implicated in semantic processing and the possibility of differential semantic context effects in the converging semantic associate paradigm suggests that this result should be interpreted with caution. With functional magnetic resonance (fMRI) measures, Schacter and colleagues (1997) have recently compared old items to related lures with both blocked and randomly intermixed presentation formats. Blood oxygenation levels in left temporoparietal cortex did not discriminate the two word types in either format. The mixed format yielded no prefrontal differences between hits and false alarms, while the possibility of motion artefacts made it difficult to determine if there was differential prefrontal activity in the blocked format. As in the PET study, numerous brain regions showed equivalent haemodynamic changes for both old words and related lures relative to a fixation baseline.

Overall, studies of brain activity using the converging semantic associate paradigm have shown a striking similarity between hits and false alarms, particularly when old and new items are intermixed during the recognition test. These results are in dramatic contrast to the large and robust ERP differences observed here with a random presentation format. Although further investigation of the conjunction lure paradigm is warranted, the discrepancy between the converging semantic associate and conjunction paradigms strongly suggests that not all false alarms are the same. The conjunction lure, syllable lure, and new items used in the present study are not semantically related to studied items, and the results suggest that false alarms to these items are generated by retrieval errors. Other authors have suggested that the related lures in the converging semantic associate paradigm are activated during the study phase (Seamon, Luo, & Gallo, 1998), so that false alarms in this paradigm may reflect encoding errors; at test, semantic lures may indeed be retrieved much like veridical memory traces and elicit similar brain activity. Although our study task was a semantic one, subjects apparently did not use that information very effectively at test and so became entrapped by the orthographic and phonological similarities of the lures. It is also interesting to note that false alarms to related lures are made with higher confidence than false alarms to unrelated words in the converging semantic associates paradigm, but we observed no confidence differences between false alarms to conjunction lures and new words. This suggests that semantic context may affect confidence in a way that familiarity per se does not.

The data from Experiment 1 all converge on the conclusion that familiarity or processing fluency for studied syllables led to a memory illusion at retrieval, but this process was not accompanied by the same LPC that accompanies retrieval of veridical memories.

EXPERIMENT 2

Experiment 1 has provided some insight about when and how memory fails in the conjunction lure paradigm, but additional information can be gleaned from examining the relations between false recognition and other cognitive processes. Experiment 2 is designed to provide such information by using neuropsychological methods in a group of older adults.

Adult age differences in recognition are weaker than those observed in recall (Craik & Jennings, 1992), but our primary interest is in utilising the variability within the elderly population to shed light on the nature of the processes involved in memory conjunction errors. There is general agreement that various cognitive functions do not decrease at the same rate with age, and that variability within a given task is typically greater within elderly than young samples (Albert, 1988; Albert, Duffy, & Naeser, 1987; Welford, 1993).

Neuropathological and neuroimaging studies indicate that prefrontal and medial temporal cortex are particularly sensitive to the normal ageing process, so that both regions are potential candidates for explanations of age-related changes in memory performance (Coffey et al., 1992; Double et al., 1996; Haug, 1985; Martin, Friston, Colebatch, & Frackowiak, 1991; Murphy et al., 1996; Raz, Torres, Spencer, & Acker, 1993; Terry, DeTheresa, & Hansen, 1987; Troncoso, Martin, Dalforrio, & Kawas, 1996). By relating older adults' performance on standardised neuropsychological tests to their experimental performance, we hope to gain insight into either the gross neuroanatomical locus and/or the basic cognitive processes underlying false recognition (for a review of the cognitive neuroscience of false memories, see Schacter, Norman, & Koutstaal, 1998). Later, we describe our approach to characterising individual differences among older adults, but first we briefly review the general background for supposing that one or both of these broadly defined brain regions may be critical for determining false alarm rates.

In a previous study using the conjunction lure paradigm, Kroll and colleagues (1996) observed similar hit rates for normal controls and patients with damage to the hippocampal system. However, patients with left hippocampal damage had false alarm rates of nearly 40% for verbal conjunction lures, as compared to about 14% for older control subjects. Patients with right hippocampal damage showed the same pattern of results for miscombined pictorial stimuli. This result supports the idea that the hippocampal formation plays a vital role in the binding of individual stimulus components into an integrated whole (Kroll et al., 1996). A handful of studies suggest that reduced recognition accuracy within normal elderly samples is due more to inflated false alarm rates than to depressed hit rates (Chao & Knight, 1997; Flicker, Ferris, Crook, & Bartus, 1989; Fulton & Bartlett, 1991; Isingrini, Fontaine, Taconnat, & Duportal, 1995; Norman & Schacter, 1997). Kroll et al.'s results might then suggest that high false alarm rates among the elderly should be attributed to age-related dysfunction of the medial temporal lobe. In contrast, other studies of patients with organic brain damage suggest that prefrontal cortex plays a critical role in determining false alarm rates. Patients with prefrontal damage show only a weak impairment in recognition memory tasks (Wheeler, Stuss, & Tulving, 1995), but this deficit is primarily due to high false alarm rates (Swick & Knight, in press). High false alarm rates in recognition tasks, and confabulation in recall tasks have both been noted in numerous case studies of patients with frontal lesions (Benson et al., 1996; Curran, Schacter, Norman, & Galluccio, 1997; Delbecq-Derousné, Beauvois, & Shallice, 1990; Fischer, Alexander, D'Esposito, & Otto, 1995; N. Kapur & Coughlan, 1980; Moscovitch, 1995; Parkin, Bindschaedler, Harsent, & Metzler, 1996; Rapscak, Polster, Corner, & Rubens, 1994; Schacter, Curran, Galluccio, Milberg, & Bates, 1996). These data then suggest that high false alarm rates among normally ageing individuals might be attributed to mild prefrontal dysfunction.

Overall, the neuropsychological literature indicates that intact medial temporal and prefrontal cortices are both necessary for accurate memory judgements. Moscovitch (1994) has proposed a general theory about the relationship between a *memory system* and a *working-with-memory* system. He argues that the medial temporal lobe is a primary component of the memory system, which is responsible for the actual encoding, storage, and retrieval of memory traces. The working-with-memory system consists primarily of prefrontal cortex, whose roles are to select input, and to monitor or interpret the output of the memory system. High false alarm rates can thus arise from generally weak memories, or a failure to assess the strength of these memories accurately. The working-with-memory system is likely to be particularly taxed in situations that involve a high degree of similarity between old and new items, as in the conjunction lure paradigm.

The results of our first experiment are most compatible with viewing false alarms as arising from a failure to assess memory output adequately. We observed an increasing false alarm rate as the test stimuli became more similar to studied items, indicating that false alarms were indeed based on some form of memory for the studied items.

However, despite the fact that brain activity clearly differentiated these similar items from those actually studied, the participants' behavioural responses did not. We interpret the ERP difference between hits and false alarms as reflecting a distinction between recollection and familiarity, but it appears that this distinction can be uncoupled from the decision or criterion-setting processes that lead to a behavioural response. In Moscovitch's (1994) framework, the failure on a false alarm trial is most likely to reside in the working-with-memory system. To the extent that this functional system is contained in prefrontal cortex, we might expect that the propensity to make false alarms will be associated with other functions ascribed to this general brain region. This prediction is tested by charactersing healthy elderly adults via their performance on neuropsychological tests that are sensitive to the presence of prefrontal lesions in patients with frank organic damage.

The proposed relationship between memory monitoring and prefrontal cortex leads to a secondary prediction about decision confidence during recognition judgements. Experiment 1 yielded the typical result of higher confidence in correct than incorrect decisions; this result indicates an intact relationship between memory strength and memory monitoring. At least one observation indicates that the subjective confidence ratings of patients with frontal lobe damage show little relationship to their actual response accuracy (Rapscak et al., 1998). If the relationship between memory strength and monitoring is weakened with advancing age, or, more specifically, a decline in prefrontal function, the correlation between accuracy and confidence might also be associated with other indices of prefrontal function.

Assessing Individual Differences in the Elderly

The present study uses a methodology developed by Glisky, Polster, and Routhieaux (1995) to categorise cognitive strengths and weaknesses among older adults. One hundred healthy elderly participants were given a battery of standardised neuropsychological tests and the scores subjected to a factor analysis. These tests are listed in Table 3. Five tests sensitive to prefrontal function in brain-damaged patients loaded on a single factor and four tests sensitive to medial temporal and/or diencephalic function in brain-damaged patients loaded on a second factor uncorrelated with the first one. Because we were interested in the differential contributions of the frontal lobes and medial temporal lobes/diencephalon that were independent of age, variance attributable to age was removed from each of the nine test scores through regression analyses (see Glisky et al., for further details). On the basis of the factor analysis, two z-scores were calculated for each subject, representing composite measures of what we will refer to as *Frontal* (F) and *Medial temporal/diencephalic* (M) functions. It is important to note that none of the tests in the frontal battery tap long-term memory; instead they test such abilities as inhibition, set switching, working memory, and strategy formation. Paired associate and other cued recall tests contributed to the M factor score. The two factor scores were then used to categorise participants as having "high Frontal" and "high Medial temporal/diencephalic" function (F+M+), "high Frontal" and "low Medial temporal/diencephalic" function (F+M-), "low Frontal" and "high Medial temporal/diencephalic" function (F-M+), or "low Frontal" and "low Medial temporal/diencephalic" function (F-M-), depending on

Table 3. *Neuropsychological Tests Loading on Frontal and Medial temporal diencephalic*

Factors
Frontal
Modified Wisconsin Card Sorting Task (Hart et al., 1988)
FAS (Benton & Hamsher, 1976)
Mental Arithmetic from Wechsler Adult Intelligence Scale-Revised (WAIS-R; Wechsler, 1981)
Backward Digit Span from Wechsler Memory Scale-Revised (WMS-R; Wechsler, 1987)
Mental Control from WMS-R (Wechsler, 1987)
Medial temporal diencephalic
Logical Memory I from WMS-R (Wechsler, 1987)
Verbal Paired Associates I from WMS-R (Wechsler, 1987)
Visual Paired Associates II from WMS-R (Wechsler, 1987)
California Verbal Learning Test-Long Delay Cued Recall (Delis et al., 1987)

whether the z-scores fell above or below zero. We used a subset of these subjects (six from each category) in the present study.

Method

Participants

Participants included 18 young adults (21–39 years old, 8 women, 10 men) and 24 healthy, community-dwelling elderly subjects (66–88 years old; 16 women, 8 men), all of whom gave informed consent. See Table 4 for demographic variables of the older participants broken down by factor score. Three additional young adults participated, but their data were excluded from the analyses due to memory performance (hits – false alarms to new words) more than two standard deviations below the mean.

Materials and Procedure

Materials included 240 of the 440 triads and 70 of the single-syllable filler words described in Experiment 1. As before, assignment of conjunction words to one of the four conditions was rotated across participants, so that each word appeared equally often in each test condition. Unlike Experiment 1, the syllable lures of Experiment 2 consisted of test items sharing either first or second syllables with study items (e.g. study PANIC, test PANDER, or study BLENDER, test PANDER). The stimuli were divided into two lists and split between two study-test cycles.

The experiment consisted of a short practice list and two study-test cycles. Participants were assigned the same study task, and words were presented the same way as in Experiment 1, except that the stimulus duration was increased from 200 to 300 msec for the older adults (stimulus onset asynchrony remained the same).

Results

Effects of Age on Performance

The proportions of two-syllable words called "old" by young and elderly participants are shown in Fig. 9. Older adults correctly classified 71% of the two-syllable words during the recognition tests, as compared to 78% for the young participants, $F(1,40) = 6.25$, $P < .02$. This small impairment in overall accuracy arises from both a slightly lower hit rate and a slightly higher false alarm rate in the elderly group, but neither the hit nor the false alarm rate showed significant age effects when analysed separately, $Fs(1,40) < 2.98$, $Ps < .09$.

Mean confidence ratings for hits, correct rejections, false alarms, and misses were analysed in an ANOVA using age, accuracy, and Old/New as variables. Not surprisingly, both old and young subjects were more confident in their correct than incorrect responses, yielding a main effect of accuracy, $F(1,40) = 111.46$, $P < .0001$. There was also an interaction between accuracy and Old/New due to the fact that old correct items (hits, mean = 2.76 out of 3) had the highest confidence ratings, followed by new correct items (correct rejections, mean = 2.45), old incorrect items (misses, mean = 2.33), and new incorrect items (false alarms, mean = 2.22). Finally, the accuracy by age interaction was also significant, $F(1,40) = 7.86$, $P < .008$. Further analyses revealed that older adults were slightly superior in their metamemory judgement, in that younger adults were a bit more confident that their false recognitions were actually correct, $F(1,40) = 3.04$, $P < .089$. There were no

Table 4. *Mean Demographic Variables of Older Adults by Factor Score*

Category	*Age*	*Education*	*Gender*	*F score*	*M score*
F+M+	73	17 years	3 males, 3 females	.68	.67
F+M–	72	15 years	1 male, 5 females	.63	–.46
F-M+	76	16 years	1 male, 5 females	–.43	.37
F-M-	75	16 years	3 males, 3 females	–.71	–.40

None of the demographic variables were significantly correlated with factor score.

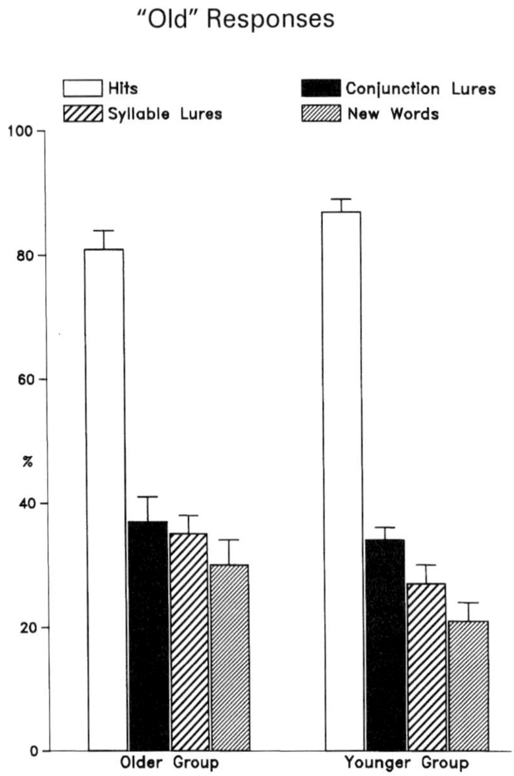

Fig. 9. *Mean percentage of items judged "old" during the recognition test (maximum = 100% in each category) of Experiment 2. Single-syllable items are not included. Error bars show standard error of the mean.*

age differences on confidence ratings for hits, correct rejections, or misses, all *F*s < 1.

Analyses of the false alarm categories in Fig. 9 revealed a significant effect of word type, $F(2,80) = 20.7$, $P < .0001$. There were no significant differences between false alarm rates for first- and second-syllable lures, *F*s < 1.0, so these were collapsed into a category of "syllable lures" in all analyses. There was no interaction between word type and age, indicating that both groups showed the same general pattern of false alarm rates (conjunction lures > syllable lures > new words). Older adults thus had no special propensity to make conjunction lure false alarms.

Effects of Neuropsychological Factor Score on Performance

A breakdown of older adults' recognition accuracy according to the neuropsychological factors is shown in Fig.10. The initial analysis evaluated overall accuracy for the two-syllable words (both hits and correct rejections as a proportion of the total trials), using the F and M factors as independent variables in a 2 × 2 ANOVA. F-participants had lower overall accuracy rates, $F(1,23) = 7.99$, $P < .01$, whereas the M score did not influence overall accuracy. An independent analysis of hit rates indicated that neither factor score yielded a significant main effect, but a somewhat lower hit rate in the F+M- group led to an interaction between the two factors, $F(1,23) = 5.73$, $P < .02$.

False alarms were examined in an ANOVA using the two neuropsychological factors and word type (conjunction lure, syllable lure, or new) as variables. This showed that the reduced overall accuracy in the low frontal groups was due to an elevated false alarm rate, $F(1,20) = 5.74$, $P < .02$. The overall false alarm rate was not influenced by the M factor. However, Fig. 10 shows that the M factor did influence the pattern of false alarms. Unlike either the young adults or the M+ older adults, both M– groups failed to show the typical gradient of false alarms. Instead, these participants displayed nearly identical false alarm rates for conjunction lures, syllable lures, and new words, leading to an interaction between the M factor score and Word Type, $F(2,40) = 3.56$, $P < .03$.

Mean confidence ratings for hits, correct rejections, false alarms, and misses were analysed in an ANOVA using F score, M score, accuracy, and Old/New as variables. Like the young adults in Experiment 1, the older adults were more confident in their correct responses than their incorrect responses, $F(1,20) = 39.06$, $P < .0001$. Our initial hypothesis was that individuals who performed well in the "frontal battery" of neuropsychological tests would also show stronger relationships between accuracy and confidence. This prediction was not supported. The F+M+ participants showed the largest differences between confidence ratings for their correct and incorrect responses, leading to a significant three-way interaction (F score ×

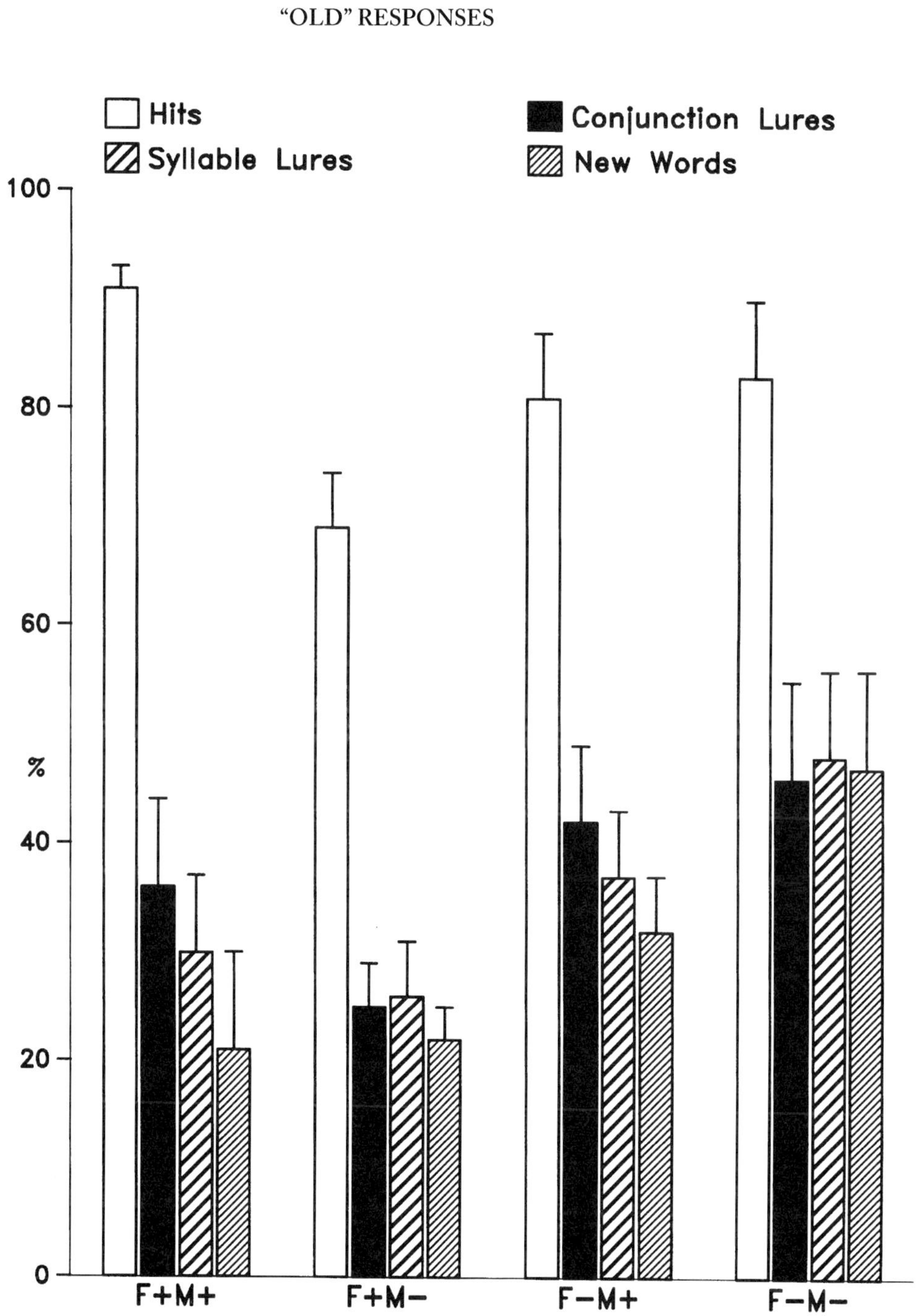

Fig. 10. *Mean percentage of items judged "old" during the recognition test (maximum 100% in each category) of Experiment 2 by neuropsychological factor score. Single-syllable items are not included. Error bars show standard error of the mean.*

M score × Accuracy), $F(1,20) = 6.04$, $P < .05$. Support for our original hypothesis would require that the F+M− group also show a stronger relationship between confidence and accuracy than the two F-frontal groups. However, an analysis comparing these three groups included only a main effect of accuracy $F(1,15) = 16.73$, $P < .001$, but no group interactions. The results thus showed that the individuals who performed the best on the entire neuropsychological test battery also had the strongest confidence/accuracy relationships.

Discussion

The behavioural results of Experiment 2 replicate those of the first experiment; both young and elderly adults overall showed a gradient of false alarm rates determined by the similarity of the recognition lures to studied items. Older adults showed slightly reduced accuracy overall, but no qualitative difference in the balance of hits to false alarms. Although there have been reports of inflated false alarm rates in elderly samples as compared to young, this finding is by no means uniform. Numerous studies also show no greater change in false alarm rate than hit rate with age (Gunter, Jackson, & Mulder, 1992; Mantyla & Backman, 1992; Mark & Rugg, 1998; Parkin & Lawrence, 1994; Swick & Knight, 1997, Trott, Friedman, Ritter, & Fabiani, 1997). Kroll et al., (1996) included control groups of older and younger adults in their study of memory conjunction errors, and they found decreased accuracy overall rather than increased false alarm rates without accompanying hit rate decreases in all but one of their conditions, and this condition appeared to have a ceiling effect insofar as the hit rates were between 95.6 and 100% even for the patient groups. Older adults did not show a disproportionate false alarm rates for conjunction lures in the current study either. This is in contrast to some studies using the converging semantic associates paradigm, which found inflated false alarm rates for older adults in the absence of depressed hit rates (Norman & Schacter, 1997; Tun, Wingfield, Rosen, & Blanchard, 1998), and points to the possibility that making a false alarm in this paradigm may involve different processes than in other paradigms.

Analyses of relationship of confidence to accuracy in the current study also revealed few differences between younger and older adults. In fact, the only age difference indicated that the older adults had somewhat better metamemory than the young when indicating their confidence level when they falsely recognised a word. Although this may seem counter-intuitive, there is quite a bit of evidence supporting the idea that the elderly are not differentially impaired on metamemory tasks (see Light, 1991, for a review).

Despite the overall similarities between older and younger adults, the neuropsychological approach employed here distinguished different patterns of memory performance among the elderly sample. The Frontal factor score, which reflects a composite of cognitive abilities excluding long-term memory, predicted overall false alarm rate. This finding meshes well with reports that patients with prefrontal lesions also show inflated false alarm rates in recognition tasks, while not exhibiting an overall memory impairment (for a comparison between frontal and hippocampal patients, see Swick & Knight, in press). This finding also lends support to Moscovitch's (1994) proposal that prefrontal cortex is critical for monitoring the output of the memory system, and making decisions about the veridicality of that output. This monitoring function is likely to be especially critical in recognition paradigms that include a high degree of similarity between new and studied items, or perhaps even long lists of studied items that increase the possibility of proactive and retroactive interference, two characteristics of the paradigm used here.

Our factor analytic approach to characterising prefrontal function in the elderly population draws on standardised neuropsychological tests generally thought to be sensitive to frontal damage. It has previously been reported that individual differences in the Frontal factor score are related to performance in another memory task known to be sensitive to prefrontal damage—source memory judgements (Glisky et al., 1995; Henkel, Johnson, & De Leonardis, 1998). More recently, we have noted that ERPs recorded at prefrontal scalp sites during a source memory paradigm differentiate healthy older adults characterised as "high Frontal" or "low Frontal" by the factor score approach (Senkfor & Van Petten, unpublished observation). These relationships between the factor analytic method and other methods in cognitive neuroscience are reassuring, but it is important to note that this statistical approach does not offer the direct anatomical link, or the anatomical precision possible in the study of patients with circumscribed lesions. It is possible that none of the tests in the frontal battery are functionally related to recognition memory, or share any anatomical substrates with recognition memory. However, the appeal of using a composite neuropsychological measure is that the tests may collectively offer a broad and stable measure of the integrity of this large brain region. To the extent that mnemonic and non-mnemonic functions of prefrontal cortex are similarly influenced by normal ageing, the observed relationships between the factor score and experimental measures of memory offer at least coarse information about the localisation of these mnemonic processes.

The Medial temporal/diencephalic factor also influenced recognition performance in a distinctive way. Participants with M scores below the mean were just as likely to judge a new word as old when it shared two, one, or no syllables with a studied item. The flat false alarm pattern in the M− group suggests that they simply did not have a good enough memory for the stimulus elements to differentiate between words composed of old and new syllables.

Although it is tempting to consider our M− group as analogous to the amnesic patient groups in other memory conjunction error studies, we feel it is inappropriate to make direct comparisons between our results and the data of Kroll et al. (1996) and Reinitz et al. (1996), because our participants' performance was in the normal range and was only slightly inferior to young participants, whereas their participants were severely impaired. Thus, differences between the current study and prior studies with varied patient groups might be accounted for in two ways. First, it is possible that the relatively small number of trials used in prior studies obscured some effects while exaggerating others. Second, the heterogeneity and severity of deficit of the groups in the various studies prohibits generalising from these groups to healthy elderly individuals. The current study takes the heterogeneity of older adults into account, and provides sufficient numbers of trials to support the conclusion that errors induced by similarity between studied and new items are most likely to be due to monitoring failures of the frontal lobes under circumstances when processing fluency creates confusion between truly old words and recombined syllables.

SUMMARY

In Experiment 1, both behavioural and ERP data indicated that so-called conjunction errors can best be explained by processing fluency during retrieval. The probability of false alarms followed the gradient of the similarity with studied words (conjunction lures > syllable lures > new words), indicating that the elevated false alarm rate to syllable lures cannot easily be attributed to faulty binding. Different classes of false alarms were accompanied by much the same brain activity, regardless of whether the item was a recombination of studied material or not. Hits and false alarms elicited different brain activity, arguing against the notion that conjunction errors are formed at encoding (or during a brief consolidation period) and later retrieved like genuine memories. Thus, although it may be possible under some circumstances to affect conjunction lure false alarm rates through an encoding manipulation, our current data point to retrieval as the time when these errors are actually generated. Experiment 1 further showed that strong memory traces lead to high confidence ratings, and that the late positive component of the ERP reflected confidence in veridical retrieval, but not false confidence when making a recognition error.

Experiment 2 indicated that although there are age differences in recognition accuracy, older adults are not disproportionately likely to recognise conjunction lures falsely. It also indicated that the neuropsychological measures tapping prefrontal cortex are most important in predicting false alarm rates. Taken together, the two experiments suggest that false alarms to conjunction lures are not similar to true recollections, but are products of faulty monitoring processes at retrieval: Items that seem familiar based on their features may generate automatic "yes" responses when there are no accurate recollections to oppose these errors.

REFERENCES

Albert, M.S. (1988). General issues in geriatric neuropsychology. In M.S. Albert & M.B. Moss (Eds.), - *Geriatric neuropsychology* (pp. 7–10). New York: Guilford Press.

Albert, M.S., Duffy, F.H., & Naeser, M. (1987). Nonlinear changes in cognition with age and their neuropsychological correlates. *Canadian Journal of Psychology, 41,* 141–157.

Allan, K., & Rugg, M.D. (1997). An event-related potential study of explicit memory on tests of cued recall and recognition. *Neuropsychologia, 35,*(4), 387–397.

Bartlett, F.C. (1932). *Remembering.* Cambridge, MA: Cambridge University Press.

Benson, D.F., Djenderedjian, A., Miller, B.L., Pachana, N.A., Chang, L., Itti, L., & Mena, I. (1996). Neural basis of confabulation. *Neurology, 46,* 1238–1243.

Bentin, S., & McCarthy, G. (1994). The effects of immediate stimulus repetition on reaction time and event-related potentials in tasks of different complexity. *Journal of Experimental Psychology: Learning, Memory and Cognition, 20* (1), 130–149.

Bentin, S., & Peled, B.S. (1990). The contribution of task-related factors to ERP repetition effects at short and long lags. *Memory and Cognition, 18,* 359–366.

Benton, A.L., & Hamsher, K. de S. (1976). *Multilingual Aphasia Examination manual.* Iowa City: University of Iowa.

Berman, S., Friedman, D., & Cramer, M. (1991). ERPs during continuous recognition memory for words and pictures. *Bulletin of the Psychonomic Society, 29,* 113–116.

Besson, M., & Kutas, M. (1993). The many facets of repetition: A cued recall and event related potential analysis of repeating words in same versus different sentence contexts. *Journal of Experimental Psychology: Learning, Memory and Cognition, 19,* 1115–1133.

Besson, M., Kutas, M., & Van Petten, C. (1992). An event-related potential analysis of semantic congruity and repetition effects in sentences. *Journal of Cognitive Neuroscience, 4,* 132–149.

Busey, T.A., Tunnicliff, L., Loftus, G.R., & Loftus, E.F. (1998). *Accounts of the confidence-accuracy relation in recognition memory.* Manuscript submitted for publication.

Chao, L.L., & Knight, R.T. (1997). Age-related prefrontal alterations during auditory memory. *Neurobiology of Aging, 18,* (1), 87–95.

Chao, L.L., Nielsen-Bohlman, L., & Knight, R.T. (1995). Auditory event-related potentials dissociate early and late memory processes. *Electroencephalograpy and Clinical Neurophysiology, 96,* 157–168.

Clark, S.E. (1997). A familiarity-based account of confidence-accuracy inversions in recognition memory. *Journal of Experimental Psychology: Learning, Memory, and Cognition, 23,* 232–238.

Coffey, C.E., Wilkinson, W.E., Parashos, I.A., Soady, S.A., Sullivan, R.J., Patterson, L.J., Figiel, G.S., Webb, M.C., Spritzer, C.E., & Djang, W.T. (1992). Quantitative cerebral anatomy of the aging human brain. *Neurology, 42,* 527–536.

Crak F.I.M., & Jennings, L.M. (1992). Human memory. In F.I.M. Craik & T.M. Salthouse (Eds.), *Handbook of aging and cognition* (pp. 51–1100). Hillsdale, NJ: Lawrence Erlbaum Associates Inc.

Craile, F.I.M., Morris, L.W., Morris, R.G., & Loewen, E.R. (1990). Relations between source amnesia and frontal lobe functioning in older adults. *Psychology and Aging, 5,* 148–151.

Curran, T., Schacter, D.L., Norman, K.A., & Galluccio, L. (1997). False recognition after a right frontal lobe infarction: Memory for general and specific information. *Neuropsychologia, 35,* (7), 1035–1049.

Deese, J. (1959). On the prediction of occurrence of particular verbal intrusions in immediate recall. *Journal of Experimental Psychology, 58,* 17–22.

Delbecq-Derousné, L, Beauvois, M.F., & Shallice, T. (1990). Preserved recall vs. impaired recognition: A case study. *Brain, 113,* 1045–1074.

Delis, D.C., Kramer, L., Kaplan, E., & Ober, B.A. (1987). *The California Verbal Learning Test.* San Antonio, TX: Psychological Corporation.

Dorfinan, J. (1994). Sublexical components in implicit memory for novel words. *Journal of Experimental Psychology, 20* (5), 1108–1125.

Double, K.L., Halliday, G.M., Krill, J.J., Harasty, J.A., Cullen, K., Brooks, W.S., Creasey, H., & Broe,

G.A. (1996).Topography of brain atrophy during normal aging and Alzheimer's disease. *Neurobiology of Aging, 17,* 513–521.

Duzel, E., Yonelinas, A.P., Mangun, G.R., Heinze, H.-J., & Tulving, E. (1997). Event related brain potential correlates of two states of conscious awareness in memory. *Proceedings of the National Academy of Sciences, 94,* 5973–5978.

Eichenbaum, K. (1994). The hippocampal system and declarative memory in humans and animals: Experimental analysis and historical origins. In D.L. Schacter & E. Tulving (Eds.), *Memory systems 1994* (pp. 147–201). Cambridge, MA: MIT Press.

Eichenbaum, H., & Bunsey, M. (1995). On the binding of associations in memory: Clues from studies on the role of the hippocampal region in paired-associate learning. *Current Directions in Psychological Science, 4,* 19–23.

Fabiani, M., & Donchin, E. (1995). Encoding processes and memory organization: A model of the von Restorff effect. *Journal of Experimental Psychology: Learning, Memory and Cognition, 21,* 224–240.

Fabiani, M., Karis, D., & Donchin, E. (1986). P300 and recall in an incidental memory paradigm. *Psychophysiology, 23,* 298–308.

Fischer, R.S., Alexander, M.P., D'Esposito, M.D., & Otto, R. (1995). Neuropsychological and neuroanatomical correlates of confabulation. *Journal of Clinical and Experimental Neuropsychology, 17,* 20–28.

Flicker, C., Ferris, S.H., Crook, T., & Bartus, R.T. (1989). Age differences in the vulnerability of facial recognition memory to proactive interference. *Experimental Aging Research, 15* (3–4), 189–194.

Francis, W.N., & Kuçera, H. (1982). *Frequency analysis of English usage: Lexicon and grammar.* Boston, MA: Houghton Mifflin.

Fulton, A., & Bartlett, J.C. (1991). Young and old faces in young and old heads: The factor of age in face recognition. *Psychology and Aging, 6* (4), 623–630.

Gardiner, J.M., & Java, R.I. (1990). Recollective experience in word and nonword recognition. *Memory and Cognition, 18,* 23–20.

Glisky, E.L., Polster, M.R., & Routhicaux, B.C. (1995). Double dissociation between item and source memory. *Neuropsychology, 9* (2), 229–235.

Gunter, T.C., Jackson, J.L., & Mulder, G. (1992). An electrophysiological study of semantic processing in young and middle-aged academics. *Psychophysiology, 29,* 38–54.

Hart, R.P., Kwentus, J.A., Wade, J.B., & Taylor, R. (1988). Modified Wisconsin Card Sorting test in elderly normal, depressed and demented patients. *Clinical Neuropsychologist, 2,* 49–56.

Haug, H. (1985). Are neurons of the human cerebral cortex really lost during aging? A morphometric examination. In J. Traber & W.H. Gispen (Eds.), *Senile dementia of the Alzheimer type.* Berlin: Springer.

Henkel, L.A., Johnson, M.K., & De Leonardis, D.M. (1998). Aging and source monitoring: Cognitive processes and neuropsychological correlates. *Journal of Experimental Psychology, 127* (3), 251–268.

Hillyard, S.A., Squires, K.C., Bauer, J.W., & Lindsay, P.H. (1971). Evoked potential correlates of auditory signal detection. *Science, 172,* 1357–1360.

Isingrini, M., Fontaine, R., Taconnat, L., & Duportal, A. (1995). Aging and encoding in memory—False alarms and decision criteria in a word-pair recognition task. *International Journal of Aging and Human Development, 41* (1), 79–88.

Jacoby, L.L. (1991). A process dissociation framework: Separating automatic from intentional use of memory. *Journal of Memory and Language, 30,* 513–541.

Janowsky, J.S., Shimamura, A.R., & Squire, L.K. (1989). Source memory impairments in patients with frontal lobe lesions. *Neuropsychologia, 27,* 1043–1056.

Jasper, H.H. (1958). The ten-twenty electrode system of the International Federation. *Electroencephalography and Clinical Neurophysiology, 10,* 371–375.

Jha, A.P., Kroll, N.E.A., Baynes, K., & Gazzaniga, M.S. (1997). Memory encoding following complete callosotomy. *Journal of Cognitive Neuroscience, 9* (1), 143–159.

Johnson, M.K., Hashtroudi, S., & Lindsay, S.D. (1993). Source monitoring. *Psychological Bulletin, 114,* 3–28.

Johnson, M.K., Nolde, S.F., Mather, M., Kounios, J, Schacter, D.L., & Curran, T. (1997). The similarity of brain activity associated with true and false recognition depends on test format. *Psychological Science, 8* (3), 250–257.

Johnson, M.K., & Raye, C.L. (in press). Cognitive brain mechanisms of false memories and beliefs. In D.L. Schacter & E. Scarry (Eds.), *Memory, brain, and belief.* Cambridge, MA: Harvard University Press.

Kapur, N., & Coughlan, A.K. (1980). Confabulation and frontal lobe dysfunction. *Journal of Neurology, Neurosurgery and Psychiatry, 43,* 461-463.

Kapur, S., Craik, F.I.M., Jones, C., Brown, G.M., Houle, S., & Tulving, E. (1995). Functional role of prefrontal cortex in memory retrieval: A PET study. *Neuroreport, 6,* 1880–1884.

Karis, D., Fabiani, M., & Donchin, E. (1984). "P300" and memory: Individual differences in the von Restorff effect. *Cognitive Psychology, 16,* 177–216.

Kroll, N.E.A., Knight, R.T., Metcalfe, L., Wolf, E.S., & Tulving, E. (1996). Cohesion failure as a source of memory illusions. *Journal of Memory and Language, 35,* 176–196.

Kutas, M., & Van Petten, C. (1994). Psycholinguistics electrified: Event-related brain potential investigations. In M. Gernsbacher (Ed.), *Handbook of Psycholinguistics* (pp. 83–143). New York: Academic Press.

Light, L.L. (1991). Memory and ageing: Four hypotheses in search of data. *Annual Review of Psychology, 42,* 333–376.

Loftus, E.F., Miller, D.G., & Burns, H.J. (1978). Semantic integration of verbal information into visual memory. *Journal of Experimental Psychology, 4,* 19–31.

Mantyla, T., & Backman, L. (1992). Aging and memory for expected and unexpected objects in real-world settings. *Journal of Experimental Psychology: Learning, Memory, and Cognition, 18,* 1298–1309.

Mark, R.E., & Rugg, M.D. (1998). Age effects on brain activity associated with episodic memory retrieval: An electrophysiological study. *Brain, 121,* 868–873.

Martin, A.J., Friston, K.J., Colebatch, J.G., & Frackowiak, R.S.J. (1991). Decreases in regional cerebral blood flow with normal aging. *Journal of Cerebral Blood Flow and Metabolism, 11,* 684–689.

Moscovitch, M. (1994). Memory and working with memory: Evaluation of a component process model and comparisons with other models. In D.L. Schacter & E. Tulving (Eds.), *Memory systems 1994* (pp. 269–310). Cambridge MA: MIT Press.

Moscovitch, M. (1995). Confabulation. In D.L. Schacter (Ed.), *Memory distortion: How minds, brains and societies reconstruct the past* (pp. 227–251). Cambridge, MA: Harvard University Press.

Moscovitch, M., & Winocur, G. (1995). Frontal lobes, memory and ageing. In J. Grafman, K.J. Holyoak, & F. Boller (Eds.), *Structure and functions of human prefrontal cortex* (pp. 119–150). New York: New York Academy of Sciences.

Murdock, B.B., & Dufty, P.O. (1972). theory and recognition memory. *Journal of Experimental Psychology, 94,* 284–290.

Murphy, D.G.M., DeCarli, C., McIntosh, A.R., Daly, E., Mentis, M.L., Pictrini, P., Szczepanik, J., Schapiro, M.B., Grady, C.L., Horwitz, B., & Rapoport, S.I. (1996). Sex differences in human brain morphometry and metabolism—an in vivo quantitative magnetic resonance and position emission tomography study on the effect of aging. *Archives of General Psychiatry, 53,* 585–594.

Neville, H.J., Kutas, M., Chesney, G., & Schmidt, A. (1986). Event-related brain potentials during the initial encoding and subsequent recognition memory of congruous and incongruous words. *Journal of Memory and Language, 25,* 75–92.

Norman, K.A., & Schacter, D.L. (1997). False recognition in younger and older adults - Exploring the characteristics of illusory memories. *Memory Cognition, 25* (6), 838–848.

Paller, K A., & Gross, M. (1998). Brain potentials associated with perceptual priming versus explicit remembering during the repetition of visual word-form. *Neuropsychologia, 36,* 559–571.

Paller, K.A., & Kutas, M. (1992). Brain potentials during memory retrieval provide neurophysiological support for the distinction between conscious recollection and priming. *Journal of Cognitive Neuroscience, 4,* 375–391.

Paller, K.A., Kutas, M., & Mayes, A.R. (1987). Neural correlates of encoding in an incidental learning paradigm. *Electroencephalography and Clinical Neurophysiology, 67,* 360–371.

Paller, K.A., Kutas, M., & McIsaac, H.K. (1998). An electrophysiological measure of priming of visual word-form. *Consciousness and Cognition, 7,* 54–66.

Parkin, A.L., Bindschaedler, C., Harsent, L., & Metzler, C. (1996). Pathological false alarm rates following damage to left prefrontal cortex. *Brain and Cognition, 32* (1), 14–27.

Parkin, A.L., & Lawrence, A. (1994). A dissociation in the relation between memory tasks and frontal lobe tests in the normal elderly. *Neuropsychologia, 32,* 1523–1532.

Paul, D.D., & Sutton, S. (1972). Evoked potential correlates of response criterion in auditory signal detection. *Science, 177,* 362–364.

Rapcsak, S.Z., Kaszniak, A.W., Reminger, S.L., Glisky, M.L., Glisky, E.L., & Comer, J.F. (1998). Dissociation between verbal and autonomic measures of memory following frontal lobe damage. *Neurology, 50,* 1259–1265.

Rapcsak, S.Z., Polster, M.R., Comer, LS., & Rubens, A.B. (1994). False recognition and misidentification of faces following right hemisphere damage. *Cortex, 30,* 565–583.

Raz, N., Torres, I.J., Spencer, W.D., & Acker, J.D. (1993). Pathoclysis in aging human cerebral cortex: Evidence from in vivo MR1 morphometry. *Psychobiology, 21,* 151–160.

Regan, D. (1989). *Human-brain electrophysiology.* New York: Elsevier.

Reinitz, M.T., & Demb, J. (1994). Implicit and explicit memory for compound words. *Memory and Cognition, 22* (6), 687–694.

Reinitz, M.T., Lammers, W.J., & Cochran, B.P. (1992). Memory-conjunction errors: Miscombination of stored stimulus features can produce illusions of memory. *Memory and Cognition, 20* (1), 1–11.

Reinitz, M.T., Morrissey, L., & Demb, J. (1994). Role of attention in face encoding. *Journal of Experimental Psychology: Learning, Memory, and Cognition, 20,* 161–168.

Reinitz, M.T., Verfaellie, M., & Milberg, W.P. (1996). Memory conjunction errors in normal and amnesic subjects. *Journal of Memory and Language, 35,* 286–299.

Roder, B.J., Faneuf, S., Burch, W., & Connors, M. (1996). *Memory for conjoined-concepts.* Poster presentation, Psychonomic Society Annual Meeting.

Roediger, H.L., III, & McDermott, K.B. (1995). Creating false memories: Remembering words not presented in lists. *Journal of Experimental Psychology: Learning, Memory, and Cognition, 21,* 803–814.

Rudy, L.W., & Sutherland, R.J. (1994). The memory-coherence problem, configural associations, and the hippocampal system. In D.L. Schacter & E. Tulving (Eds.), *Memory systems 1994* (pp. 19-146). Cambridge, MA: MIT Press.

Rugg, M.D., & Doyle, M.C. (1992). Event-related potentials and recognition memory for low- and high-frequency words. *Journal of Cognitive Neuroscience, 4,* 69–79.

Rugg, M.D., & Doyle, M.C. (1994). Event-related potentials and stimulus repetition in direct and indirect tests of memory. In H.J. Heinze, T.F. Munte, & G.R. Mangun (Eds.), *Cognitive electrophysiology* (pp. 124–138). Boston, MA: Birkhauser.

Sanquist, T.F., Rohrbaugh, J.W., Syndulko, K., & Lindsley, D.B. (1980). Electrocortical signs of levels of processing: Perceptual analysis and recognition memory. *Psychophysiology, 17,* 568-576.

Schacter, D.L., Buckner, R.L., Koutstaal, W., Dale, A., & Rosen, B.R. (1997). Late onset prefrontal activity during true and false recognition: An event-related fMRI study. *Neuroimage, 6,* 259–269.

Schacter, D.L., Curran, T., Galluccio, L., Milberg, W.P., & Bates, LF. (1996). False recognition and the right frontal lobe: A case study. *Neuropsychologia, 34* (8), 793–808.

Schacter, D.L., Harbluk, J.L., & McLachlan, D.R. (1984). Retrieval without recollection: An experimental analysis of source amnesia. *Journal of Verbal Learning and Behavior, 23,* 593–611.

Schacter, D.L., Norman, K.A., & Koutstaal, W. (1998). The cognitive neuroscience of constructive memory. *Annual Review of Psychology, 49,* 289–318.

Schacter, D.L., Reiman, E.M., Curran, T., Yun, L.S., Bandy, D., McDermott, K.B., & Roediger, H.L. III (1996). Neuroanatomical correlates of veridical and illusory recognition memory: Evidence from positron emission tomography. *Neuron, 17,* 267–274.

Seamon, J.G., Luo, C.R., & Gallo, D.A. (1998). Creating false memories of words with or without recognition of list items. Evidence for nonconscious processes. *Psychological Science, 9,* 20–26.

Senkfor, A.J., & Van Petten, C. (1998). Who said what? An event-related potential investigation of source and item memory. *Journal of Experimental Psychology: Learning, Memory, and Cognition, 24,* 1005–1025.

Smith, M.E. (1993). Neurophysiological manifestations of recollective experience during recognition memory judgements. *Journal of Cognitive Neuroscience, 5,* 1–13.

Smith, M.E., & Guster, K. (1993). Decomposition of recognition memory event-related potentials yields target, repetition, and retrieval effects. *Electroencephalography and Clinical Neurophysiology, 86,* 335-343.

Swick, D., & Knight, R.T. (1997). Event-related potentials differentiate the effects of aging on word and nonword repetition in explicit and implicit memory tasks. *Journal of Experimental Psychology: Learning, Memory, and Cognition, 23,* 123–142.

Swick, D., & Knight, R.T. (in press). Contributions of prefrontal cortex to recognition memory: Electrophysiological and behavioral evidence. *Neuropsychology.*

Terry, R.D., DeTheresa, R., & Hansen, L.A. (1987). Neocortical cell counts in normal human adult aging. *Annals of Neurology, 21,* 530–539.

Troncoso, L.C., Martin, L.J., Dalforno, G., & Kawas, C.H. (1996). Neuropathology in controls and demented subjects from the Baltimore longitudinal study of aging. *Neurobiology of Aging, 17,* 365–371.

Trott, C.T., Friedman, D., Ritter, W., & Fabiani, M. (1997). Item and source memory: Differential age effects revealed by event-related potentials. *Neuroreport, 8,* 3373–3378.

Tulving, E., Kapur, S., Markowitsch, H.J., Craik, F.I.M., Habib, R., & Houle, S. (1994). Neuroanatomical correlates of retrieval in episodic memory: Auditory sentence recognition. *Proceedings of the National Academy of Science, 91,* 2012–2015.

Tulving, E., Markowitsch, H.J., Craik, F.I.M., Habib, R., & Houle, S. (1996). Novelty and familiarity activations in PET studies of memory encoding and retrieval. *Cerebral Cortex, 6,* 71–79.

Tun, P.A., Wingfield, A., Rosen, M.J., & Blanchard, L. (1998). Response latencies for false memories: Gist-based processes in normal aging. *Psychology and Aging, 13* (2), 230–241.

Underwood, B.J., Kapelak, S.M., & Malmi, R.A. (1976). of discrete verbal units in recognition memory. *Journal of Experimental Psychology: Human Learning and Memory, 2,* 293–300.

Underwood, B.J., & Zimmerman, J. (1973). The syllable as a source of error in multisyllable word recognition. *Journal of Verbal Learning and Verbal Behavior, 12,* 338–344.

Van Petten, C., & Kutas, M. (1988). The use of event-related potentials in the study of brain asymmetries. *International Journal of Neuroscience, 39,* 91–99.

Van Petten, C., & Senkfor, A.J. (1996). Memory for words and novel visual patterns: Repetition, recognition, and encoding effects in the event-related brain potential. *Psychophysiology, 33,* 491–508.

Wechsler, D. (1981). *Wechsler Adult Intelligence Scale—Revised manual.* New York: Psychological Corporation.

Wechsler, D. (1987). *Wechsler Memory Scale—Revised manual.* New York: Psychological Corporation.

Welford, A.T. (1993). The gerontological balance sheet. In J. Cerella, J. Rybash, W. Hoyer, & M.L. Commons (Eds.), *Adult information processing: Limits on loss* (pp. 3–10). New York: Academic Press.

Wheeler, M.A., Stuss, D.T., & Tulving, E. (1995). Frontal lobe damage produces episodic memory impairment. *Journal of the International Neuropsychologica Society, 1,* 525–536.

Wilding, E.L., & Rugg, M.D. (1996). An event-related potential study of recognition memory with and without retrieval of source. *Brain, 119,* 889–905.

COGNITIVE NEUROPSYCHOLOGY, 1999, 16 (3/4/5), 489–508

False Memories and Source Monitoring

Rahul M. Dodhia and Janet Metcalfe
Columbia University, New York, USA

This article investigates the relation between misremembering and source judgments in both the misleading information paradigm and the false memory paradigm. A computational model, CHARM (Composite Holographic Associative Recall Model), is used to simulate source monitoring in both paradigms. Despite the fact that CHARM stores memories in a composite memory trace, it is shown that the model can account for source judgements, and can explain the discrepancy between the source judgement and the recognition data in the misleading information paradigm. It also can account for the basic phenomena of the false memory paradigm, wherein thematically related items induce a memory for a nonpresented but prototypical critical item. In two experiments linking these two research lines, we presented the critical item in a different list from that used to induce the false memory effect. Although the model predicted that the presentation of the critical item should increase the false memory effect, its presentation inhibited false memories instead—but only with particular word lists and in certain treatment combinations. It seems likely that the presence of the critical item in an alternate list allowed people to use an exclusionary rule to inhibit the false memories. Such a rule would be straightforward to implement in CHARM, and could allow the model to account for this false memory suppression effect.

INTRODUCTION

Although misremembering may be produced in a number of different ways, there are two basic paradigms that have enjoyed extensive experimental investigation, and which are considered here. The first is the classic *misleading information paradigm*, in which misinformation is actually presented to the person, and it is this presented information that is the cause of the person's memory errors. The second is the *false memory paradigm*, in which the misremembered information is not presented. Instead, the false memories result from inferences or constructions that the person creates internally, and then later mistakes for events that happened externally. In this article, we will address both of these misremembering paradigms. It has been shown, in the classic misleading information paradigm, that if people are asked to make judgements concerning the origin or source (Johnson, Hashtroudi, & Lindsay, 1993) of the would-be misleading information they are sometimes able to sharpen their focus, and discount the misleading information by attributing it to its correct source. Thus, in at least one of these paradigms, source judgements can be used to enhance people's memory, and eliminate false information (Lindsay & Johnson, 1989; Zaragoza & Koshmider, 1989). We investigate whether such judgements might also be efficacious in the other paradigm.

Requests for reprints should be addressed to Janet Metcalfe, Department of Psychology, 401 Schermerhorn Hall, Columbia University, New York, 10027, USA (E-mail: metcalfe@paradox.psych.columbia.edu).

This research was supported by National Institute of Mental Health Grant MH 48066 to Janet Metcalfe. We thank Lisa Schwartz for her help with Experiment 2. We also thank Walter Mischel, Kenneth A. Norman, Henry L. Roediger III, and Daniel L. Schacter for their helpful comments on an earlier version of the manuscript.

In the misleading information paradigm (of which there are a number of variants) an incident, such as a crime, is witnessed and then later, if he or she is in the experimental condition, the person is given some misleading information about some detail in the incident. For example, if the person originally saw a car go through a red light, it might later be suggested that the vehicle had been a van. When given a two-alternative forced choice test including the correct object and the misleading suggestion, people who received the misleading information performed worse than did people who received no misleading information (Loftus, 1979). The CHARM model has been used, in the past, to model situations such as this (Metcalfe, 1990). It explained these, and related, findings in terms of the implications of retrieving a superimposed representation that contains both the original event (the car) superimposed on the misleading suggestion (the van). The effect is analogous to a TV screen showing simultaneously two different programmes, or to a photograph that has been double-exposed. When those two exact alternatives are retrieved and contrasted in this superimposed manner, at the time of test, the person has difficulty distinguishing them, and so performance suffers—as has been shown empirically.

A number of researchers have criticised and modified the original version of the misleading information paradigm. When the lures given at the time of test are not identical to the misleading item that was first suggested, people who received the misleading suggestion usually performed at about the same level as did control participants (e.g. McCloskey & Zaragoza, 1985; cf. Payne, Toglia, & Anastasi, 1994). The CHARM model—employing a composite memory trace—can predict these data (Metcalfe, 1990). Only the misleading item is superimposed on the correct item at time of retrieval, so other items tend not to interfere with the correct item (unless, of course, they are sufficiently similar to the original item, the suggested item, or both, so that confusion occurs because of a discriminability problem). There are a number of other experimental variants on this basic misleading information paradigm (see, for example, Belli, 1989; Ceci, Ross, & Toglia, 1987; Chandler, 1989; Christiaansen & Ochalek, 1983; Kroll & Timourian, 1986; Loftus & Hoffman, 1989; Tversky & Tuchin, 1989) to which the CHARM model has been applied with some success. The composite retrieval characteristic of the model has allowed it to account for all of the major recognition and recall findings reported in this paradigm, except for one.

The only major experimental finding within the classic misleading information paradigm to which the model has not been applied, as pointed out by Lindsay (1991), is source monitoring. Rather than being tested for only for simple recognition or recall, in the source monitoring paradigm, people are asked to remember and report the source of the memory probe item. This paradigm is of especial interest for three reasons. First, judgements of source are a key component to people's episodic memory. Second, these judgements allow people to clarify and improve their memory performance, and greatly offset their susceptibility to misleading information (Lindsay & Johnson, 1989). The third reason for our interest is that the manner in which the CHARM model retrieves a representation with information from multiple sources superimposed, would seem, at first blush, to disallow it from making source judgements. Much of the explanatory power of the CHARM model stems from the construct of a composite trace—including the basic explanation for the misleading information effect itself. The challenge to CHARM, then, is that it would seem that a model that uses a composite trace as a core construct (as opposed, say, to the more traditional separate-trace models) might seem intuitively to be unable to distinguish the sources. In the first section of this article, we will show, though, that CHARM can handle the basic source-monitoring results without difficulty.

In the second major section of this article we turn to the other misremembering paradigm. Roediger and McDermott (1995, and see Deese, 1959) have investigated a paradigm for creating false memories, in which the false memories are not explicitly implanted by an outside source, as in the classic paradigm; instead, the participant appears to create them by some internal process. Participants are presented with a list of semantic associates of a critical item. They do not study the critical item itself but, nevertheless, exhibit false memory for it at test. For example, a person might be presented with a list of semantically associated words such as *hill, valley, climb,* etc., and then be tested on a critical item such as *mountain.* This paradigm, which has been of great interest recently, will be described in greater detail later in the paper.

In the classic misleading information paradigm people can use source information to differentiate suggested from true memories about a particular scene (Lindsay & Johnson, 1989; Zaragoza & Koshmider, 1989). We conjectured that source judgements might also be useful in the false memory paradigm. To investigate this possibility, our first step was to model the effect of source-monitoring in the misleading information paradigm within the CHARM (composite, holographic, associative, recall, and recognition memory) model (Metcalfe Eich, 1982, 1985; Metcalfe, 1990, 1991a,b, 1993a,b, 1997; Metcalfe, Cottrell, & Mencl, 1992). We then showed that this simple model is able to account for the basic phenomena within the false memory paradigm. Finally, we used CHARM's source monitoring predictions to investigate the impact of the presence of source information in the false memory paradigm.

MODELLING SOURCE JUDGEMENTS WITH *CHARM* IN THE MISLEADING INFORMATION PARADIGM

Lindsay and Johnson (1989) conducted an experiment in the misleading information tradition, in which they showed that memory could be ameliorated by asking participants for source judgments. In their experiment, the participants viewed an initial event—a picture taken from a magazine. They then read a text that was a description of the picture but which included some misleading information (as well as other information). Then participants were either asked to make old/new recognition judgements about whether each of the probe items was in the original picture they had seen (in a manner similar to that used in the classic paradigm), or they were given a source judgement task. In the latter task, they were asked to say whether a given item was seen only in the picture, was only in the text, was in both the picture and the text, or was entirely new. To equate between the recognition judgement and the source judgement conditions, the probability of saying that an item was seen in the picture (as given directly in the recognition judgement case) was taken, in the source judgement condition, to be the sum of the probabilities of saying that it was in the picture only and that it was in both.

Technically the two tests were asking the same question: Was the probe in the picture? Nevertheless, the results were quite different. Misled participants given the recognition test were much more likely to false alarm to the misleading items that were presented only in the text than were their matched controls who were given no misleading suggestions. In the source judgement condition, though, misled participants were perfectly well able to say that these items were only in the text, and they did not exhibit a tendency to claim that they had been in the picture. These results, of course, are of practical interest. But they raise an interesting theoretical question as well: Can a model that produces a superimposed retrieved item account for this discriminative ability? And if it can, how does it do it?

In this section we will first demonstrate that there are conditions, mapping onto the experimental situation in a straightforward manner, that allow the CHARM model to produce both the recognition results and the source monitoring results. Not surprisingly, the model is unable to produce both patterns of data—those for recognition and for source judgement—if it does exactly the same thing. So examination of exactly how the model produced the two different sets of data is of interest.

Source Simulations of CHARM

Items are represented in CHARM as vectors, and the elements of these vectors correspond to the features of the items. The elements are sampled from a standard normal distribution and the vectors are usually normalised to make mathematical analysis easier. The vectors created in this way are independent of each other, so the similarity of one random vector to another, as measured by their dot product, is 0. The similarity of one vector to another can be manipulated, however, by setting their dot product to some fraction greater than 0. Items are associated by the operation of convolution, and the resulting vector is superimposed onto an existing trace, which is initialised to be a noisy random vector. Items can be retrieved from the trace by correlating it with a probe vector. The resulting vector is a combination of all the items with which the probe had been associated. This retrieved vector is then sent off to a decision routine that distinguishes among yes/no recognition, forced-choice recognition, recall, and so on, as dictated by the constraints of the situation. In yes/no recognition, the retrieved vector is matched to the probe itself. If the dot product is greater than a preset criterion, the probe is considered as having been recognised. In multiple-choice recognition, the retrieved item is matched to each of the presented alternatives, and the one that matches best is given as the selection chosen, as long as it exceeds a criterion (if, in the experiment, the option to not answer is given). In recall, the retrieved vector is matched to each of the vectors in the lexicon. The vector that is recalled is the vector that provides the largest dot product with the retrieved vector, if the dot product is above a preset criterion.

In our first set of simulations, every item was assumed to have source information linked to it, via the associative operation of convolution. Source information consists of the perceptual and other sensory details that are the setting in which an event occurs. For modelling purposes, **Source**, **S**, is abstracted into "features" just as content information is. For the purposes of demonstrating the detailed predictions of the model, context or source, and content will be represented in the following way: If someone sees a picture of a car, this will be considered to be encoded in the trace **Trace**, as:

$$\mathbf{Trace} = \mathbf{Car}*\mathbf{Car} + \mathbf{Car}*\mathbf{Source}_{\text{Picture}},$$

where **Car** is a vector representing the mental representation of the car, $\mathbf{Source}_{\text{Picture}}$ is a vector giving the mental representation of the picture source, and "$*$" is the operation for convolution. When the cue **Car** is given, retrieval occurs by correlating (#) the **Trace** with **Car**. In general, the result of retrieval by any cue, **Q**, which is correlated with an association between any two vectors such as **X**$*$**Y**, is that **Y** is retrieved to the extent that **Q** is similar to **X**, and **X** is retrieved to the extent that **Q** is similar to **Y**, and the two components are added to one another. This occurs for all associations in the composite memory trace (and all retrieved components are added together). Thus, in the present case, the result of correlating the cue **Car** with the **Trace** is a vector which contains both **Car** and $\mathbf{Source}_{\text{Picture}}$, specifically:

$$\begin{aligned}\mathbf{Car}\#\mathbf{Trace} &= \mathbf{Car}\#[(\mathbf{Car}*\mathbf{Car}) + (\mathbf{Car}*\mathbf{Source}_{\text{Picture}}] \\ &= 2\mathbf{Car} + \mathbf{Source}_{\text{Picture}} \qquad (1)\end{aligned}$$

Since the source of the car memory is returned in the retrieved vector, this vector can be used to make a source judgment. The source of an item is judged to be retrieved if the dot product of the source vector in question and the retrieved vector is above a set criterion.

In Lindsay and Johnson's (1989) experiments the first factor was type of study group—Control or Misled. The second factor was type of test—Recognition or Source Judgement. In phase 1, both groups looked at a slide containing various items, thus encoding them in a pictorial context. In phase 2, both groups read a narrative describing the slide, encoding items in a textual context. The Control group read a narrative that was completely faithful to the slide, but the Misled group read a narrative that had additional information in it, items that had not appeared in the slide. In phase 3, participants from both groups received either a yes/no recognition test or a source judgement test. The test items consisted of items that had appeared only in the slide (Picture Only), items that had appeared in both the slide and the narrative (Picture and Text), items that had appeared in the misleading narrative only (Text Only) and items that had neither appeared in the slide nor the narrative (New).

Method

To model this situation, a lexicon of 10 vectors of 63 elements each was created. Vectors 1 and 2 were designated W and were associated with the picture source S_p only. Vectors 3 and 4 were designated X, and were associated with both the picture source S_p and the text source S_t, vectors 5 and 6 were designated to be Y and were associated with the text source S_t only, vectors 7 and 8 were designated Z and reserved to be new. Two additional items were added into the composite trace as noise, but were not tested. Four sets of this lexicon were created, each with different random vectors. To avoid repetition and enhance clarity, the traces below are shown with only one set of vectors. In the simulation all four sets were used. Two other vectors were also created—they were source vectors, specifically Picture Source S_p and Text Source S_t. These were simply set up as independent random vectors.

Two traces were constructed, one for each of the study groups. The Control trace (T_c) was constructed as follows:

$$T_c = W*W + W*S_p + X*X + X*S_p + X*X + X*S_t + \text{noise}$$

The Misled trace (T_m) was constructed as follows:

$$T_m = W*W + W*S_p + X*X + X*S_p + X*X + X*S_t + Y*Y + Y*S_t + \text{noise}$$

The test items W, X, Y, and Z were each correlated with the traces. An item was classified as having been recognised if its similarity (measured by a dot product) to the vector it retrieved from the trace was above a criterion of 1.2. To enact the source judgement the probe was correlated with the trace and the vector that was retrieved was matched with the picture context and with the text context. If the dot product of either match was above 0.8, then the model recognised the probe as having occurred in the corresponding context. If both matches were above criterion, then the probe was recognised as having appeared twice, once in each context. If neither match was above criterion, then the probe was assumed to be new. The simulation was replicated 500 times, with different random vectors each time.

Results and Discussion

As can be seen from Fig. 1, the model, like people, produced a high rate of false "attribution to picture," in the recognition task only, to those items that were presented in the text only and were not given in the picture. In the source judgements task, however, this error was attenuated, both in people's judgements and in the model.

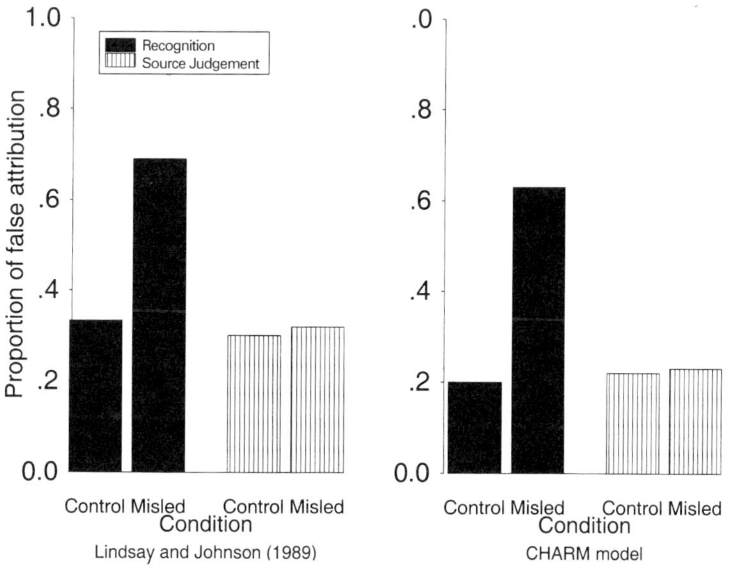

Fig. 1. *A comparison between Lindsay and Johnson (1989) and CHARM of the mean proportion of false attribution to "Picture" of "Text Only" items.*

The reason the model did this was that the recognition decision was based on matching the item retrieved to the probe only (as has been the method of recognition used in many past simulations with CHARM, e.g. Metcalfe, 1991a), and it did not consider the source. When only the recognition of the probe itself is considered, and the source is disregarded, a high false alarm rate to items presented in the non/pictorial context arises. In contrast, under the source judgement instructions, the model was specified to match the retrieved item to both the picture and the text source, and to make attribution decisions based on the extent of those matches. If the retrieved vector failed to match the picture source it would not be attributed to the picture. Because the source retrieved by the model for the misleading item probes was the text and not the picture (because it had never been associated with the picture, but had been associated with the text), the model did not have a high rate of misattribution of these probes to the picture. It is notable that, in both the recognition and the source judgment conditions, the item that was retrieved by the model was actually the same and the source information was present. In the recognition condition it was not considered in the decision, however, whereas it was in the source judgement condition.

Figure 2 shows the pattern of data concerned with attribution to the picture source, in the experiment and the model, for all probe items rather than only for the critical misleading items. The match of the model to the experimental data was good. Figure 3 shows the distribution of attribution to "new," both in the model and in the experiment.

Increased Emphasis on Source in Recognition Instructions

Lindsay and Johnson (1989) conducted a second experiment, related to the first, in which their concern was that people had not understood the recognition instructions. Perhaps the participants may have just thought that they were to call the items old if they had occurred at all in the experiment. Thus, in the follow-up experiment they emphasised that people were to say old *only* if the item occurred in the picture, and not otherwise. When Lindsay and Johnson clarified and emphasised that occurrence in the picture was crucial, they found that this manipulation had an effect in decreasing the false alarms to the items that were presented in the text but not in the picture context. In CHARM, by allowing the source assessment procedure to come into play in the recognition condition, we were easily able to simulate Lindsay and Johnson's follow-up experiment. As we will argue, when we discuss our own experiments, participants may sometimes use only a simple recognition process (which some researchers call a "familiarity" judgement, though this too involves retrieval in CHARM) when the context in which the probe was experienced is requested, but they may also, under certain circumstances, voluntarily use the source monitoring procedure to check their responses.

Source Judgements When the Misleading Items are Related to Original Items

An experiment related to that of Lindsay and Johnson (1989) was also conducted by Zaragoza and Koshmider (1989); in it, participants were presented with a series of slides followed by a narrative describing them. Unlike the Lindsay and Johnson experiments, though, in which the misleading items were unrelated additions, the misleading items in Zaragoza and Koshmider's experiment were highly related to particular original items. For example, a screwdriver in the slides would be replaced with a hammer in the narrative. Participants then received a source monitoring test in which the test items were presented as slides, rather than as text. Test probes could be either original test items or misleading test items. Participants had to decide whether they had seen each test probe in the picture, in the text only, or, if they could not remember the source, then whether the item was consistent or inconsistent with what they had seen in the experiment.

We conducted simulations of this paradigm in CHARM. The main difference between the previous simulations and these ones was that the misleading items, which were themselves autoconvolved and added into the composite memory

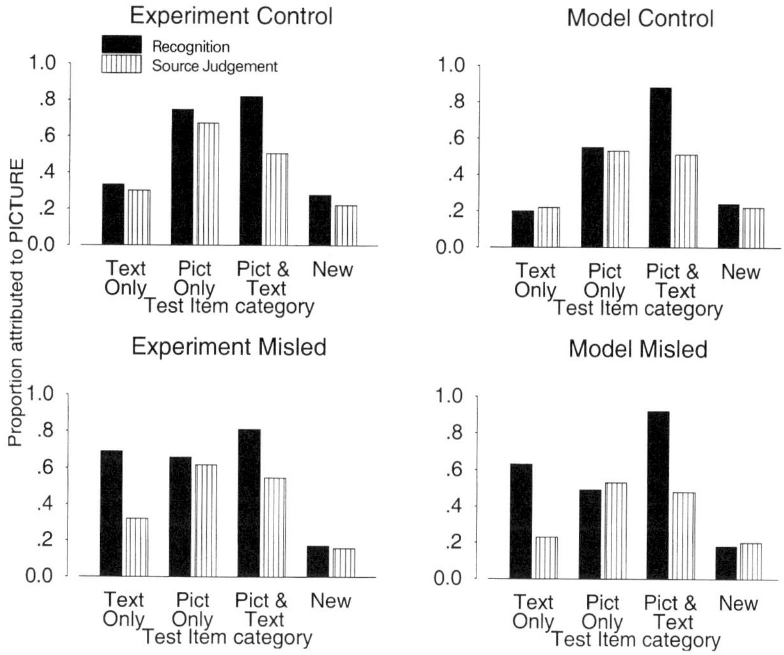

Fig. 2. *A comparison between Lindsay and Johnson (1989) and CHARM of the mean proportion of false attribution to "Picture" of all test items.*

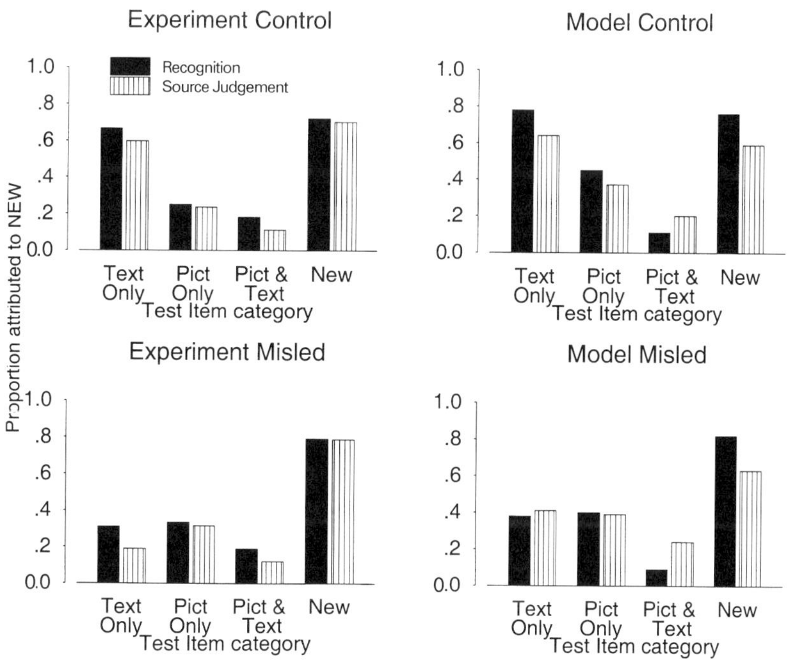

Fig. 3. *A comparison between Lindsay and Johnson's (1989) experiment and CHARM predictions of the mean proportion of false attribution to "New" of all test items.*

trace, and which were also convolved with a vector representing the narrative context, in this case were vectors that had considerable feature overlap with the vectors entered into the composite memory trace in association with the original context. The results of these simulations will not be reported in detail, except to say that they produced results that were consistent with the data reported by Zaragoza and Koshmider. Thus, regardless of whether the misleading items are related or unrelated to the original items, source judgements are useful in improving performance. The simple mechanisms in the CHARM model, used to account for these differences between recognition and source judgements, are sufficient to account for the results found experimentally.

The logic of incorporating source information into memory encoding and decisions, in at least one of these three forms, can also be implemented other models, such as those of Hintzman (1988), Ayers and Reder (1998), or Reyna and Brainerd (1995). These models have very different conceptual bases from CHARM, but can plausibly handle these source monitoring data. It is especially pleasing, though, that models relying on a composite memory trace can account for the source monitoring results since the nature of the composite trace and composite retrieval—which have many interesting conceptual spin-offs—makes this capacity unintuitive for this class of models.

THE FALSE MEMORY PARADIGM

The second half of this article focuses on the second paradigm for misremembering—the false memory paradigm—in which people are presented with a variety of related items, and tend to false alarm on critical items that were not presented, but which are highly related to those items that were. For example, a person might be presented with a list of items including *sugar, cake, honey,* and *chocolate.* Later they would be tested with the critical (unpresented) item *sweet,* which is a high associate of the presented items. Roediger and McDermott (1995) reported false alarm rates in recognition ranging from 58% to 81% for such critical items, though Roediger, Gallo, Watson, and Balota (1998) have recently shown much more variability. Robinson and Roediger (1997) showed that the rate of false attributions increases monotonically with increases in the number of associates in the study list. Norman and Schacter (1997) showed that older adults are more vulnerable to these kind of false memories than are younger adults.

Perhaps surprisingly, given the data with older adults, Korsakoff and non-Korsakoff amnesics showed reduced levels of false memories (Schacter, Verfaellie, Anes, & Racine, 1998). Interestingly enough, as the level of remembrance for true memories increased, the Korsakoff amnesics also showed an increase in their level of false memories. In the same experiment, though, with normal controls, as the level of true memory increased, the rate of false alarming to the critical item decreased.

Several experiments have shown that repetition of the study list (with normals) results both in an increase in true memory and a decrease in false memories (McDermott, 1996). Furthermore, other manipulations that increase the distinctiveness of the items in the to-be-remembered list also decrease the probability of false memories. Israel and Schacter (1997) showed that the pictorial encoding of the inducing list items—which were presented in the form of line drawings—decreased the false memory effect. However, there is some indication that neither repetition nor pictorial encoding are effective in obviating the effect in elderly subjects (Kensinger & Schacter, this issue; Koutstaal & Schacter, 1997; Schacter, Kaszniak, Kihlstrom, & Valdiserri, 1991).

CHARM and False Memories

The most straightforward way to handle the false memory paradigm in CHARM is to consider it to be a special case of prototype formation, which has been modelled formally in CHARM (Metcalfe Eich, 1982; and see Metcalfe, 1991b). In that paradigm, as in the false memory paradigm, a number of items that are highly similar to one another—call them I_1, I_2, I_3, I_4, etc., and to an item that might be called either a "critical item" in the false memory paradigm) or a prototype—call it $\mathbf{I}_p$ (for prototype)—are autoassociated and added into the composite trace. Thus, the composite trace is:

$$\mathbf{T} = \mathbf{I}_1*\mathbf{I}_1 + \mathbf{I}_2*\mathbf{I}_2 + \mathbf{I}_3*\mathbf{I}_3 + \mathbf{I}_4*\mathbf{I}_4 + \ldots + \text{noise} \quad (2)$$

The predictions of the model, in this situation, are straightforward. If $\mathbf{I}_p$ is used as the retrieval cue, each of the encoded **I***'s* will be retrieved as a function of their similarity to $\mathbf{I}_p$. Furthermore, they will all be superimposed (see Metcalfe, 1991b, for some illustrations of superimposed representations going back to Galton's (1878) seminal work on composite photography and "family resemblance"). $\mathbf{I}_p$, then, will retrieve something that closely resembles a prototype, and if that resultant retrieved item is matched to $\mathbf{I}_p$, itself, the extent of match can be very high indeed, depending upon the similarity of the encoded items ($\mathbf{I}_1$, $\mathbf{I}_2$, etc.) to $\mathbf{I}_p$, and also upon how many such items were encoded. If very few related items were entered into the trace, then the generalisation to the critical item will be low, but as more and more highly/related items are added into the composite trace the generalisation to the critical item increases. This finding in the model (see Metcalfe Eich, 1982, for simulations) corresponds nicely to Robinson and Roediger's (1997) findings.

It also follows that if people are remembering very few of the presented items, they may have encoded only a few items. Even though a large number of the related items might have been presented, if only a few of those items were encoded and entered into the trace, then the situation is the same as if only a few related items were presented. In the model, when one item is encoded in the list, and an item that is similar to it is presented as the cue, the retrieved item will match the cue item as a function of the degree of similarity between the two, but there is no convergent generalisation from multiple items. Similarly, with only a few encoded items, there may be insufficient information in the composite trace to support the generalisation to the critical items, and no false memory effect will be manifest. Thus some degree of true memory is needed if people are to demonstrate false memories, since the "false" memories themselves depend upon superimposed retrieval of the true memories. As the level of overall memory increased with the amnesics in Schacter et al.'s (1998) study, presumably the number of encoded items increased, allowing generalisation to the false memory. Thus, the finding that amnesics may fail to show a false memory effect with low levels of true memory, but then show the false memory effect with higher levels of true memory, may be strongly related to the finding of Robinson and Roediger (1997)—that false memories increase with an increase in the number of associates presented. Furthermore, as the inducing items are made more and more similar to one another and to the critical item, the model predicts that false memory for the critical item should also increase.

At the other extreme, if the individual items in the list are extremely well discriminated, that is, they are either not highly related to one another, or if they are encoded such that their distinctive features are emphasised, the false memory effect should be offset. This can be captured in the model either by using items that are not highly similar to one another (see Metcalfe Eich, 1982, for simulations), or by allowing a high proportion of distinctive features (and not just the most typical features) to be encoded by a selective feature-sampling process (see Metcalfe, 1991b, for details of feature sampling in the model, and some of the implications). High levels of distinctive encoding could allow discrimination of the critical item from the presented items. Thus, at extremely high levels of learning of the individual items—as long as that learning entailed emphasis on the distinctive features—the false memory effect may disappear. (There are conditions under which the false memories may not disappear, however. The explanation forwarded here is that, with many presentations, people are intentionally forging distinctive mental representations that distinguish the presented items from one another and from the critical item. Looking for, and encoding, the differences among the items is likely to be under voluntary control, however, and if the participants in the experiment are not doing it, but are simply strengthening the canonical representational forms of the presented items, then high levels of true memory may still give rise to high levels of false memory, as in the experiments conducted on ageing people, cited earlier.)

This interpretation is consistent with that of Schacter, Israel, and Racine (1999).

There are other experimental manipulations that appear to give rise to distinctive encodings, where distinctive means that the features that are different across items are particularly emphasised. Pictures may evoke a more distinctive and unique event encoding than do words. Several experiments have shown that pictorial encoding is less likely to evoke false memories than is verbal encoding (Israel & Schacter, 1997; Schacter et al., 1999). The idea that the difference between pictures and words, in this paradigm, is a function of the distinctiveness of the two kinds of materials, leaves open the possibility that one might be able to choose pictures to be nondistinctive, in which case they may be as good as words at producing false memories. The disappearance of the false memory effects at high levels of memory, then, is for reasons quite different from those accounting for its failure to occur at very low levels of memory.

Theoretical Predictions about False Memories and Source

There may be other situations that could allow a person to discriminate a false memory from events that were present in the episode under study. Our hypothesis, in the present experiment, was that source information may provide a clue that, at least under some circumstances, may serve as discriminative information.

The paradigm investigated here was devised to produce potentially paradoxical effects. We thought that by presenting the critical item itself we might, under some very constrained situations, set the stage for people to inhibit false memories concerning that item. However, although these were our expectations, they were *not* the straightforward predictions of CHARM, and so this paradigm holds especial interest for us. The paradigm was one in which the human participants (and the model) were presented with two lists. One list contained the highly related items like those usually used to induce a false memory effect. We will call this list the Inducing List. In the Other List we either presented (in the Experimental Condition) or did not present (in the Control Condition) the critical item.

To instantiate this situation in the model, each of the related items in the Inducing List is autoconvolved, and also convolved with the Inducing List source vector, and all of these convolutions are added into the composite memory trace. Thus, the situation resembles that given in Equation 2, except that each item is also convolved with its list source vector. The items in the Other List are also autoconvolved and each is convolved with an item representing the Other List source. In the equation given below, though (because, aside from the critical item itself, the content of the vectors in the other list is irrelevant) we will simply call these associations that comprise the associations from the Other List "noise". The Inducing List Source is notated S_i (for inducing); the source vector representing the Other List is notated S_o (for other). In the Experimental Condition the critical item, which is notated as I_p (or prototype item, as given in Equation 2) is encoded as a member of the Other List. In the control condition the critical item is not encoded at all. Schematically, then, the experimental trace, T_e, and the control trace, T_c, are as follows:

$T_e = I_1{*}I_1 + I_1{*}S_i + I_2{*}I_2 + I_2{*}S_i + I_3{*}I_3 + I_3{*}S_i + \ldots +$ noise (from the rest of the Inducing List and from preexperimental sources) $\ldots + I_p{*}I_p + I_p{*}S_o +$ noise (from Other List)

$T_c = I_1{*}I_1 + I_1{*}S_i = I_2{*}I_2 + I_2{*}S_i + I_3{*}I_3 + I_3{*}S_i + \ldots +$ noise (from the rest of the Inducing List and from preexperimental sources) $\ldots +$ noise (from Other List)

The crucial difference between the two traces is in whether or not the critical item itself ($I_p{*}I_p$), as well as its association to the Other List source vector ($I_p{*}S_o$), is or is not included

At time of retrieval, the critical item, I_p is correlated with the composite trace, and, under recognition instructions, the vector that is thereby retrieved is compared to the probe (as is usual in recognition in the model). The match between the retrieved item and the critical item probe, in the Control Condition, is high (by virtue of all the highly related items retrieved from the Inducing List). But the match between the retrieved item and the critical item probe, in the Experimental Condition, is even higher, because in addition to all of the information retrieved in the Control Condition, the presented critical item itself is also retrieved. Thus CHARM—like all other models of simple recognition—predicts that under conditions of recognition—as long as people are only considering the information about the content of the item itself and are disregarding source information, the probability of saying "yes" to the critical item should be higher in the experimental condition than in the control condition.

What about the predictions when the task is source monitoring? The answer is straightforward if people are making a judgement as given in the simulations presented in the first section of this article. In the Control Condition, there is a great deal of retrieved information converging on the Inducing List as the source of the critical item, since each of the inducing items was associated with the Inducing List Source vector. There is no information pointing to any other source for the critical item. Thus, the model predicts that people should think that the critical item came from the Inducing List, and not from the Other List or from both lists. The model will sometimes allow that the source is "neither" if the resonance criterion is not reached.

In contrast, in the Experimental Condition, while all of the information pointing to the Inducing List as the source is present in the Experimental Condition as it was in the Control Condition, in addition, the presented critical item was associated with the Other List source, and hence, via this association the probe also retrieves the Other List source. Given that both of these sources are retrieved, then, the model predicts that people should give all three responses—Inducing List, Other List, and especially BOTH lists—as the source of the critical item.

Thus, to summarise, the predictions of the model were that under recognition conditions, people should be more likely to affirm that the critical item was in the Inducing List if it was presented in another list. The experimental condition should produce higher false recognition of the critical item than should the Control Condition. If asked for the source of the critical item in the Control Condition, people should say it was from the Inducing List. In the Experimental Condition they should say that it was present in both the Inducing List and the Other List.

Experiments 1 and 2

We ran two separate experiments, both of which conform to the basic design such that the critical item is presented in the alternative list in the Experimental Condition, or is not presented in the Control Condition. The results of these experiments will be presented individually because certain interactions appear in one experiment and not in the other. The first experiment was run on the computer, using PsyScope; the second was run on flash cards. The second experiment was conducted because the first experiment did not allow us to investigate the fate of the exact same materials in the experimental and control conditions. Roediger et al. (1998) have shown that there can be extreme differences in results in the false memory paradigm as a function of the exact word lists used, and so we were concerned (correctly, as it turns out) that this aspect of the experiment be carefully controlled before reaching any conclusions. In the first experiment participants were tested both for source judgements and for yes/no recognition. In the second experiment we tested only for yes/no recognition.

Methods

Participants. Participants were students in an Introductory Psychology course at Columbia University, who received partial course credit for participating in this experiment, or were paid volunteers (also Columbia University students) who were given $10 for their efforts. There were 67 participants in Experiment 1 and 26 in Experiment 2. Data from two participants, in Experiment 1, were eliminated because these individuals did not follow the instructions.

Design. Participants studied two lists in every trial. Each list consisted of seven associated "inducing" words that were related to a critical item and two words that were unrelated to the general theme of the list. In the Experimental Conditions, one of these two words was the critical word for the alternative list. In the Control Conditions, both of these words were unrelated both to the theme of the list in which they were presented and to the theme of the alternative list. The two lists were not related to each other. Thus, each participant was tested on what was basically a 2 × 2 within-subjects design. The two factors were: Presentation of Critical Item (presented in the alternate list in the Experimental Condition or not presented in the Control Condition) and Test List (either List 1 or List 2).

Test List 1 means that the inducing words—*cake, sugar, honey,* etc.—were presented in List 1, and that subjects were instructed, in recognition, to say yes only to words that had occurred in List 1. On experimental trials, the critical word "*sweet*" would be presented in the second list; on control trials nothing else related to the first list would be presented in the second list. Conversely, Test List 2 implies that List 2 was the inducing list and that the critical item appeared—if the particular trial in question was one in the Experimental Condition—in the first list.

In Experiment 1, 33 participants were tested exclusively on a yes/no recognition task and 32 participants received exclusively a 4-choice source judgement task. In Experiment 2, all participants were tested on yes/no recognition only.

There were several other factors included, for control purposes, in the first experiment. A between-participants factor was Trial Type. For 33 participants, the list pairs comprising each trial were structured such that on each trial only one critical item was presented. The other 32 participants saw trials in which both lists contained critical items, or neither contained critical items. These two methods of linking the two lists were initially conducted as separate mini-experiments and run sequentially during the semester, but they are presented here as one experiment since there were no effects of this variable. Another factor was the Set of Materials used. Set B reversed the ordering of pairs of linked lists that were used in Set A, such that the lists that were first in Set A were second in Set B. The word lists that were used in each treatment combination in Set A were also rotated, as a block, to a different treatment combination in Set B. Although this materials manipulation did put different critical items into different treatment combinations, it did not provide a direct contrast on the same materials between the experimental manipulation. (This necessary control condition was implemented in Experiment 2). Finally, each of the four main experimental conditions was replicated six times within each participant, and the "critical item" data are proportions based on six observations.

In Experiment 2, the 48 lists from Experiment 1 were randomly repaired. Six such pairs were assigned to each of the four treatment combinations—Experimental Condition Test List 1, Experiment Condition Test List 2, Control Condition Test List 1, Control Condition Test List 2. In Set B the exact lists that had been used in the Experimental Conditions in Set A (except that the critical words were now replaced by random, unrelated words) were used in the corresponding Control Conditions, and the exact lists that had been in the two Control Conditions in Set A were used in the corresponding Experimental conditions in Set B. Thus, if in Set A, in some trial the "sweet" list had been presented first and the "chair" list second in the Experimental Condition Test List 1 (such that the word "sweet" was presented in the second list), the related trial in Set B would again have the "sweet" list presented first, the "chair" list presented second, and the first list would again be tested. However, now this trial would be in the Control Condition, and the critical word "sweet" would *not* be presented in the study lists.

Materials. Twenty-four lists were constructed using the materials of Roediger and McDermott (1995), and 24 additional lists were formed from the University of Florida associate norms database (Nelson, McEvoy, & Schreffier, 1994). Each list consisted of the seven highest associates of a critical item. Two unrelated words were also inserted into the list. In half of the lists, one of the unrelated words was the critical item. This item always occupied one of the middle three positions in the 7-item list, in Experiment 1, and was on average in position 6 in Experiment 2. In the computer-generated experiment List 1 words were always presented in blue at the top of the screen, and were surrounded by a thick oval border. List 2 words were in red and in a different font from the List 1 words. They appeared at the bottom of the screen and were surrounded by a rectangular border. In Experiment 2, List 1 items were always presented on blue cards and List 2 items on pink cards. These contextual differences were intended to help participants discriminate between the two lists.

In Experiment 1, the test lists consisted of 12 words: the critical item for both lists, two old List 1 words, two old List 2 words, a new word that was a low associate (the 8th-ranked associate) of the critical item related to List 1, a new word that was a low associate of the critical item related to List 2, and four new unrelated words. The order of these words within the test list was randomised across trials and across participants. In the yes/no task, List 1 was assigned to be called "old" in half the trials, and List 2 was "old" in the other half. Counterbalancing across all the within-particpants factors was maintained during this assignation.

In Experiment 2, eight words on each trial were used as test probes: the critical items from Lists 1 and 2, two presented exemplars from each of the two lists, and two unrelated new words.

Procedure. In Experiment 1 the trials were presented on a computer monitor. Participants received the following instructions verbally:

> You will be doing the same task over 24 trials. For each trial, this is what you will do: First, click the mouse button to begin the trial. Then you will see a list of words appearing at the top of the screen. They will be in blue, and will appear one by one, rather quickly. After the list of blue words is over, you will see a number in the middle of the screen. Count backwards, and aloud, in steps of 3 from this number. For example, if you see 100, you would say, "97 ... 94 ... 91... and so on." Then the red list will begin. Words will appear at the bottom of the screen, one by one, in red. After this list is over, you will do the counting backwards task again. Then you will see a third list of words. Instructions on the screen will inform you about what to do. In half the trials, you will have to click on the "Yes", button if you saw the word in the blue list, and click "No" otherwise. In the other half of the trials, you will have to click on the "Yes" button if you saw the word in the red list, and click "No" otherwise. Remember, the instructions on the screen will inform you about which list you are supposed to say "Yes" to. After this test is over, you can begin the next trial.

Then they went through a practice trial before beginning the 24 experimental trials. Participants began each trial by clicking on a mouse button. List 1 then appeared, one word at a time, at a rate of 2.5sec per word. At the end of the list, participants saw a number in the middle of the screen and counted backwards aloud from this number in steps of three for 16 seconds. This task was meant to minimise rehearsal of the list they had just studied. Then List 2 started, and the words appeared at the same rate as in List 1. The counting backwards task was repeated after this list, and then the instructions for the test appeared on the screen.

The instructions for recognition were: "For each of the following words, click on the 'yes' button only if the word previously appeared in the blue [red] list. Otherwise click 'no'." Blue was always List 1 and red was always List 2. These instructions appeared in blue if they were for List 1, and in red if they were for List 2. The test words appeared one at a time and participants used the mouse to choose between "yes" and "no." Participants could then begin the next trial, or take a break for a few seconds.

The participants performing the source judgement task received these instructions: "Please indicate in which list(s) the following words appeared." They then used the mouse to click on one of four buttons as each test word was presented. The buttons were labelled "Blue only", "Red only", "Blue and Red", "Neither."

The procedure was similar in Experiment 2, except that subjects were only asked for recognition. At the end of List 2, on each trial, they were presented with the instruction card indicating which list they were to remember.

Experiment 1 Results

Recognition. The main finding of interest was that the presentation of the critical item was found to inhibit false memories to that item. The main effect of Presentation of Critical Item [$F(1,29) = 9.61$, $MSe = 0.39$], was significant. There was also a main effect of Test List, [$F(1,29) = 7.85$, $MSe = 0.46$], such that the false memory effect was stronger when List 2 was tested than when List 1 was tested. These main effects were qualified by the interaction between them [$F(1,29) = 4.52$, $MSe = 0.36$], such that participants were more likely to show false memory suppression, attributable to presentation of the critical item, when List 1 was tested than when List 2 was tested. This interaction is shown in Fig. 4.

In half of the trials, when the critical item was actually presented, the recognition instructions tested not the Inducing List, but the Other List. The person would, under these instructions, be correct to call the presented critical item old. Under these conditions, the probability of calling the critical item old, when it occurred in List 2, was 0.60. When it occurred in List 1 the probability of calling the critical item old in this condition was .40. The difference between the two conditions was significant [$t(32) = 4.61$].

This result may simply indicate that items appearing in List 2 were better remembered—enjoying a recency effect. However, there was no analogous difference between other old items presented in either List 1 or List 2, as is

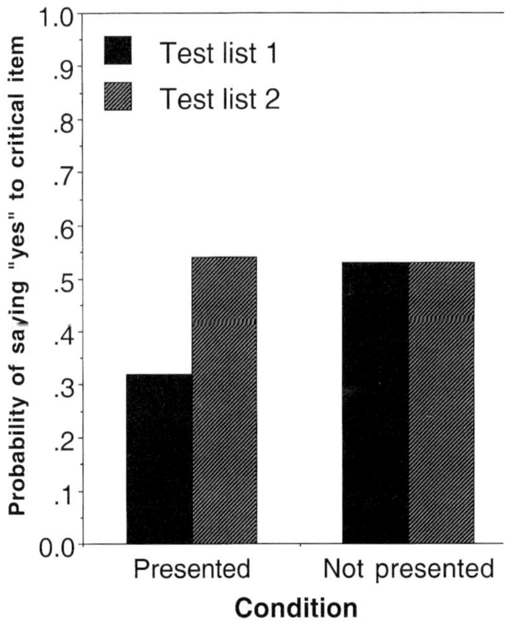

Fig. 4. *Proportion of "yes" responses to the critical item in the recognition task in Experiment 1, as a function of Test List.*

shown in Table 1. Thus, the simple recency effect explanation of the difference in the memorability of the critical items seems unlikely. The alternative, and more active, explanation for this difference is that after having experienced a large number of related words in one list, participants may have experienced the critical item, presented afterwards in a list that had a different theme, as an unexpected solution to a puzzle. Indeed, some participants reported to the experimenter, at time of debriefing, that they experienced surprise at the critical item word having been sometimes presented in the wrong list—after the list in which its compatriots were presented—and especially noted its occurrence.

The enhanced memory for the second list critical items might be related to the false memory inhibition effect in this experiment. It is notable that the critical items that were remembered better were also the items that produced false memory inhibition. Perhaps it is necessary that the actual presentation of the critical item itself remembered crisply, (presumably also with the information that it occurred in a context different from the inducing list) if it is to be useful in inhibiting the false memory.

Source Judgements. When attribution to the inducing list was considered in isolation in the source judgement data, there was a main effect of the Presence of the Critical Item, such that when the critical item was present in the alternative list there was an inhibition effect. People were less likely to say that the critical item had been in the Inducing List when it had been presented in the Other List than when it had not been presented at all [$F(1,31) = 19.58$, $MSe = 0.02$]. People were also less likely to attribute the critical item to the Inducing List if they were tested for List 1 than if they were tested for List 2 [$F(1,31) = 40.93$, $MSe = 0.03$]. There was an interaction between the Presence of the Critical Item and Test List [$F(1,31) = 4.81$, $MSe = 0.02$], such that the false memory inhibition effect due to the presence of the critical item in the alternate list was larger when the test list was List 1 than when it was List 2. These results are shown in Fig. 5.

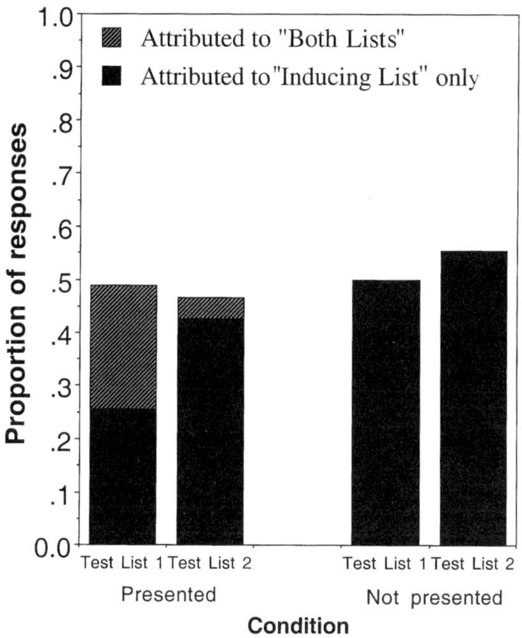

Fig. 5. *Proportion of false attribution of the critical item in the source judgement task.*

Figure 5 also shows the proportion of attributions to "both lists." People never made an attribution to both lists in the control conditions, that is, when the critical item was not presented in the alternative list. The main effect of Presence of the Critical Item was significant [$F(1,31) = 35.98$, $MSe = 0.01$]. The attribution to both lists was greater when the first list was tested than when the second list was tested [$F(1,31) = 52.92$, $MSe = 0.01$]. In addition, the interaction between the Presence of the Critical Item and the Test List was significant [$F1,31) = 37.66$, $MSe = 0.01$].

As can be seen by comparing Fig. 4 and 5, the "both" judgements in the source judgement task did not seem to translate into what seems like the logical affirmation that the critical item *had* in fact been presented in the first list, as well as the second, in the recognition task. Instead, the items that were thought to have occurred in both lists seem to have been subtracted out of the simple recognition judgements, such that the source judgments made to "Inducing List only" correspond closely to the recognition data. It is as if when participants felt, in the source monitoring task, that the critical item had been present in both lists, this assessment led to the conclusion, in the recognition task, that the item had *not* occurred in the first list.

Other Test Items. Table 1 gives the attribution to the Inducing List for the other five test items: the old words from List 1 and List 2, the extra list low associates of List 1 and List 2, and the new words. Tables 2 and 3 show the attribution of old List 1 words and old List 2 words, respectively, to each of the four possible choices in the source judgment task. New items were rejected (attributed to Neither) at levels ranging from .97 to .99 in all conditions.

Experiment 2 Results

As was the case in Experiment 1, in Experiment 2 there was a significant false memory inhibition effect such that presenting the critical items in the alternate list decreased the chance that people would false alarm to those same critical items as members of the Inducing List [$F(1,24) = 9.08$, $MSe = 0.41$]. However, this inhibition effect was dependent upon interactions with the set of items used. There was an effect of Test List [$F(1,24) = 9.51$, $MSe = 0.45$], an interaction between Set and Presentation of the Critical Item [$F(1,24) = 4.73$, $MSe = 0.21$], and a large and significant three-way interaction among Set, Test List, and Presentation of the Critical Item [$F(1,24) = 23.05$, $MSe = 0.55$]. As is shown in Fig. 6, the words in Set B exhibited an inhibition pattern like that found in Experiment 1. However, as is also shown in Fig. 6, Set A produced a different pattern, unlike that found in the first experiment.

To make the interpretation of the results clearer, we rearranged the presentation of the triple interaction data to show what happened with each of the fours groups of word lists, first when presented in the Experimental Condition (with one group of participants) then in the Control Condition (with other participants). A listing of the 24 critical words, divided into these 4 groups, are given on the abscissa of Figure 7. As can be seen from the data given in the figure, the first two word groups showed the inhibition effect when the critical word

Table 1. *Proportion of Attributions to the Inducing List in the Yes/No Recognition Task (Expt. 1)*

	Experimental Condition			
	Inducing List is List 1		*Inducing List is List 2*	
Test Item	*Critical Item Absent*	*Critical Item Present*	*Critical Item Absent*	*Critical Item Present*
Old List 1 words	.68	.74	.09	.07
Old List 2 words	.10	.09	.67	.73
List 1 low associate	.05	.06	.02	.02
List 2 low associate	.02	.02	.04	.05
New words	.04	.02	.01	.02

Table 2. *Attribution Fate of Old List 1 Words in the Source Judgement Task (in Proportions) (Expt. 1)*

	Experimental Condition			
	Inducing List is List 1		*Inducing List is List 2*	
Test Item	*Critical Item Absent*	*Critical Item Present*	*Critical Item Absent*	*Critical Item Present*
List 1	.77	.79	.79	.79
List 2	.03	.03	.02	.03
Both	.00	.00	.01	.00
Neither	.20	.17	.18	.17

Table 3. *Attributions of Old List 2 Words in the Source Judgement Task (in Proportions) (Expt. 1)*

	Experimental Condition			
	Inducing List is List 1		*Inducing List is List 2*	
Test Item	*Critical Item Absent*	*Critical Item Present*	*Critical Item Absent*	*Critical Item Present*
List 1 only	.04	.04	.06	.07
List 2 only	.77	.79	.74	.75
Both lists	.00	.01	.00	.02
Neither list	.19	.16	.21	.16

was presented, whereas the last two groups did not. We have spent many hours pondering the reasons for this particular breakdown, and have found no obvious explanation. It is notable, though, that Roediger et al. (1998) reported that there are large and apparently idiosyncratic differences among particular words in the probability of production of the basic false memory effect. At the present time, we know of no coherent explanation for either of these findings.

In summary, then, in both Experiment 1 and Experiment 2 we found inhibition of the false memory effect when the critical word was presented in an alternate list. However, the effect is conditional and rather fleeting—occurring in the first experiment only when the critical word came after the Inducing List, and in the second experiment only for a subset of the word lists. It is possible that the appearance of the inhibition effect depends on the salience of the presented critical word, as well as

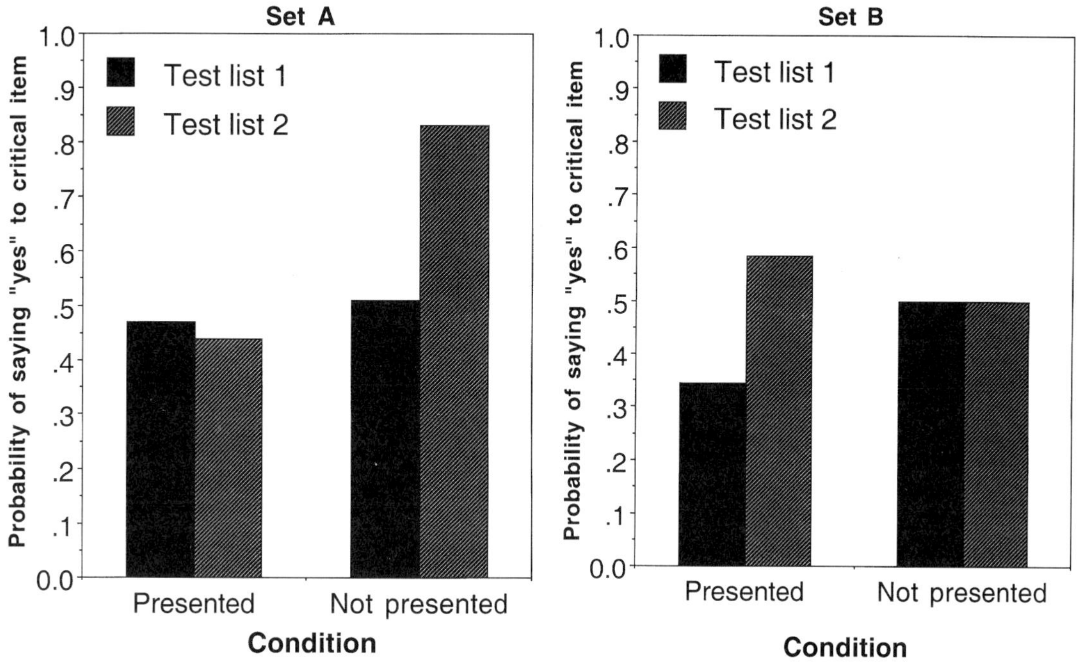

Fig. 6. *Proportion of "yes" responses to the critical item in the recognition task in Experiment 2, as a function of Set and Test List.*

on the participant registering that it is out of the context of the Inducing List. This conjecture, while appealing, would require further empirical investigation.

CONCLUSION

People appear, at least under some conditions, to be able to use source information to sharpen and improve their memories in both of the misremembering situations investigated in this article. In the misleading information paradigm, when asked, they are able to use source information to indicate that the misleading information did not actually occur in the event in question. Similarly, in the false memory paradigm, in which a memory is induced by a number of related items, the salient presence of the real critical item in a context other than that of the inducing list itself can sometimes be used to suppress false alarms to that critical item that is only induced (see Johnson & Raye, 1981; and Johnson, Kounios, & Reeder, 1994 for discussions of reality monitoring). In the latter case, the exact circumstances both of when the critical item is presented, and of which particular words are used, appear to be important. Even so, it seems that the highly salient and memorable occurrence of the critical item in the wrong context may allow people to disconfirm it as a member of the inducing list.

A phenomenon similar to the one observed here—that people reject an item based on the fact that they remember it as having occurred in the wrong context—can be found in the Jacoby (1991) exclusion condition of the process dissociation paradigm. In that paradigm, participants were explicitly told that if they remember an item as having occurred in a particular list it means that it definitely did not occur in the other list. Although the participants in our experiment were not told this, and did, in fact, subscribe incorrectly to the double presentation of the critical item in two lists when they were asked for source judgements, the paradigm we used did conform, in some respects, to Jacoby's process dissociation paradigm (Jacoby, 1991; Jacoby & Kelley, 1992; Jacoby, Toth, &

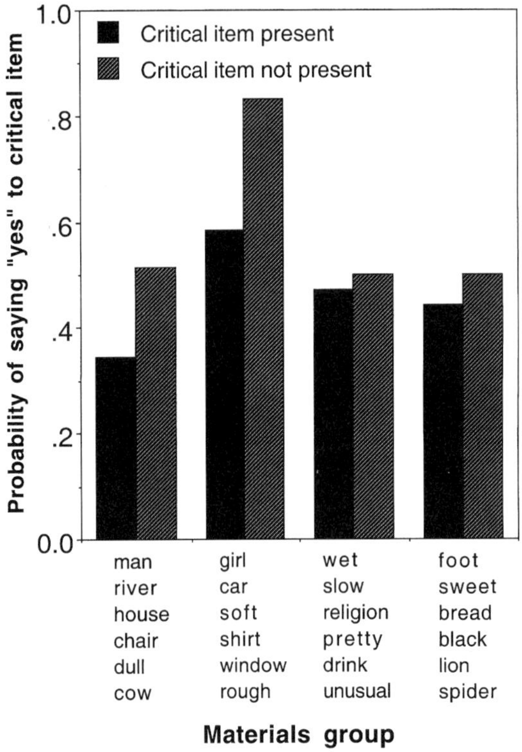

Fig. 7. *The inhibition effect in Experiment 2, as a function of the particular lists used.*

Yonelinas, 1993; Yonelinas & Jacoby, 1996), insofar as items never *actually* occurred in both lists.

It is possible that participants, under our recognition instructions, used the exclusion logic to their advantage in this experiment—deciding that an item was not in the inducing list if he or she remembered that it was in the alternate list. The source monitoring data seem to weigh against this explanation, at least on the face of it. People, in the source judgement task, freely told us that they thought (incorrectly) that many of the critical items had been presented in *both* lists. Had they been using a strict exclusion rule, even on the source judgement task, they presumably would not have subscribed to the "both" option. On the other hand, participants often mentioned at time of debriefing that, although it had seemed as if certain items that had been presented in both lists, they had responded under the hypothesis that this phenomenology was illusory, and hence they had used an exclusion rule. We could easily model the exclusion rule in CHARM, and hence account for the data in these experiments. Such a rule would have something of a post hoc quality, given the instructions in the experiments, but even so, if it is the rule people were using, it would be entirely reasonable to include it in the model in this situation.

REFERENCES

Ayers, M.S., & Reder, L. (1998). A theoretical review of the misinformation effect: Predictions from an activation-based memory model. *Psychonomic Bulletin and Review, 5,* 1–21.

Belli, R.F. (1989). Influences of misleading postevent information: Misinformation interference and acceptance. *Journal of Experimental Psychology: General, 118,* 72–85.

Ceci, S.J., Ross, D.F., & Toglia, M.P. (1987). Suggestibility of children's memory: Psycholegal implications. *Journal of Experimental Psychology: General, 117,* 201–203.

Chandler, C.C. (1989). Specific retroactive interference in modified recognition tests: Evidence for an unknown cause of interference. *Journal of Experimental Psychology: Learning, Memory, and Cognition, 15,* 256–265.

Christiaansen, R.E., & Ochalek, K. (1983). Editing misleading information from memory: Evidence for the coexistence of original and postevent information. *Memory & Cognition, 11,* 467–475.

Deese, J. (1959). On the prediction of occurrence of particular verbal intrusions in immediate recall. *Journal of Experimental Psychology, 58*(1), 17–22.

Galton, F. (1878). Composite portraiture. *Nature, 18,* 97–100.

Hintzman, D.L. (1988). Judgments of frequency and recognition memory in a multiple-trace memory model. *Psychological Review, 95,* 528–551.

Israel, L., & Schacter, D.L. (1997). Pictorial encoding reduces false recognition of semantic associates. *Psychonomic Bulletin and Review, 4,* 577–581.

Jacoby, L.L. (1991). A process dissociation framework: Separating automatic from intentional uses of memory. *Journal of Memory and Language, 30,* 513–541.

Jacoby, L.L., & Kelley, C.M (1992). A process-dissociation framework for investigating unconscious influences: Freudian slips, projective tests, subliminal perception, and signal detection theory. *Current Directions in Psychological Science, 1,* 174–179

Jacoby, L.L., Toth, J.P., & Yonelinas, A.P. (1993). Separating conscious and unconscious influences of memory: Measuring recollection. *Journal of Experimental Psychology: General, 122,* 139–154.

Johnson, M.K., Hashtroudi, S., & Lindsay, D.S. (1993). Source monitoring. *Psychological Review, 114,* 3–28.

Johnson, M.K., Kounios, L, & Reeder, J. (1994). Time-course studies of reality monitoring and recognition. *Journal of Experimental Psychology: Learning, Memory, and Cognition, 20,* 1409–1419.

Johnson, M.K., & Raye, C.L. (1981). Reality monitoring. *Psychological Review, 88,* 67–85.

Kensinger, E.A., & Schacter, D.L. (this issue). When true memories suppress false memories: Effects of ageing. *Cognitive Neuropsychology, 16,* 399–415.

Koutstaal, W., & Schacter, D.L. (1997). Gist-based false recognition of pictures in older and younger adults. *Journal of Memory and Language, 37,* 555–583.

Kroll, N.E., & Timourian, D.A. (1986). Misleading questions and the retrieval of the irretrievable. *Bulletin of the Psychonomic Society, 24,* 165–168.

Lindsay, D.S. (1991). CHARMed, but not convinced: Comment on Metcalfe (1990). *Journal of Experimental Psychology: General, 120,* 101–105.

Lindsay, D.S., & Johnson, M. (1989). The eyewitness suggestibility effect and memory for source. *Memory & Cognition, 17,* 349–358.

Loftus, E.F. (1979). *Eyewitness testimony.* Cambridge, MA: Harvard University Press.

Loftus, E.F., & Hoffman, H.G. (1989). Misinformation and memory: The creation of new memories. *Journal of Experimental Psychology: General, 118,* 100–104.

McCloskey, M., & Zaragoza, M.S. (1985). Misleading postevent information and memory for events: Arguments and evidence against memory impairment hypotheses. *Journal of Experimental Psychology: General, 114,* 1–16.

McDermott, K.B. (1996). The persistence of false memories in list recall. *Journal of Memory and Language, 35,* 212–230.

Metcalfe, J. (1990). A composite holographic associative recall model (CHARM) and blended memories in eyewitness testimony. *Journal of Experimental Psychology: General, 119,* 145–160.

Metcalfe, J. (1991a). Recognition failure and the composite memory trace in CHARM. *Psychological Review, 98,* 529–553.

Metcalfe, J. (1991b) Composite memories. In W. Hockley & S. Lewandowsky (Eds.) *Relating theory and data. Essays on human memory in honor of Bennet B. Murdock* (pp. 399–423). Hillsdale, NJ: Lawrence Erlbaum Associates Inc.

Metcalfe, J. (1993a). Novelty monitoring, metacognition, and control in a composite holographic associative recall model: Implications for Korsakoff amnesia. *Psychological Review, 100,* 3–22.

Metcalfe, J. (1993b). Monitoring and gain control in an episodic memory model: Relation to P300 event-related potentials. In A.F. Collins, S.E. Gathercole, M.A. Conway, & P.E. Morris (Eds.), *Theories of Memory* (pp. 327–354) Hove, UK: Lawrence Erlbaum Associates Ltd.

Metcalfe, J. (1997). Predicting syndromes of amnesia from a Composite Holographic Associative Recall/Recognition Model (CHARM). *Memory, 5,* 233–253

Metcalfe, J., Cottrell, G.W., & Mencl, W.E. (1992). Cognitive binding: A computational-modeling analysis of a distinction between implicit and explicit memory. *Journal of Cognitive Neuroscience, 4,* 289–298.

Metcalfe Eich, J. (1982). A composite holographic associative recall model. *Psychological Review, 89,* 627–661.

Metcalfe Eich, J. (1985). Levels of processing, encoding specificity, elaboration, and CHARM. *Psychological Review, 91,* 1–38.

Nelson, D.L., McEvoy, C.L., & Schreiber, T.A. (1994). *The University of South Florida word association, rhyme and word fragment norms.* Unpublished manuscript.

Norman, K.A., & Schacter, D.L. (1997). False recognition in younger and older adults: Exploring the characteristics of illusory memories. *Memory & Cognition, 25,* 838–848.

Payne, D.G., Toglia, M.P., & Anastasi, S. (1994). Recognition performance-level and the magnitude of the misinformation effect in eyewitness memory. *Psychonomic Bulletin and Review. 1,* 376–382.

Reyna, V.F., & Brainerd, C.J. (1995). Fuzzy-trace theory: An interim synthesis. *Learning and Individual Differences, 7,* 1–75.

Robinson, K.J., & Roediger, H.L. (1997). Associative processes in false recall and false recognition. *Psychological Science, 8,* 231–237.

Roediger, H.L., Gallo, O.A., Watson, J.M., & Balota, D.A. (1998). *Eliminating and enhancing illusory memories.* Presentation given at the Annual Meeting of the Psychonomic Society, Nov. 21, Dallas, Texas.

Roediger, H.L., & McDermott, K.B. (1995). Creating false memories: Remembering words not presented in lists. *Journal of Experimental Psychology: Learning, Memory. and Cognition, 21,* 803–814.

Schacter, D.L., Israel, L., & Racine, C. (1999). Suppressing false recognition in younger and older adults: The distinctiveness heuristic. *Journal of Memory and Language, 40,* 1–24.

Schacter, D.L., Kaszniak, A.W, Kihlstrom, J.F, & Valdiserri, M. (1991). The relation between source memory and aging. *Psychology and Aging, 6,* 559–568

Schacter, D.L., Verfaellie, M., Anes, M. D., & Racine, C. (1998). When true recognition suppresses false recognition: Evidence from amnesic patients. *Journal of Cognitive Neuroscience, 10,* 668–679.

Tversky, B., & Tuchin, M. (1989). A reconciliation of the evidence on eyewitness testimony: Comments on McCloskey and Zaragoza. *Journal of Experimental Psychology: General, 118,* 86–91.

Yonelinas, A.P., & Jacoby, L.L. (1996). Response bias and the process-dissociation procedure. *Journal of Experimental Psychology: General, 125,* 422–434.

Zaragoza, M.S., & Koshmider, J.W. (1989). Misled subjects may know more than their performance implies. *Journal of Experimental Psychology: Learning, Memory, and Cognition, 15,* 246–255.

COGNITIVE NEUROPSYCHOLOGY, 1999, 16 (3/4/5), 509–512

SUBJECT INDEX

